Patrick Palacci, Ingvar Ericsson

Esthetic Implant Dentistry

Soft and Hard Tissue Management

Esthetic Implant Dentistry

Soft and Hard Tissue Management

Edited by
Patrick Palacci, DDS

Contributing editor
Ingvar Ericsson, LDS, Odont Dr

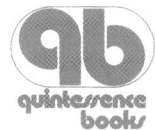

qb
quintessence books

Chicago, Berlin, London, Tokyo, Paris,
São Paulo, Barcelona, Moscow, Prague, and Warsaw

Library of Congress Cataloging-in-Publication Data

Esthetic implant dentistry : soft and hard tissue management / edited by Patrick Palacci
and Ingvar Ericsson.
                                p. ; cm.
    Includes bibliographical references and index
    ISBN 0-86715-392-X
    1. Dental implants. I. Title: Optimal implant positioning and soft and hard tissue management. II. Palacci,
Patrick. III. Ericsson, Ingvar.
        [DNLM: 1. Dental Implantation. 2. Periapical Tissue. WU 640 E79 2000]
    RK667.I45 E88 2000
    617.6'9—dc21   00-041523

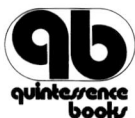

© 2001 Quintessence Publishing Co, Inc

2nd reprinting, 2006
Quintessence Publishing Co, Inc
4350 Chandler Drive, Hanover Park, IL 60133, USA
www.quintbook.com

Layout and design by Jean Veltcheff, Marseille, France, and Fredrik Persson, Göteborg, Sweden

Printed in Germany

Contents

Foreword   7

Per-Ingvar Brånemark

Preface   9

Contributors   11

Introduction   13

Ingvar Ericsson

Chapter 1   **Implant Integration and Stability**   15

Lars Sennerby

Chapter 2   **Biology and Pathology of Peri-implant Soft Tissue**   33

Ingvar Ericsson

Chapter 3   **Practical Guidelines Based on Biomechanical Principles**   47

Bo Rangert, Franck Renouard

Chapter 4   **Implant Placement Philosophy**   69

Patrick Palacci, Ingvar Ericsson

Chapter 5   **Anterior Maxilla Classification**   89

Patrick Palacci, Ingvar Ericsson

Chapter 6   **Optimal Implant Positioning**   101

Patrick Palacci

Chapter 7   **Minor Bone Augmentation Procedures**   137

Peter Moy, Patrick Palacci

Chapter 8   **Peri-implant Soft Tissue Augmentation Procedures**   159

Patrick Palacci

Chapter 9   **Rationale for the Use of Different Prosthetic Components**   203

Hans Nilson, Ingvar Ericsson, Patrick Palacci

Chapter 10   **One-stage Surgery and Early Functional Loading**   219

Ingvar Ericsson

Foreword

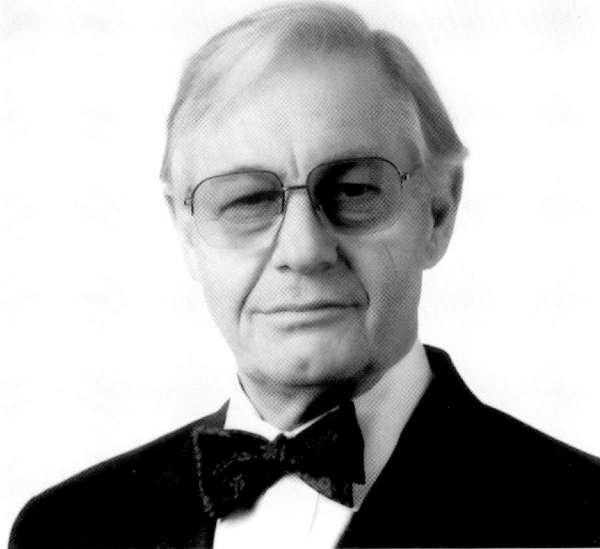

The increasing development of sophisticated components and procedures to replace teeth according to the osseointegration principle carries a risk related to superoptimization of the final therapeutic result. There is convincing evidence that anchorage of artificial substitutes for teeth can be predictably provided according to a carefully controlled recipe. Clinical predictability has been verified in carefully controlled multicenter studies all over the world. More recently, simplified technological alternatives in surgery and prosthetics have allowed for greater cost efficiency, making oral rehabilitation more agreeable to patients' expectations.

Once the anchorage function of teeth can be replaced and the masticatory function restored, another aspect of repair of edentulism should be considered. How far should one go to bring the patient back to original natural teeth? Is there a limit to achievable *restitutio ad integrum*?

Philosophically, there are two approaches to this question. First, if technically possible, would it be beneficial for the patient? Second, are reasonably safe procedures available to achieve a lasting mechanical retention for a third dentition as a final goal?

In health care, one should always consider the patient's desire for reasonable restoration in the quality of life that is often severely impaired by the loss of one, several, or all teeth. Clinical experience indicates that for some patients there is a strong motivation to restore not only anchorage but also hard and soft tissue topography and function to their original conditions.

This book describes and documents how to enable patients to incorporate prosthetic teeth into their body and mind without experiencing this feeling of looking like a foreign body. It is important that this book is based on long-term clinical ambitions, methodological development, and scientific documentation to provide a predictable treatment modality for these particular oral invalids.

Per-Ingvar Brånemark, MD, PhD

Preface

In early 1990, several distinguished clinicians and researchers were invited to contribute to Dr Palacci's first book, *Optimal Implant Positioning & Soft Tissue Management for the Brånemark System*, published in 1995. The book was an immediate success and especially appreciated by clinicians.

Several years ago we began to revise the text and expand the material. Several well-known experts in the field, researchers and clinicians from Europe and the United States, have contributed to the revised edition, *Esthetic Implant Dentistry: Soft and Hard Tissue Management*.

This book presents current guidelines for optimizing the functional and esthetic result of the "third dentition." Minor bone augmentation procedures are described with their specific indications for optimizing implant positioning and creating adequate soft tissue support. The papilla regeneration technique is presented with specific modifications related to single-tooth replacements and anterior ridge augmentation.

The latest prosthetic developments using the Brånemark implant system to achieve optimal precision and esthetics are presented. Finally, the early functional loading concept based on current research and clinical experience is discussed.

We greatly appreciate the work and cooperation of the contributors and also gratefully acknowledge the excellent collaboration of Quintessence.

Patrick Palacci, DDS

Ingvar Ericsson, LDS, Odont Dr

Contributors

Ingvar Ericsson, LDS, Odont Dr
Department of Prosthetic Dentistry
Malmö University
Malmö, Sweden

Private practice
Göteborg, Sweden

Peter Moy, DMD
Visiting Professor and Codirector, Dental
    Implant Center
University of California at Los Angeles
Los Angeles, California

Private practice
Los Angeles, California

Hans Nilson, LDS
Associate Professor of Prosthetic Dentistry
Umeå University,
Umeå, Sweden

Patrick Palacci, DDS
Visiting Professor
Boston University
Boston, Massachusetts

Private practice
Marseille, France

Bo Rangert, Mech Eng, PhD
Chief Scientist, Implants
Nobel Biocare AB
Göteborg, Sweden

Associate Professor of Biomechanical
    Engineering
Rensselaer Polytechnic Institute
Troy, New York

Franck Renouard, DDS
Private practice
Paris, France

Lars Sennerby, LDS, PhD
Professor
Department of Biomaterials/Handicap
    Research
Göteborg University
Göteborg, Sweden

Introduction

Ingvar Ericsson, LDS, Odont Dr

Titanium implants have been used for many years with good long-term success in the rehabilitation of totally and partially edentulous patients (see, for example, Adell et al 1981, 1990; Albrektsson et al 1986; Ericsson et al 1986, 1990; Jemt et al 1989; van Steenberghe et al 1990; Arvidson et al 1992; Albrektsson 1993; Jemt and Lekholm 1993, 1995; Lekholm et al 1994; Makkonen et al 1997; Palmer et al 1997). The Brånemark implant system was introduced 30 to 35 years ago (Brånemark et al 1969), and the principle of osseointegration, or "direct anchorage of an implant by the formation of bony tissue around the implant without the growth of fibrous tissue at the bone-implant interface" (Dorland's 1994), was emphasized (Albrektsson et al 1986; Albrektsson 1993). This implant methodology provided not only a scientific foundation for implant stability but also predictable long-term clinical success (see, for example, Adell et al 1981, 1990; Ericsson et al 1986, 1990; Jemt et al 1989; van Steenberghe et al 1990; Jemt and Lekholm 1993, 1995; Lekholm et al 1994).

The esthetic outcome of this treatment has sometimes been neglected, but during the last decade the topic has received more attention, mainly in response to demands of patients (especially partially edentulous patients). Surgeons and periodontists have learned to optimize the placement of implant pillars in regard to both position and angulation in order to produce the best possible esthetic outcome. Optimal placement sometimes necessitates soft and/or hard tissue augmentation. Furthermore, improved knowledge of the anatomy, composition, and behavior of the peri-implant mucosa

has resulted in the ability to optimize the final architecture of the peri-implant soft tissue. For example, clinicians can now create a papillalike soft tissue anatomy surrounding implants. Hence, the treatment team cannot only imitate the anatomy of the original teeth but also create a soft tissue outline that corresponds as much as possible to the original.

Another important aspect of dental implant treatment is biomechanics. Long-term results may be influenced by the loading conditions of the prostheses and especially by the stress level of the individual implants; overload can lead to biological and/or mechanical complications (Rangert et al 1995). Restorations in partially edentulous arches are more susceptible to bending overload than are full-arch restorations because of the former's more linear implant configuration (Rangert and Sullivan 1993). Treatment of partially edentulous arches is becoming more frequent, and biomechanical considerations will correspondingly increase in importance.

Therefore, to minimize the risk of bending overload, as well as to optimize the final esthetic outcome, Brånemark system implants are now available in three different diameters (narrow, regular, and wide platform) (Herrman and Rangert 1997). However, as indicated, there is no conflict between biomechanical requirements for optimal treatment results on the one hand and esthetic and biological demands on the other. This book presents some guidelines for optimizing the functional and esthetic results of the "third dentition" by refining implant placement and soft tissue management based on the current knowledge of the involved tissues as well as of biomechanics.

References

Adell R, Eriksson B, Lekholm U, Brånemark P-I, Jemt T. A long-term follow-up study of osseointegrated implants in the treatment of totally edentulous jaws. Int J Oral Maxillofac Implants 1990;5:347–359.

Adell R, Lekholm U, Rockler B, Brånemark P-I. A 15-year study of osseointegrated implants in the treatment of the edentulous jaw. Int J Oral Surg 1981;6:387–416.

Albrektsson T. On long-term maintenance of the osseointegrated response. Aust Prosthodont J 1993;7:15–24.

Albrektsson T, Zarb G, Worthington P, Eriksson RA. The long-term efficacy of currently used dental implants: A review and proposed criteria of success. Int J Oral Maxillofac Implants 1986;1:11–25.

Arvidson K, Bystedt H, Frykholm A, von Konow L, Lothigius E. A 3-year clinical study of Astra dental implants in the treatment of edentulous mandibles. Int J Oral Maxillofac Implants 1992;7:321–329.

Brånemark P-I, Breine U, Adell R, Hansson B-O, Ohlsson Å. Intra-osseous anchorage of dental prostheses, I. Experimental studies. Scand J Plast Reconstr Surg 1969;3:81–100.

Dorland's Illustrated Medical Dictionary, ed 28. Philadelphia: Saunders, 1994:1198.

Ericsson I, Glantz P-O, Brånemark P-I. Tissue integrated implants ad modum Brånemark in the rehabilitation of partially edentulous jaws. In: Laney WR, Tolman DE (eds). Tissue Integration in Oral, Orthopedic and Maxillofacial Reconstruction. Chicago: Quintessence, 1990:174–187.

Ericsson I, Lekholm U, Brånemark P-I, Lindhe J, Glantz P-O, Nyman S. A clinical evaluation of fixed-bridge restorations supported by the combination of teeth and osseointegrated titanium implants. J Clin Periodontol 1986;13:307–312.

Herrman I, Rangert B. Dependable documentation sustains clinical performance: Only clinical follow-up can ensure predictable treatment results. Global Forum 1997;11:4–5.

Jemt T, Lekholm U. Oral implant treatment in posterior partially edentulous jaws: A 5-year follow-up report. Int J Oral Maxillofac Implants 1993;8:635–640.

Jemt T, Lekholm U. Implant treatment in edentulous maxillae: A 5-year follow-up report on patients with different degrees of jaw resorption. Int J Oral Maxillofac Implants 1995;10:303–311.

Jemt T, Lekholm U, Adell R. Osseointegrated implants in the treatment of partially edentulous patients: A preliminary study on 876 consecutively placed fixtures. Int J Oral Maxillofac Implants 1989;4: 211–217.

Lekholm U, van Steenberghe D, Herrman I, Bolender C, Folmer T, Gunne J, et al. Osseointegrated implants in the treatment of partially edentulous jaws: A prospective 5-year multicenter study. Int J Oral Maxillofac Implants 1994;9:627–635.

Makkonen TA, Holmberg S, Niemi L, Olsson C, Tammisalo T, Peltola JA. A 5-year prospective clinical study of Astra Tech dental implants supporting fixed bridges or overdentures in the edentulous mandible. Clin Oral Implants Res 1997;8:469–475.

Palmer RM, Smith BJ, Palmer PJ, Floyd PD. A prospective study of Astra single tooth implants. Clin Oral Implants Res 1997;8:173–179.

Rangert B, Krogh PHJ, Langer B, van Roeckel N. Bending overload and fixture fracture: A retrospective clinical analysis. Int J Oral Maxillofac Implants 1995;10:326–334.

Rangert B, Sullivan R. Biomechanical principles preventing prosthetic overload induced by bending. Nobelpharma News 1993;7:4–5.

van Steenberghe D, Lekholm U, Bolender C, Folmer T, Henry P, Herrman I, et al. The applicability of osseointegrated oral implants in the rehabilitation of partial edentulism: A prospective multicenter study on 558 fixtures. Int J Oral Maxillofac Implants 1990;5:272–281.

Chapter 1

Implant Integration and Stability

Lars Sennerby, LDS, PhD

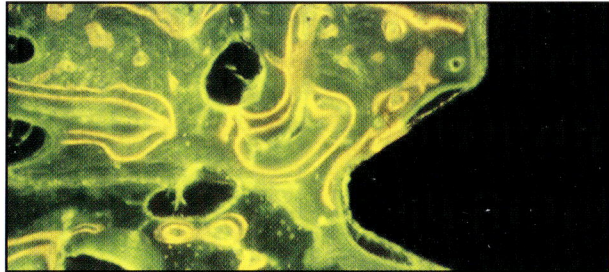

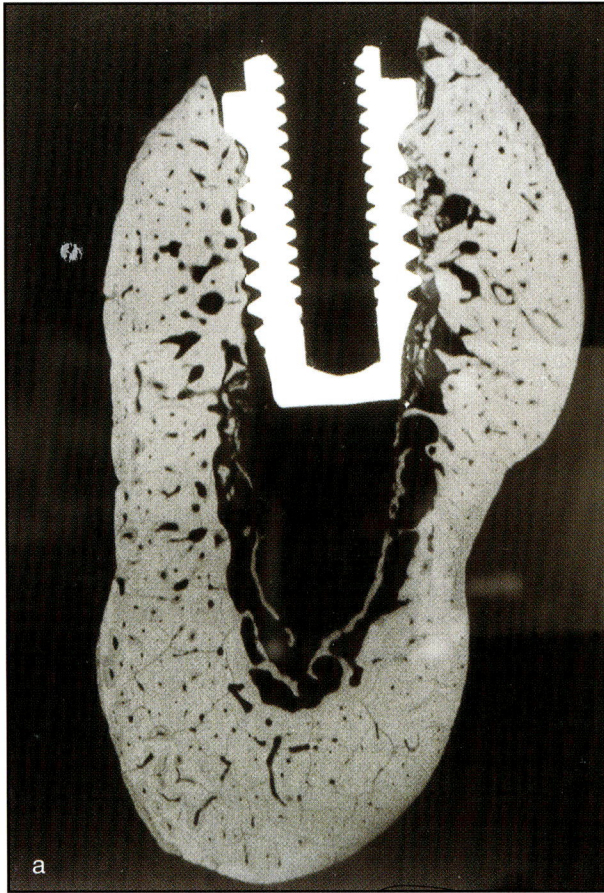

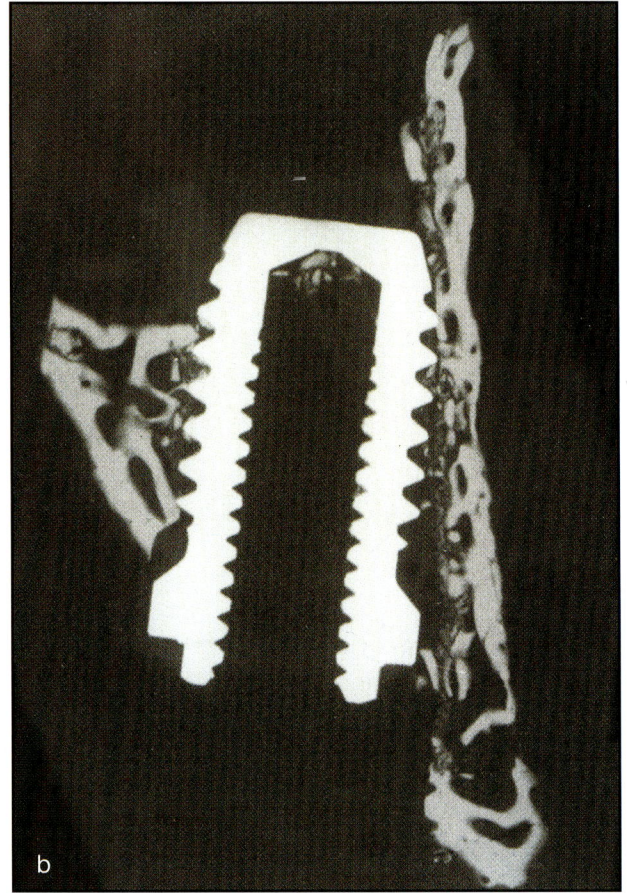

Fig 1-1 Microradiographs of specimens taken immediately after implant placement in human cadavers. *(a)* Mandibular specimen with dense cortical bone surrounding an implant of presumably high primary stability. *(b)* Maxillary specimen with only a small amount of mineralized tissue and a very thin cortical layer distinguishable.

The clinical manifestation of osseointegration is absence of implant mobility; thus, achieving and maintaining implant stability are prerequisites for successful long-term function of bone-anchored prostheses. From a structural and morphological point of view, implant stability is the result of contact between bone and the implant's surface. In principle, however, this stability is governed by additional factors related to the implant, the host, and the clinician. Primary stability, achieved at implant placement, is mainly determined by the mechanical properties of the jaw bone and influenced by the surgical technique and the design of the implant, especially in relatively soft bone (Fig 1-1). After primary healing, secondary stability is determined by the biological response to surgical trauma and healing conditions, as well as to the implant material. Ultimately, bone formation and remodeling at the implant interface lead to an increased degree of bone-implant contact (Fig 1-2). However, following traumatic surgery, preloading, infection, or the use of a nonbiocompatible implant material, the tissue response may result in bone resorption, decreased implant stability, and in some instances fibrous encapsulation and total loss of stability—that is, implant failure (Fig 1-3). The long-term prognosis and maintenance of implant

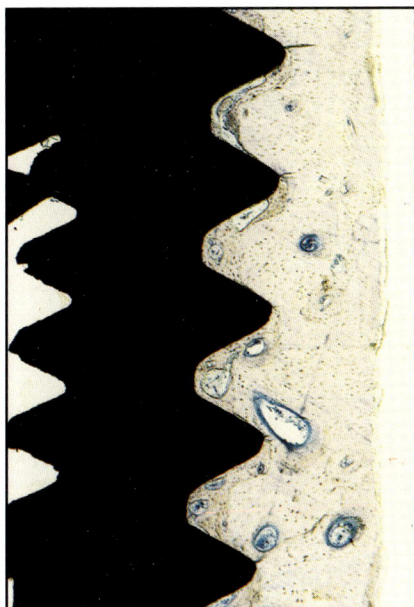

Fig 1-2 Light micrograph of an implant retrieved 6 months after placement in the posterior mandible. The implant is surrounded by dense cortical bone. Within the implant threads is bone formation, and a large portion of the surface is in direct contact with the newly formed bone.

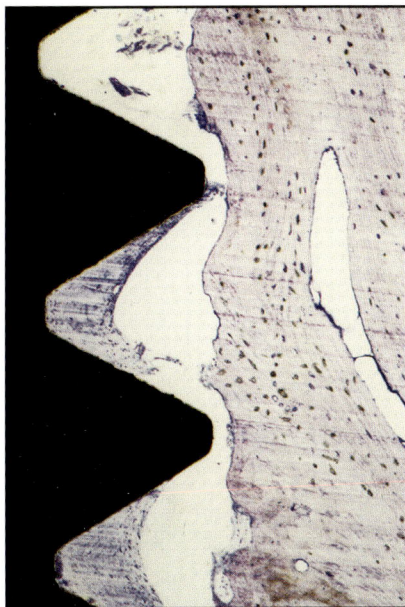

Fig 1-3 Light micrograph of a clinically mobile, failed implant. A layer of fibrous scar tissue separates the surface from bone tissue.

stability for Brånemark implants depend mainly on mechanical factors such as the degree of anchorage and loading conditions, although peri-implant infections may also affect stability.

Bone Tissue

Structure of bone

Bone is a rigid form of connective tissue with unique mechanical and biological properties. For example, it can heal without scar formation, and it can adapt to load conditions by changing structure. Bone is made up of both cortical (compact) and cancellous (trabecular, spongy) bone (Fig 1-4), which have distinct three-dimensional structures and thus different mechanical properties. Mature cortical bone consists of densely packed sheets of lamella, including concentric (osteons, haversian systems with vessel channels), interstitial, and parallel lamellae, whereas mature cancellous bone is a meshwork of bars and spicules of bone lamella, ie bone trabeculae. Cancellous bone consists of 70% soft tissue—mostly bone marrow—whereas cortical bone is up to 95% mineralized. Cortical bone is 10 to 20 times stiffer than cancellous bone, which

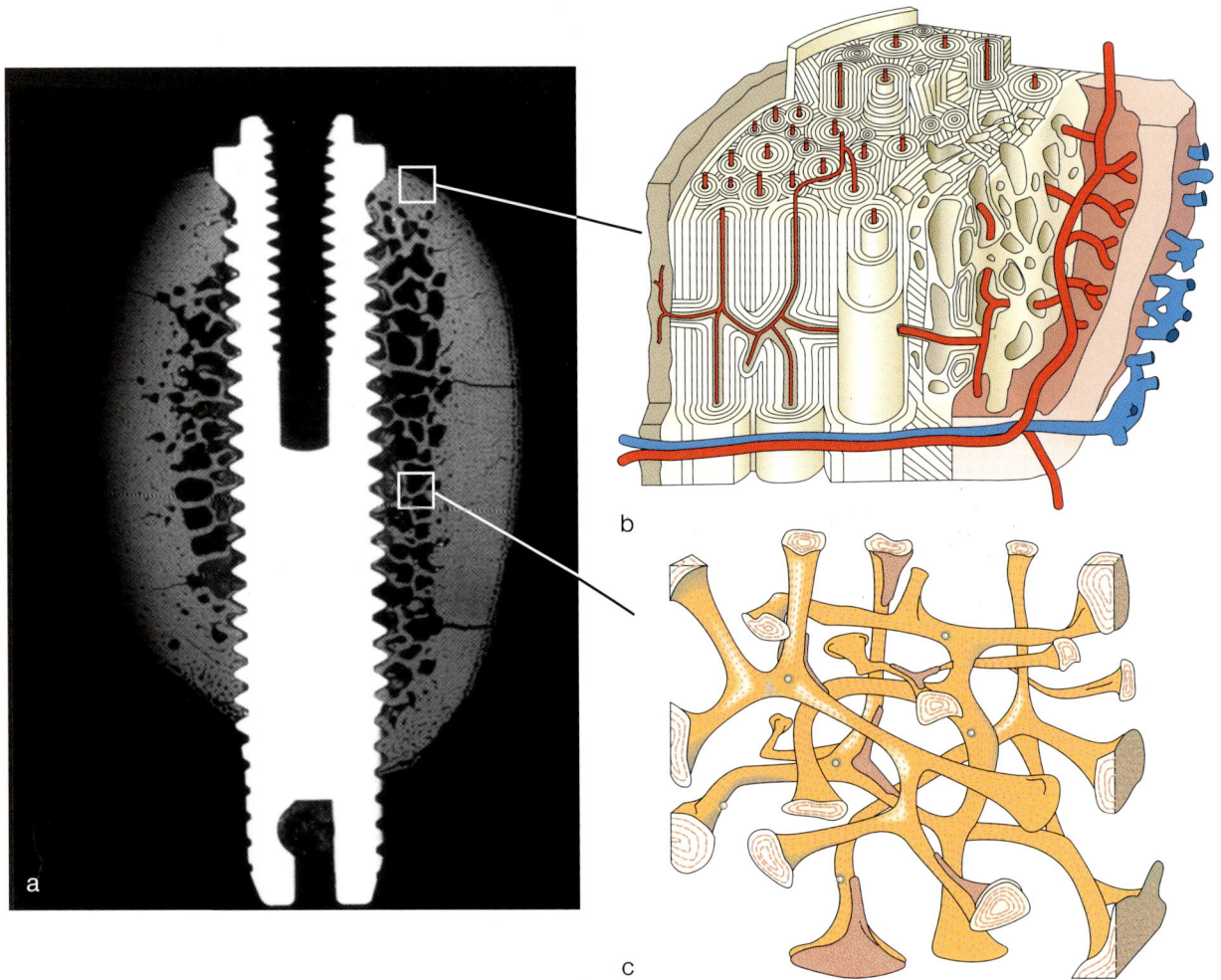

Fig 1-4 *(a)* Implant placed in bone. *(b)* The cortical bone consists of densely packed lamellae and vessel channels. *(c)* The porous cancellous bone consists of bone trabeculae and bone marrow tissue.

explains why it supports implants better than cancellous bone.

Mineralized bone can be classified as woven (fiber or primary) or lamellar (secondary), depending on the stage in development or healing. Woven bone is formed at an early stage and consists of loosely, irregularly packed collagen fibers, large scattered osteocyte lacunae, and minerals. It will eventually be replaced by lamellar bone, which has an organized structure and consists of smaller osteocyte lacunae and mineralized fiber bundles. Woven bone is softer than lamellar bone because of differences in structure and degree of mineralization. However, the mechanical properties of a unit of woven bone improve with time as a result of remodeling and lamellar bone replacement. For these reasons, lamellar bone provides better mechanical support for an implant than woven bone.

The mandible is basically a tubular long

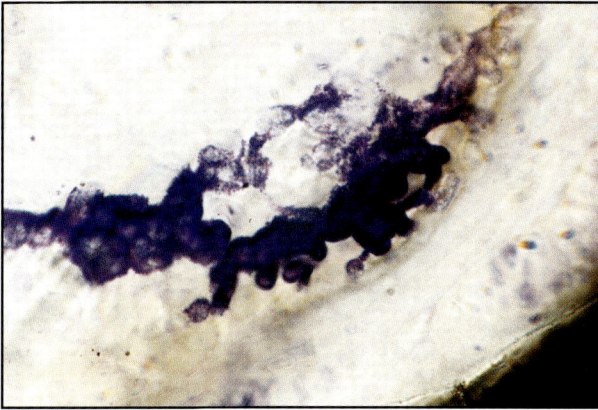

Fig 1-5 Light micrograph showing early bone formation near an implant 7 days after insertion in a rabbit tibia. Differentiated mesenchymal stem cells have started to produce mineralized tissue in a collagen matrix.

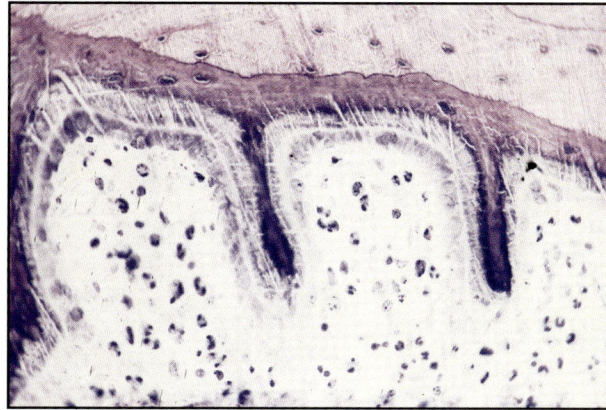

Fig 1-6 Light micrograph showing appositional bone formation 7 days after placement of an implant in a rabbit tibia. Active osteoblasts are producing osteoid, and a demarcation line appears between newly formed and old bone, as well as between the osteoblast-osteoid seam and new bone.

bone composed of an outer cortical layer surrounding central cancellous bone of various densities. The strength of the mandible is related to its dense cortical bone (see Fig 1-1a), which is thicker anteriorly at the lower border and posteriorly at the upper border. In contrast, the maxilla is composed of a thin outer cortical layer and a core of cancellous bone of various densities (see Fig 1-1b).

Bone formation

The three stages of bone formation are endochondral, intramembranous, and appositional. In endochondral bone formation, a cartilage template is formed that will later be replaced by bone; long bones, the base of the skull, and the bones of the vertebral column are formed by endochondral ossification. The vault of the skull, the facial bones, and the pelvis are formed via intramembranous ossification. This stage of bone formation starts with an aggregation of undifferentiated mesenchymal stem cells that then differentiate into osteoblasts and form osteoid in a collagen matrix (Fig 1-5). The osteoid is subsequently mineralized, and when the osteoblast is trapped into the mineralized bone, it becomes an osteocyte. Some osteoblasts flatten onto the bone surface; these are transformed to bone-lining cells, also known as surface osteocytes or resting osteoblasts. In appositional bone formation, osteoblasts produce bone on existing bone surfaces (Fig 1-6); this type of ossification occurs in periosteal enlargement of bones during development and growth and during bone modeling and remodeling.

Bone tissue undergoes constant remodeling throughout the life of the bone. Osteoclasts are the cells responsible for resorption of bone and are attracted to specific sites by lining cells. Cortical bone remodeling occurs by means of creeping substitution by bone-metabolizing units (BMUs) or by cutting the filling cones. Osteoclasts cut canals into the bone through which vessels and osteoblasts will follow, laying down new lamellar bone.

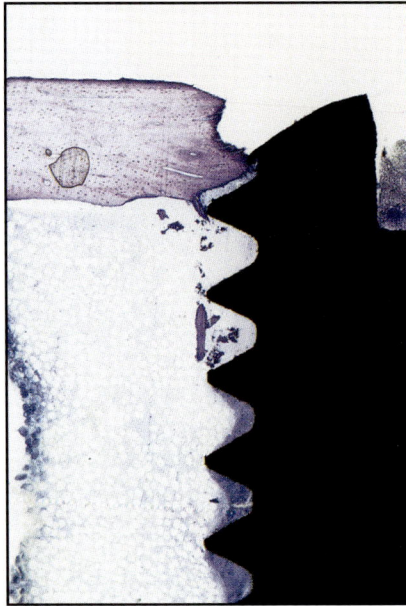

Fig 1-7 Light micrograph of an implant 3 days after placement in a rabbit tibia. The interface area consists of bone fragments displaced from the drilling procedure, a hematoma, and bone marrow tissue. This resolution level shows no signs of bone formation or resorption.

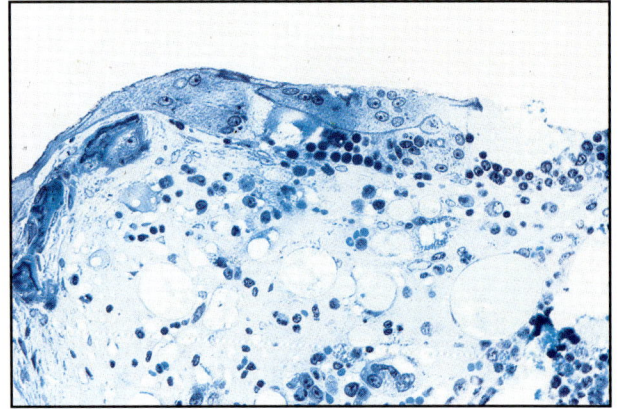

Fig 1-8 Light micrograph showing multinucleated giant cells attaching to an implant surface 7 days after implant placement in a rabbit tibia.

Remodeling of trabecular, endosteal, and periosteal bone surfaces is similar to that of cortical bone except that the osteoclasts lie on the surface of the bone, creating cavities known as Howship's lacunae.

Bone healing

Trauma (for example, fracture, osteotomy, or implant placement) initiates a preprogrammed healing process to repair the fracture/defect and return the bone to its original form via remodeling/modeling. The events of healing resemble those involved in the development of bone. In intramembranous bone, healing can be divided into the following phases: (1) formation of a hematoma, (2) release and activation of mediators from the injured tissues and the circulating blood, (3) accumulation of inflammatory and mesenchy-mal stem cells, (4) revascularization and formation of a granulation tissue, (5) tissue degradation by macrophages and giant cells, (6) cell differentiation to osteoblasts, (7) formation of woven bone, and (8) remodeling/modeling.

Integration of Implants

Surgical placement of an implant results in a varying degree of contact between bone and the implant. The interface area consists of bone, marrow tissue, and a hematoma mixed with bone fragments from the drilling procedure (Sennerby et al 1993a) (Fig 1-7). As in the healing of a defect or fracture, after implant placement inflammatory and mesenchymal stem cells migrate from adjacent

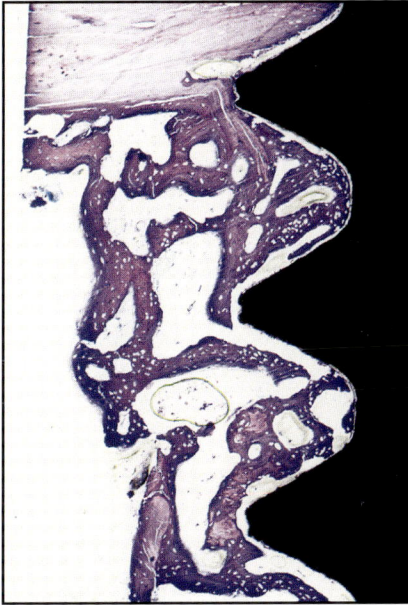

Fig 1-9 Light micrograph demonstrating extensive bone formation and condensation into the implant threads 14 days after placement in a rabbit tibia.

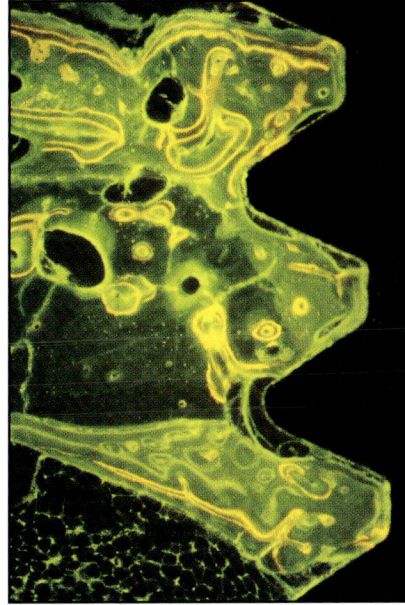

Fig 1-10 Fluoroscopy of a ground section 12 weeks after implant placement in a rabbit tibia. Tetracycline administered 1 week prior to killing the rabbit has been incorporated in bone formation sites, which indicates extensive remodeling of the interface bone. The formation of secondary osteons is evident.

vessels and the marrow stroma toward the interface area. The hematoma is replaced by proliferating vessels and loose connective tissue. Multinucleated giant cells cover the implant surfaces that face nonmineralized tissue (Fig 1-8). This classic sign of a foreign body reaction may indicate that bone encapsulation of an implant is a foreign body reaction of bone. However, these cells decrease in number with time and an increasing amount of bone-implant contact.

In the early phase of healing, woven bone is formed by osteoblast seams at the surfaces of trabecular and endosteal cortical bone surrounding the implant. Extensive remodeling—that is, resorption followed by bone forma-

tion—in the cortical bone near the implant surface results in an increased number of secondary osteons and woven bone formation in voids between the implant and the cut surface of the bone. The newly formed bone approaching the implant surface leads to bone condensation both into the implant threads and toward the implant surface (Fig 1-9). Consequently, the amount of bone in the threads and the degree of bone-implant contact increase with time. In the late phase of healing, lamellar bone replaces woven bone in a process of creeping substitution (Fig 1-10). The first phase of bone healing has been calculated to take 4 to 16 weeks, whereas the remodeling process may take 4 to 12 months

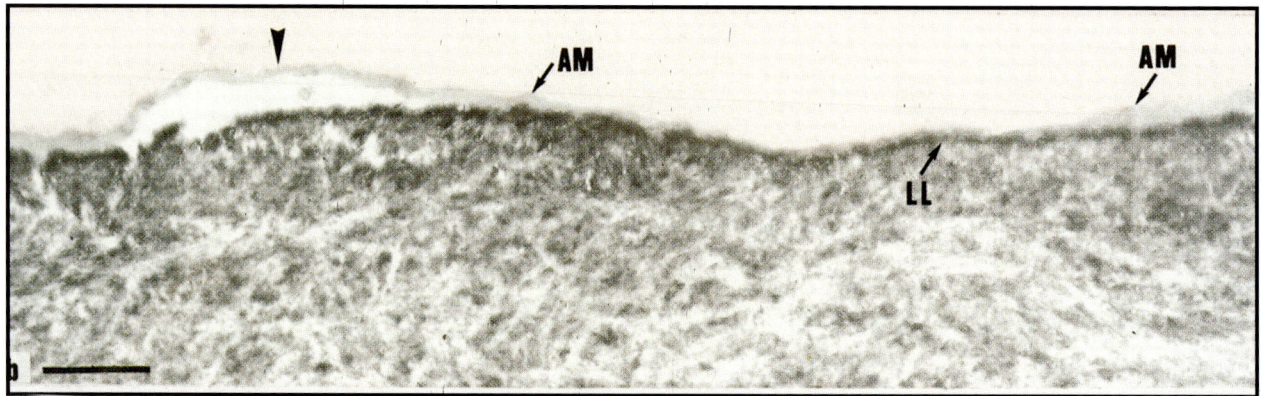

Fig 1-11 Transmission electron micrograph of the bone-titanium interface 1 year after placement in a rabbit tibia. Two layers can be distinguished: *(1)* an amorphous layer (AM) between the implant surface and the bone tissue below and *(2)* an electron-dense layer (lamina limitans, LL) at the border between the mineralized bone and the amorphous layer.

or longer in humans (Roberts et al 1994). Thus, complete healing probably takes longer than the conventional 3 to 6 months.

Although bone seems to be in intimate contact with titanium implants on the light microscope level, ultrastructural studies in both animals and humans indicate the presence of an unmineralized zone between the implant surface and the mineralized tissues. Linder et al (1983) and Albrektsson et al (1986) placed titanium-coated polycarbonate implants in rabbit tibiae and described a zone resembling ground substance with a thickness of 20 to 50 nm. Sennerby et al (1991, 1992, 1993b) reported on two main features of this interface area: *(1)* a 100- to 400-nm-thick amorphous unmineralized layer separating the implant surface from the mineralized bone and *(2)* a 100-nm-wide electron-dense line (lamina limitans) present at the border between the mineralized bone and the non-calcified amorphous layer (Fig 1-11). These findings indicate that implant fixation does not depend on a true chemical bond between bone and titanium. Instead, the clinical stability of an implant depends on a mechanical interlocking of mineralized bone and both the irregularities on the implant surface created by the turning procedure and macroscopic undercuts such as holes and bone chip chambers.

Implant Stability

Implant stability depends on the nature of the contact between bone and implant surface. Although accurate clinical measurement of implant stability has not been possible, the degree of anchorage obviously influences the long-term results of osseointegrated implants. Clinical follow-up studies have shown that short implants fail more often than longer ones. Many studies have found poor bone quality to be a risk factor. For instance, Jaffin and Berman (1991) reported failure rates of up to 40% in type 4 bone (according to Lekholm and Zarb 1985) during a 5-year follow-up period.

Manufacturers and researchers thus have been focusing on the "soft bone" problem and have presented solutions related mainly to implant design and surface. Moreover, recent research based on long experience with osseointegrated implants has demonstrated that no healing periods are needed under certain conditions; bone healing prior to loading is not always a prerequisite for long-term success.

Techniques to evaluate the bone-implant interface and stability

Development of a simpler and more successful osseointegration technique involves experimental models and techniques to evaluate relevant parameters. A number of experimental and clinical methods to estimate implant stability in bone have been developed.

Donath and Breuner (1982) and Donath (1988) introduced a technique that enabled the preparation of approximately 10-µm-thick undecalcified sections of intact bone-implant interface for light microscopy (see Figs 1-7, 1-9, and 1-10). Histomorphometry has been extensively used to analyze such ground sections; the bone tissue response to threaded implants is described according to the amount of bone-metal contact and the bone area within the threads.

Johansson and Albrektsson (1987) introduced the removal torque test to describe the stability and fixation of experimental threaded implants in rabbit bone. This destructive test measures the torsion force (Ncm) needed to rupture the bone-implant interface. The researchers showed that the removal torque for commercially pure titanium implants is related to the amount of bone-metal contact, which was interpreted as being a consequence of the healing process (bone formation and maturation at the implant surface). The technique has since been used in biocompatibility studies and has proved to be a valuable tool for describing the bone tissue response to various materials and surface

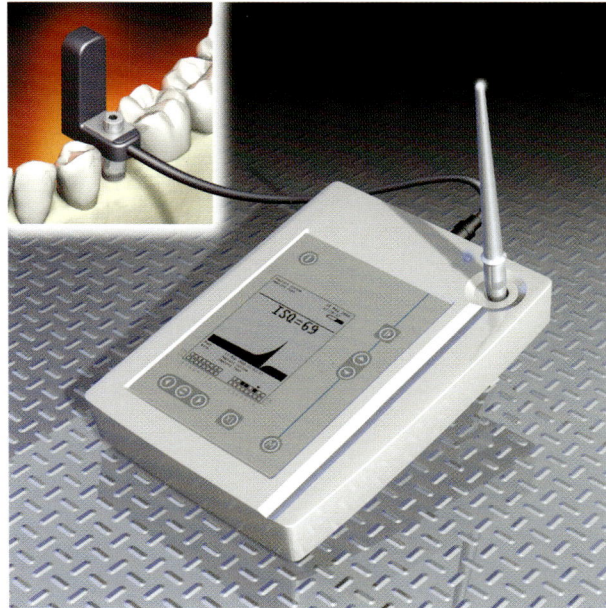

Fig 1-12 Transducer and instrument for RFA measurements.

modifications (Johansson 1991; Morberg 1991; Wennerberg 1996).

Resonance frequency analysis (RFA), developed by Meredith (1997), is a relatively new and promising noninvasive method to evaluate implant stability and osseointegration. Resonance frequency analysis measures stability by applying a microscopic bending load, the most relevant type of clinically applied functional load. The technique uses an L-shaped transducer attached to the implant or abutment (Fig 1-12). Using a frequency response analyzer, a personal computer, and dedicated software, the transducer beam is excited over a frequency range (typically 5 to 15 kHz), its response is measured, and the resonance frequency (RF) of the system is recorded. The RF is determined by two parameters: the degree of stiffness at the implant-bone interface and the level of bone surrounding the transducer. Because the stiffness of the implant components and the transducer are constant, it is the stiffness of

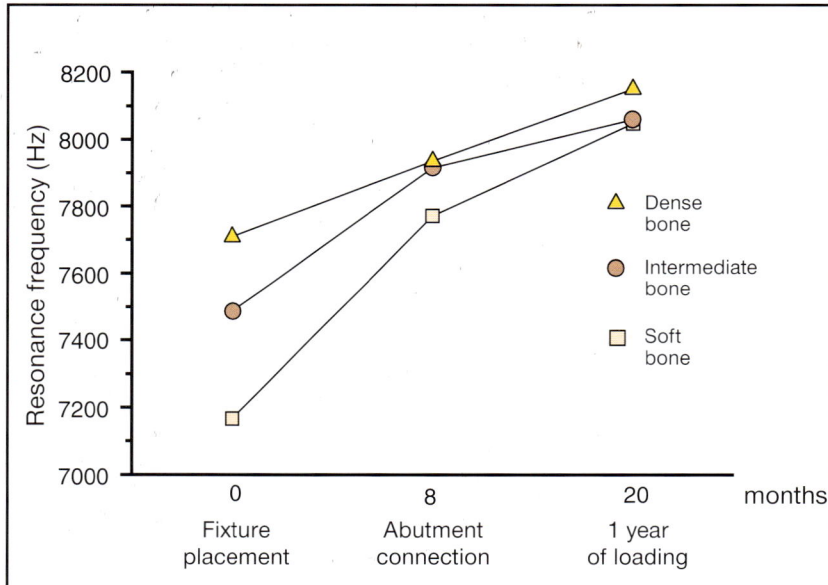

Fig 1-13 Changes of RF and implant stability with time for maxillary implants placed in soft, medium, and hard bone densities. Statistically significant differences are seen in initial stability; however, after 8 and 20 months there are no differences between the three groups because of bone formation, remodeling, and maturation at the bone-implant interface.

the surrounding implant-tissue interface that is relevant. If the implant-tissue interface stiffness is high, the RF will be high, which also indicates high implant stability. Resonance frequency analysis has provided valuable information from direct measurements of experimental and clinical implants in various situations. The data obtained have increased the understanding of how osseointegration and implant stability develop in different situations.

Bone quality, healing time, and implant stability

One obvious way to increase stability after implant surgery is to allow the surrounding bone to heal before loading; this is one of several reasons why a two-stage technique originally was advocated by Brånemark (1977). How much time is needed to reach sufficient stability is not known, but empirical healing periods of 3 and 6 months have resulted in favorable long-term results for mandibular and maxillary implants, respectively.

Clinical and in vitro work using the RFA technique have demonstrated a correlation between primary stability and bone density as assessed by cutting torque measurements (Friberg et al 1999b). It is not surprising that implants in soft-quality bone showed a lower primary stability than implants in denser bone (Fig 1-13). Furthermore, the stability of implants in soft bone increased more than that of implants in denser bone from placement to abutment connection. Twenty months after placement, all implants had reached a similar degree of stability irrespective of bone quality and primary stability. The results indicate that the healing process around an implant in soft bone, which consists mainly of trabecular bone, results in a change in bone quality in relation to the implant surface. It is also likely that loading has a positive influence. From a structural point of view, this change is most likely due to a condensation of trabecular bone to a lamina dura–like structure at the implant interface (Fig 1-14), as described radiographically by Strid (1985). The results indicate that long healing periods

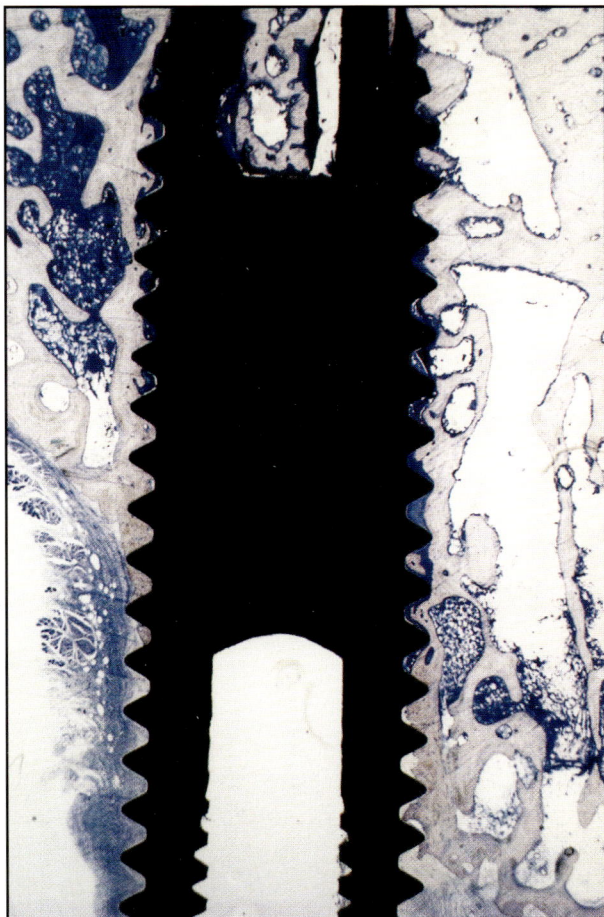

Fig 1-14 Light micrograph of a clinically retrieved maxillary implant showing condensation of the bone trabeculae toward the implant surface.

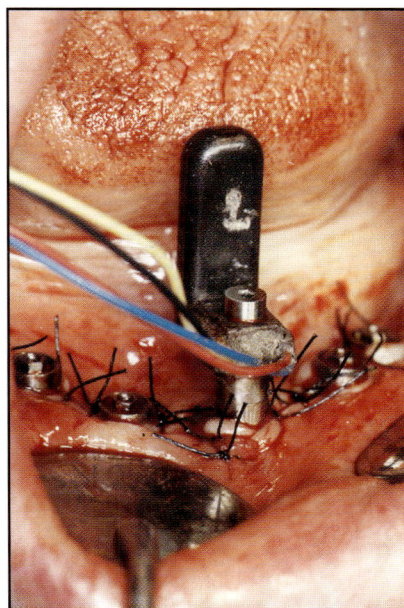

Fig 1-15 Resonance frequency analysis transducer attached to a one-stage implant in the mandible.

may be needed for implants placed in soft bone with low primary stability.

The RFA technique has also been used to study implant stability in dense bone. A group of 15 patients with edentulous mandibles were each treated with five one-stage implants placed between the mental foramina (Friberg et al 1999a) (Fig 1-15). The implants were allowed to heal for 15 weeks before a fixed partial denture was connected. Resonance frequency analysis measurements were per-

formed at surgery and 1, 2, 6, and 15 weeks after implant placement. A slight decrease of resonance frequency because of some marginal bone resorption was observed during the 15 weeks of healing. A final registration after 1 year of loading revealed no further change in RF or marginal bone resorption (Fig 1-16). The findings support the correlation of direct or early loading of implants with high primary stability. The healing and osseointegration that most probably occurred around

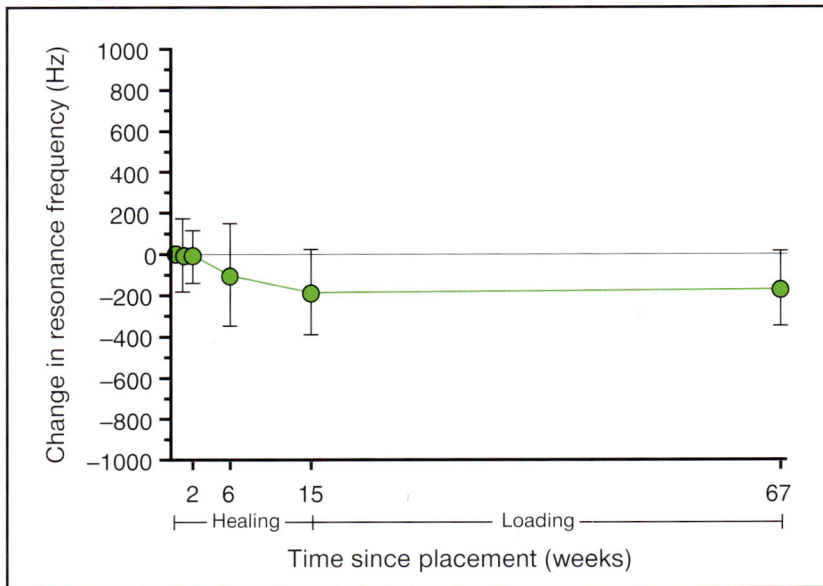

Fig 1-16 Changes of RF and implant stability with time for one-stage implants in the mandible. A statistically significant decrease is seen after 15 weeks, which is explained by some marginal bone loss. No changes appear from 15 weeks to the first annual check-up.

these implants did not measurably affect their stability, because the primary stability was already very high.

These clinical and in vitro studies show that the mechanical properties of the jaw bone dictate the primary stability of an implant and the length of the healing period needed to reach sufficient stability. Moreover, the data also justify the use of a two-stage procedure in medium to soft bone and suggest that healing periods longer than 6 months may be needed with low primary stability. Most important, the results indicate that total treatment time can be dramatically reduced for many patients. If suitable candidates can be identified at implant placement—for instance, by using the RFA technique—the treatment can be simplified without compromising the long-term results.

Influence of surface topography on implant stability

Experimental studies have yielded extensive evidence that more bone is found at the sur-face of implants with rough surfaces than smoother surfaces. Several studies also have demonstrated higher removal torque values for rough implants, which would indicate a better bone response to such surfaces. Wennerberg (1996) used a laser technique to make noncontact measurements of surface roughness. Sa, which describes the average deviation from a reference plane in three dimensions, was recognized as a useful parameter. In a series of experimental studies using histomorphometry and removal torque tests, Wennerberg (1996) found that implants with an Sa of about 1.5 μm performed better than those with smoother or rougher surfaces. Experimental investigations in animals and humans have reported benefits of using rougher implant surfaces (Buser et al 1991; Buser et al 1999; Lazzarra et al 1999; Ivanoff et al in press). In a recent study, 26 pairs of machined and titanium dioxide (TiO_2)-grit-blasted microimplants were placed in the jaws of patients (Ivanoff et al, unpublished data). Histomorphometry after 3 to 8 months of healing revealed more bone for the rougher implants.

If there is a relationship between histomorphometric findings, removal torque tests, and the clinical success of an implant design, implants with a rough surface should perform better clinically. However, in spite of the experimental data, to date no clinical evidence supports the assertion that implants with a rough surface perform better. Clinical documentation shows that rough screw-shaped implants may perform at least as well as machined ones and that rough cylindrical implants show continuous marginal bone resorption and high long-term failure rates. In a 2-year clinical study, Karlsson et al (1997) compared machined and TiO$_2$-grit-blasted screw implants and could not find any statistically significant difference between the two implants. Åstrand et al (1999), who also compared machined and TiO$_2$-grit-blasted implants in a randomized comparative prospective study for 1 year, reported a higher failure rate for the machined implants but no statistically significant differences between patients treated with the two implants. In a retrospective clinical study, Sullivan et al (1997) studied the survival of acid-etched implants (Osseotite) over 3 years. The overall failure rate was low, but further analysis of the data showed that the failure rate in soft bone (type 4) was about 37%. In spite of their own results, the authors concluded that their implant worked especially well in soft-quality bone.

The use of RFA in experimental studies has failed to find higher primary or secondary stability of implants with a rough surface (gritblasted or acid-etched) in contrast with the results of the removal torque studies. The reason is probably that the torque test measures the strength of the bone-implant interface in shear whereas RFA measures the stiffness of the bone-implant interface in bending, which probably better reflects the applied functional loads in the clinical situation. It can be speculated that if there were clinical benefits to using rough implant surfaces, they would be most often seen in soft-quality bone. The lack of clinical data to support the superiority of rough surfaces may be explained by the fact that no controlled comparative clinical studies in soft-quality bone have been performed.

Influence of surgical technique and implant design on implant stability

Ivanoff et al (1997) demonstrated a relationship between implant diameter and removal torque. Thus, loosening of wider implants requires a higher removal torque, a characteristic that may also indicate better clinical function. However, a negative relationship between implant survival and implant diameter was found in a retrospective clinical study in which 5-mm implants failed more often than standard implants over a 3- to 5-year period. The reason was probably that most 5-mm implants were short (6 mm) and were used as rescue implants in situations where standard implants could not be placed with sufficient primary stability. Although other clinical studies have shown more favorable results, there is no evidence that wide implants are better than standard-diameter implants. Like roughsurfaced implants, wide implants are probably as good, but not better than, standard ones when used under similar conditions.

The high failure rates observed in type 4 bone may be explained by the fact that pretapping initially was used in all bone qualities. Because of the "soft bone problem," most surgeons today use self-tapping implants or place standard implants as self-tapping implants in soft-quality bone. Wider implants, smaller drill diameters, or both are often used to compress the bone for good primary stability. In a cadaver study, O'Sullivan et al (unpublished data) demonstrated a dramatic difference in the primary stability of standard implants when pretapping was used or omitted (Fig 1-17). The results suggested that tapping in soft bone should be abandoned. The

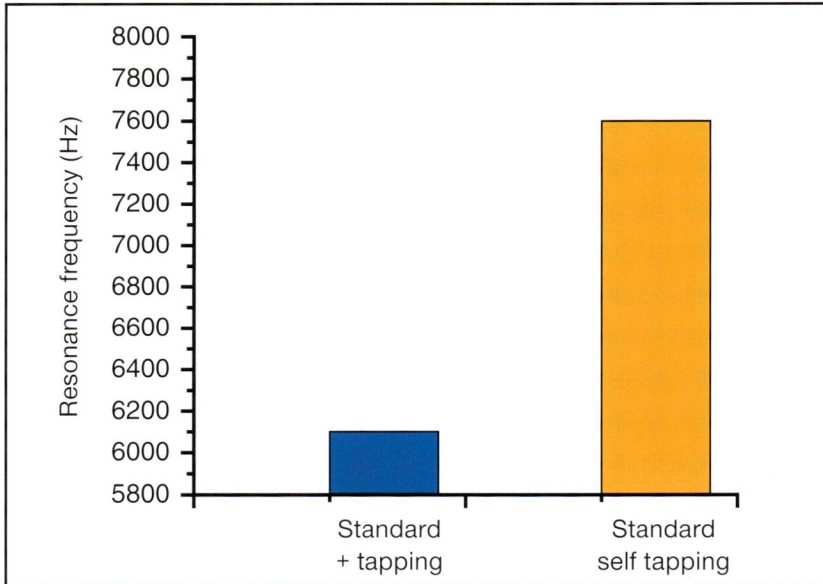

Fig 1-17 Initial stability for standard implants in type 3 cadaver bone with and without pretapping.

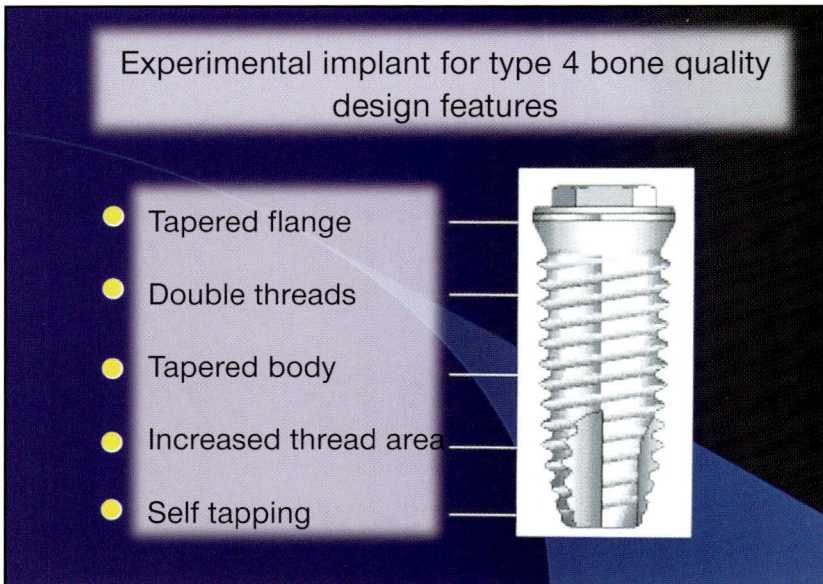

Experimental implant for type 4 bone quality design features

- Tapered flange
- Double threads
- Tapered body
- Increased thread area
- Self tapping

Fig 1-18 Design features for the Mark IV Brånemark implant.

findings also underscore the importance of surgical technique in obtaining good primary stability in soft bone.

A novel implant design for soft-quality bone has been developed and evaluated. The idea of the design is to eliminate surgical variations in implant placement, resulting in optimal pri-mary stability in soft bone. The design includes a slight taper (1 degree) and double threads (Fig 1-18). During insertion, the tapered design results in lateral compression of the bone; increased stiffness of the interfacial bone; and an increase in primary stability, as evaluated by RFA in both in vitro and ani-

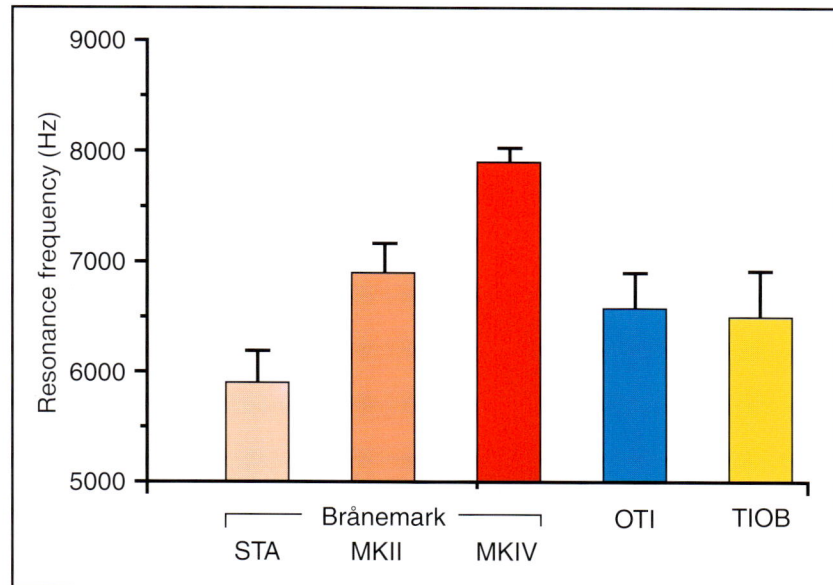

Fig 1-19 Initial stability for five implant designs placed in type 4 cadaver bone. STA indicates standard Brånemark implant; MKII, Mark II Brånemark implant; MKIV, Mark IV Brånemark implant; OTI, 3i Osseotite implant; and TIOB, Astra Tech TiOBlast implant.

mal experiments. The double threads enable quicker installation and result in less wobbling during placement. In a cadaver study by O'Sullivan et al (2000), it was evident that all implant designs (standard with and without tapping, Mark II, and Mark IV) showed high primary stability in type 2 bone, but differences became evident with softer-quality bone (Fig 1-19). The new Mark IV design showed the highest insertion torque, as well as the highest primary stability, in type 4 bone. One possible problem with the Mark IV design is that lateral compression may result in a negative tissue response and bone resorption during healing. In a recent animal study, however, placement of this new implant resulted in a higher primary stability as compared with the standard design (unpublished data). Furthermore, there were no signs of negative tissue response to the tapered design over time. However, although the experimental data suggest better stability and clinical results with the new design, to date no clinical studies support this suggestion.

Conclusions

Data from experimental and clinical studies of osseointegration and implant stability suggest that osseointegration is a consequence of bone healing initiated by surgical trauma and the excellent biocompatibility of titanium. Recent studies indicate that RFA can be used clinically to assess implant stability and osseointegration. Based on the results of RFA, a two-stage procedure provides better stability of implants in bone of medium to poor quality (types 3 and 4) but may not lead to increased stability in denser bone (types 1 and 2). Thus, although osseointegration occurs in response to surgical trauma, it is not always needed before loading. In the future the RFA technique may be used to identify patients in whom one-stage and early-loading protocols would not compromise long-term results.

References

Albrektsson T, Hansson HA. An ultrastructural characterisation of the interface between bone and sputtered titanium or stainless steel surfaces. Biomaterials 1986;7:201–205

Åstrand P, Engquist B, Dahlgren S, Engquist E, Feldmann H, Gröndahl K. AstraTech and Brånemark system implants: A 5-year comparative study: Results after one year. Clin Implants Dent Rel Res 1999;1:17–26.

Brånemark P-I. Osseointegrated implants in the treatment of the edentulous jaw. Experience from a 10-year period. Stockholm: Almquist and Wiksell, 1977.

Buser D, Nydegger T, Oxland T, Cochran DL, Schenk RK, Hirt HP, et al. Interface shear strength of titanium implants with a sandblasted and acid-etched surface: A biomechanical study in the maxilla of miniature pigs. J Biomed Mater Res 1999;45: 75–83.

Buser D, Schenk RK, Steinemann S, Fiorellini JP, Fox CH, Stich H. Influence of surface characteristics on bone integration of titanium implants: A histomorphometric study in miniature pigs. J Biomed Mater Res 1991;25:889–902.

Donath, K. Die Trenn-Dünnschliff-Technik zur Herstellung histologischer Präparate von nicht schneidbaren Geweben und Materialien. Der Präparator 1988;34:197–206.

Donath K, Breuner GA. A method for the study of undecalcified bones and teeth with attached soft tissue. J Oral Pathol 1982;11:318–325.

Friberg B, Sennerby L, Lindén B, Gröndahl K, Lekholm U. Stability measurements of one-stage Brånemark implants during healing in mandibles: A clinical resonance frequency study. Int J Oral Maxillofac Surg 1999a;28:266–272.

Friberg B, Sennerby L, Meredith N, Lekholm U. A comparison between cutting torque and resonance frequency measurements of maxillary implants: A 20-month clinical study. Int J Oral Maxillofac Surg 1999b;28:297–303.

Ivanoff CJ, Hallgren C, Wennerberg A, Widmark G, Sennerby L. Histologic evaluation of the bone integration of TiO_2 grit blasted and turned microimplants in humans (in press).

Ivanoff CJ, Sennerby L, Johansson C, Rangert B, Lekholm U. Influence of implant diameters on the integration of screw implants: An experimental study in rabbits. Int J Oral Maxillofac Surg 1997; 26:141–148.

Jaffin RA, Berman CL. The excessive loss of Brånemark fixtures in type IV bone: A 5-year analysis. J Periodontol 1991;62:2–4.

Johansson C, Albrektsson T. Integration of screw implants in the rabbit: A 1 year follow up of removal torque of titanium implants. Int J Oral Maxillofac Implants 1987;2:69–75.

Johansson CB. On Tissue Reactions to Metal Implants [thesis]. Göteborg, Sweden: Univ of Göteborg, 1991.

Karlsson U, Gotfredsen K, Olsson C. Single-tooth replacement by osseointegrated Astra Tech dental implants: A 2-year report. Int J Prosthodont 1997;10:318–324.

Lazzarra RJ, Testori T, Trisi P, Porter S, Weinstein R. A human histologic analysis of Osseotite and machined surfaces using implants with 2 opposing surfaces. Int J Periodontics Restorative Dent 1999;9:117–129.

Lekholm U, Zarb GA. Patient selection and preparation. In: Brånemark P-I, Zarb GA, Albrektsson T (eds). Tissue-integrated Prostheses: Osseointegration in Clinical Dentistry. Chicago: Quintessence, 1985:199–209.

Linder L, Albrektsson T, Brånemark PI, Hansson HA, Ivarsson B, Jönsson J, et al. Electron microscopic analysis of the bone-titanium interface. Acta Orthop Scand 1983;54:45–52.

Meredith N. On the clinical measurement of implant stability and osseointegration [thesis]. Göteborg, Sweden: Univ of Göteborg, 1997.

Morberg P. On bone tissue reactions to acrylic cement [thesis]. Göteborg, Sweden: Univ of Göteborg, 1991.

O'Sullivan D, Sennerby L, Meredith N. Measurements comparing the initial stability of five designs of dental implants: A human cadaver study. Clin Implants Dent Rel Res 2000;2:35–92.

Roberts E, Garetto L, Brezniak, N. Bone physiology and metabolism. In: Misch C (ed). Contemporary Implant Dentistry. St Louis: Mosby–Year Book, 1994:327–368.

Sennerby L, Thomsen P, Ericson LE. Early bone tissue response to titanium implants inserted in rabbit cortical bone, I. Light microscopic observations. J Mater Sci Mater Med 1993a;4:240–250.

Sennerby L, Thomsen P, Ericson LE. Early bone tissue response to titanium implants inserted in rabbit cortical bone, II. Ultrastructural observations. J Mater Sci Mater Med 1993b;4:494–502.

Sennerby L, Thomsen P, Ericson LE. Structure of the bone-titanium interface in rabbits. J Mater Sci Mater Med 1992;3:262–271.

Sennerby L, Thomsen P, Ericson LE, Lekholm U, Åstrand P. Structure of the bone-titanium interface in retrieved clinical dental implants. Clin Oral Implants Res 1991;2:103–111.

Strid KG. Radiographic procedures. In: Brånemark P-I, Zarb GA, Albrektsson T (eds). Tissue Integrated Prostheses. Osseointegration in Clinical Dentistry. Chicago: Quintessence, 1985.

Sullivan DY, Sherwood RL, Mai TN. Preliminary results of a multicenter study evaluating a chemically enhanced surface for machined commercially pure titanium implants. J Prosthet Dent 1997;78: 379–386.

Wennerberg A. On Surface Roughness and Implant Incorporation [thesis]. Göteborg, Sweden: Univ of Göteborg, 1996.

Chapter 2

Biology and Pathology of Peri-implant Soft Tissue

Ingvar Ericsson, LDS, Odont Dr

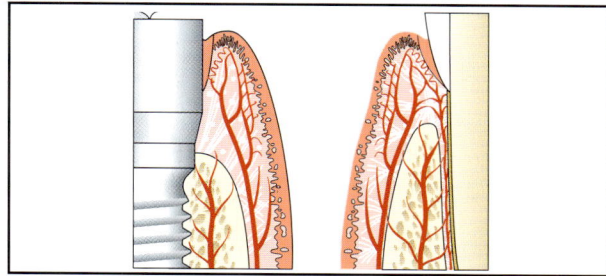

Teeth are anatomically unique, as they are the only structures of the body that penetrate a lining or covering epithelium. Teeth and dental implants are two examples of structures that pierce the integument. Whereas proper anchorage of an implant in the bone (osseointegration) is a prerequisite for the implant's stability, long-term retention of an implant seems to depend on the proper epithelial and connective tissue attachment to the titanium surface (that is, a complete soft tissue seal protecting the bone from the oral environment) (Brånemark 1985; Gould 1985; Ten Cate 1985; McKinney et al 1985; Carmichael et al 1989).

It has been proposed that the free marginal gingiva and the peri-implant mucosa share many clinical and histological features (Adell et al 1986; Lekholm, Adell, et al 1986; Lekholm, Ericsson, et al 1986; Akagawa et al 1989; Seymour et al 1989). Adell et al (1986) and Lekholm, Adell, et al (1986) performed biopsies on the soft tissue surrounding successful implant sites in edentulous patients who had been treated with the Brånemark implant system. The authors reported that this peri-implant mucosa frequently lacked inflammatory lesions, and when present, the lesions were minute and located adjacent to and along a junctional epithelium. Lekholm, Ericsson, et al (1986) examined clinically healthy and slightly inflamed gingiva and peri-implant mucosa obtained from partially edentulous patients enrolled in an individually designed maintenance care program; the authors concluded that the two types of tissue harbored inflammatory-cell infiltrates with similar locations and extensions.

Several animal and in vitro experiments have demonstrated similarities between the gingiva and the peri-implant mucosa with respect to both epithelial structures and connective tissue components (Gould et al 1981; Schroeder et al 1981; Jansen et al 1985; McKinney et al 1985; Hashimoto et al 1988;

van Drie et al 1988; Buser et al 1989). However, the absence of a root cementum layer on the implant surface creates basic differences between implants and teeth in regard to connective tissue fiber orientation and attachment (Buser et al 1989). How the soft tissue seal at implant sites contributes to its functional success has not yet been completely evaluated. However, well-controlled experimental studies in this field have been performed by a research team at Göteborg University in Sweden (Berglundh et al 1991, 1992, 1994; Ericsson and Lindhe 1993; Ericsson et al 1992; Leonhardt et al 1992; Lindhe et al 1992; Marinello et al 1995; Berglundh and Lindhe 1996; Abrahamsson et al 1998).

Healthy Peri-implant Mucosa

Berglundh et al (1991) compared clinically healthy (normal) peri-implant mucosa and free marginal gingiva using the beagle model with respect to structure and composition. Histological analysis revealed that each of the two soft tissue units had a keratinized oral epithelium and a junctional epithelium with a length of approximately 2 mm. The height of the gingival supracrestal connective tissue portion was approximately 1 mm; the collagen fiber bundles were oriented in a fan shape, originating from the acellular root cementum (Figs 2-1 and 2-2). Titanium implants lack root cementum, however, so the collagen fiber bundles in the peri-implant mucosa run mainly parallel to the implant surface and originate from the bone surface (Figs 2-3 and 2-4).

This observation is supported by Listgarten et al (1992), who placed in dog mandibles epoxy resin replicas of dental implants coated with a layer of pure titanium 90 to 120 nm thick. Biopsy specimens were analyzed using light and electron microscopy. The supracre-

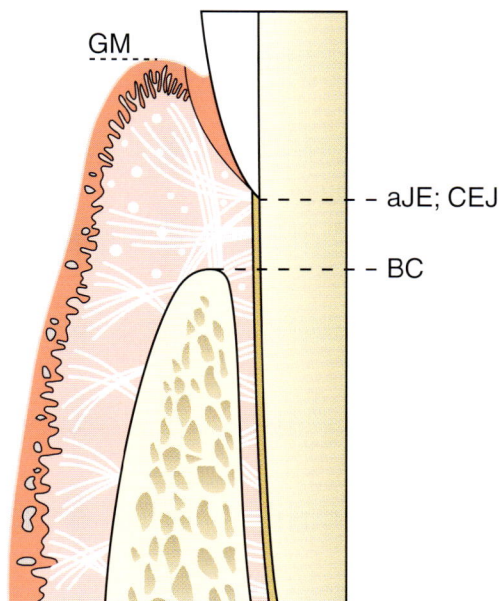

Fig 2-1 Anatomy of clinically healthy soft and hard tissue surrounding teeth. GM indicates gingival margin; aJE, apical termination of the junctional epithelium; CEJ, cementoenamel junction; and BC, marginal bone crest.

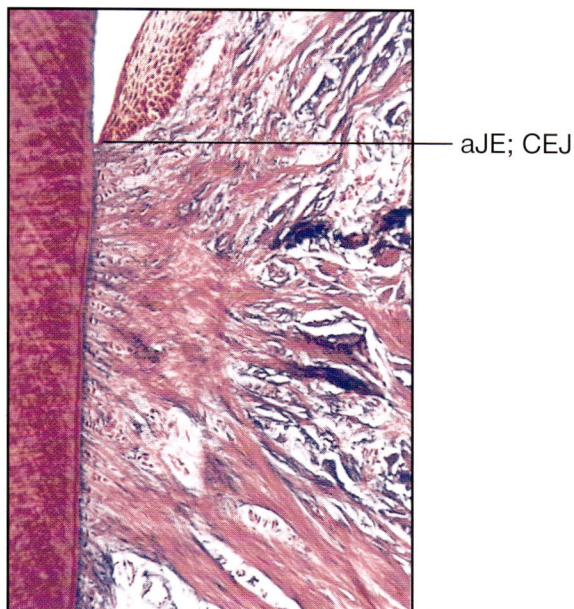

Fig 2-2 Supracrestal connective tissue attachment at teeth. aJE indicates apical termination of the junctional epithelium and CEJ, cementoenamel junction.

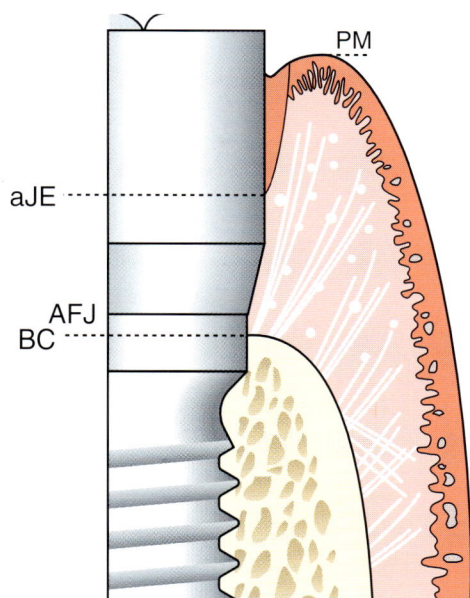

Fig 2-3 Anatomy of clinically healthy soft and hard tissue surrounding Brånemark titanium dental implant. PM indicates peri-implant soft tissue margin; aJE, apical termination of the junctional epithelium; AFJ, abutment-fixture junction; and BC, marginal bone crest.

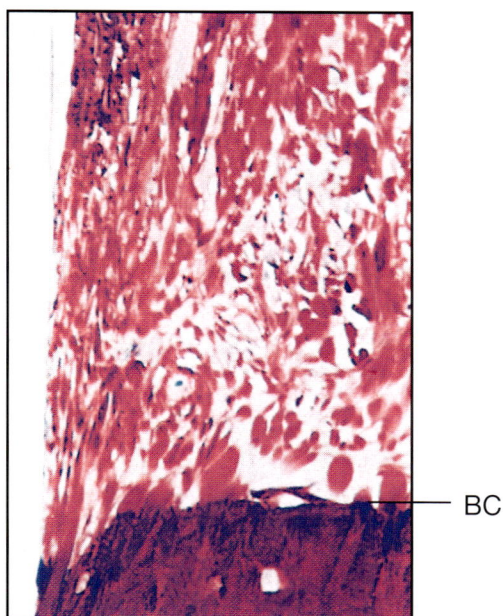

Fig 2-4 Apical portion of the supracrestal connective tissue at titanium implants. The empty space to the left represents the titanium implant surface. BC indicates marginal bone crest.

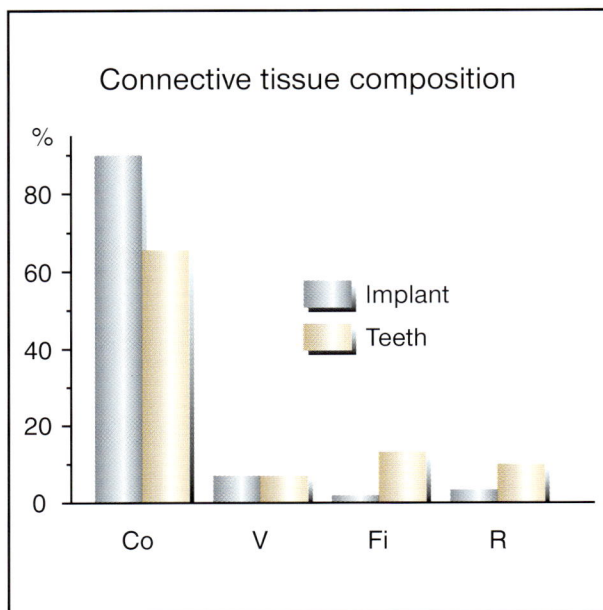

Fig 2-5 Composition of the supracrestal connective tissue at implants and teeth. Co indicates collagen; V, vessels; Fi, fibroblasts; and R, residual tissue.

stal implant surface facing the connective tissue, defined coronally by the apical cells of the junctional epithelium and apically by the bone surface, was found to be approximately 2 mm in height, or about two times the height of the gingival supracrestal connective tissue attachment (see Figs 2-1 and 2-3) (Berglundh et al 1991). Within this epithelium-free zone a reaction must have occurred between the connective tissue and the titanium dioxide abutment surface that in one way or another limited the proliferation possibility of the junctional epithelium. Evidently, this zone of interaction is not apprehended as a wound surface, a characteristic that must have a significant effect on the adhesion of the peri-implant mucosa to the titanium abutment, and thus also on the soft tissue defense against exogenous irritation.

A qualitative analysis of the portion of the connective tissue subjacent to the junctional epithelium and within the supracrestal region

revealed that the peri-implant mucosa contained significantly more collagen and fewer fibroblasts than corresponding gingival connective tissue (Fig 2-5). Furthermore, it has been demonstrated that the characteristics described regarding adaptation and dimensions of the peri-implant mucosa are also valid when the Brånemark system is used as a one-stage implant system (Ericsson et al 1996), that is, using the nonsubmerged technique. Thus, it is obvious that once initial stability has been obtained for the fixture part of the implant following placement, a proper soft tissue seal will form around the implant pillar whether or not the implant was initially submerged.

In a dog experiment, Berglundh and Lindhe (1996) further studied the dimensions of the mucosa-implant attachment. In conjunction with the second-stage surgery (abutment connection), the height of the ridge mucosa at the test implants was reduced to approximately 2 mm, whereas at the contralateral control sites the thickness of the mucosa was maintained at approximately 4 mm (Fig 2-6). Mechanical plaque control was performed during the next 6 months, resulting in clinically healthy peri-implant mucosa at all experimental sites. At the termination of this 6-month period, tissue biopsies were harvested and prepared for histological examination. The microscopic analysis revealed that the interface between the soft tissue and the titanium implant surface was similar at the test and control sites. In both situations the soft tissue seal consisted of (1) an approximately 2-mm-long junctional epithelium and (2) a zone of connective tissue 1.3 to 1.8 mm high. Although following abutment connection the ridge mucosa at the test and control sites differed in thickness (height), the resulting peri-implant soft tissue seal was almost identical. At sites where the volume of the mucosa was reduced, the healing process consistently included bone resorption (angu-

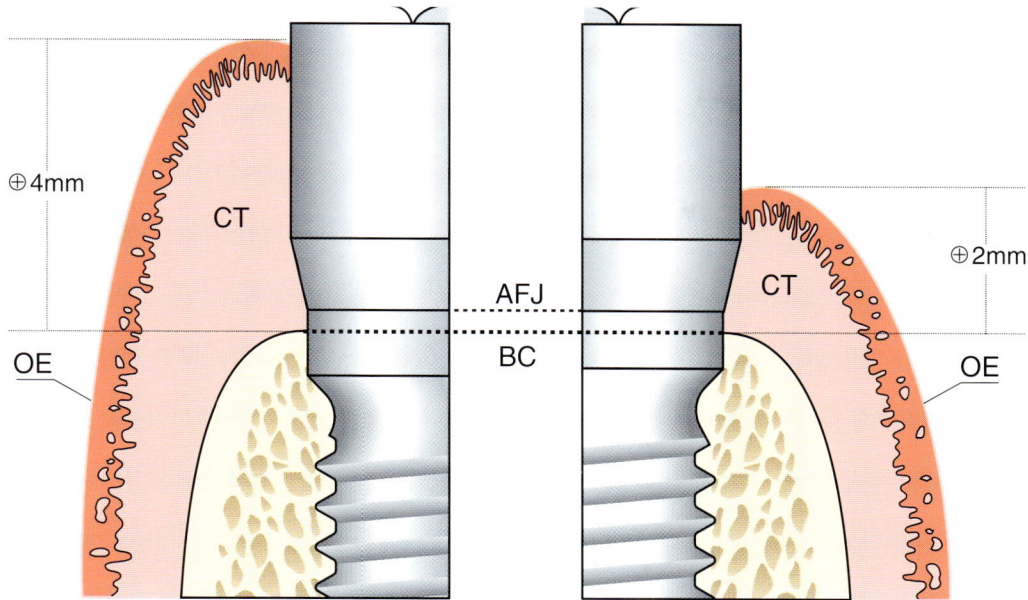

Fig 2-6 Volume of the mucosa reduced to approximately 2 mm at the test sites *(right)*; volume of the mucosa maintained at approximately 4 mm at the control sites *(left)*. CT indicates connective tissue; AFJ, abutment-fixture junction; BC, marginal bone crest; and OE, oral epithelium.

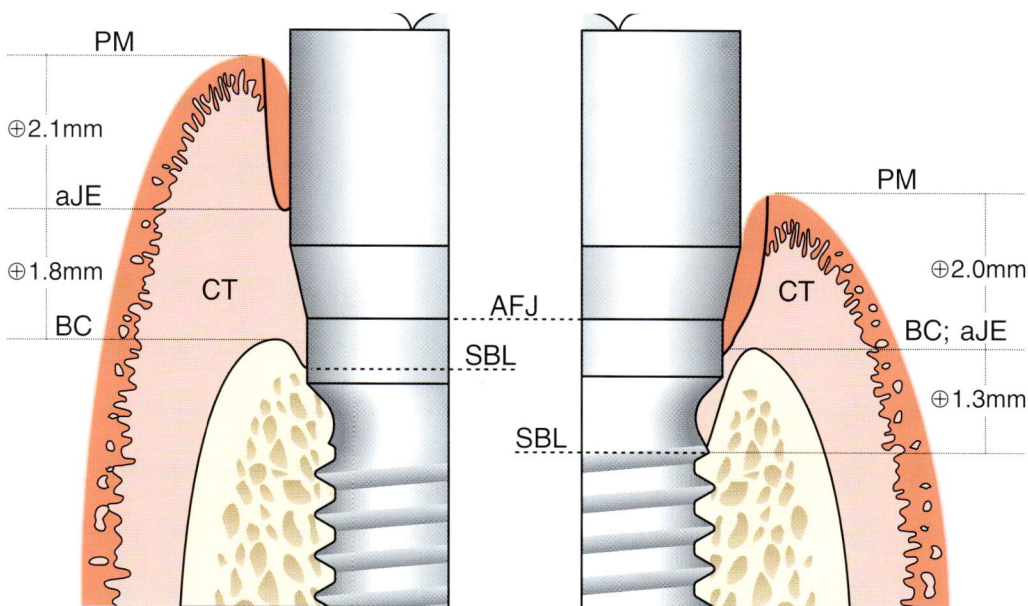

Fig 2-7 Peri-implant mucosa at both the test site *(right)* and control site *(left)* had a junctional epithelium approximately 2 mm high and a zone of connective tissue of approximately 1.5 mm facing the titanium implant surface. PM indicates peri-implant soft tissue margin; aJE, apical termination of the junctional epithelium; AFJ, abutment-fixture junction; BC, marginal bone crest; CT, connective tissue; and SBL, supporting bone level.

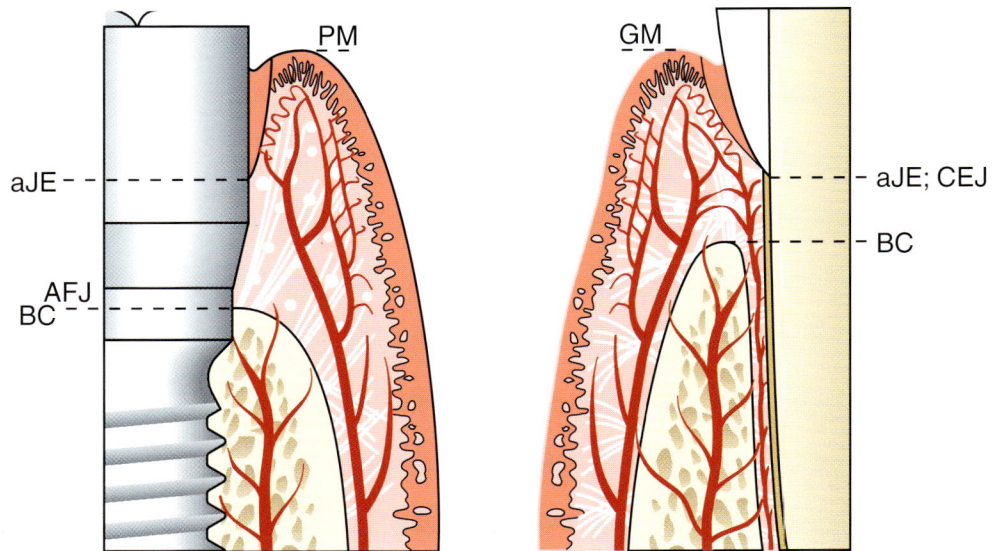

Fig 2-8 Vascular topography of the peri-implant soft and hard tissue *(left)* and of the periodontium *(right)*. PM indicates peri-implant soft tissue margin; aJE, apical termination of the junctional epithelium; AFJ, abutment-fixture junction; BC, marginal bone crest; GM, gingival margin; and CEJ, cementoenamel junction.

lar bone defect) to create a soft tissue seal that was about 3 mm high (Fig 2-7). Berglundh and Lindhe conclude "that a certain minimum width of the peri-implant mucosa is required, and that bone resorption may take place to allow a proper soft tissue attachment to form." Furthermore, they suggest "that once the implant is exposed to the oral environment and in function, a mucosal attachment of a certain minimum dimension is required to protect osseointegration."

Abrahamsson et al (1998) have reported from experiments using the dog model that abutments fabricated of commercially pure titanium or aluminum-based sintered ceramic (Al_2O_3) create proper conditions for mucosal healing and a subsequent proper soft tissue seal. In contrast, the authors also observed that following abutment connection, abutments made of gold alloy or dental porcelain resulted in improper tissue healing character-

ized by bone resorption and soft tissue recession.

Berglundh et al (1994) studied the vascular topography of the periodontium and the peri-implant soft and hard tissue using the beagle model. The authors observed that the gingiva and the supracrestal connective tissue adjacent to teeth are supplied by *(1)* supraperiosteal vessels lateral to the alveolar process and *(2)* vessels from the periodontal ligament. The peri-implant mucosa, in contrast, was found to be supplied by terminal branches of larger vessels originating from the periosteum of the bone at the implant site. In both situations, the blood vessels built a characteristic "crevicular plexus" lateral to the junctional epithelium (Egelberg 1966). Adjacent to teeth, the supracrestal connective tissue portion demonstrated rich vascularization, whereas at the corresponding implant sites very few, if any, vessels were observed (Fig 2-8). These observations

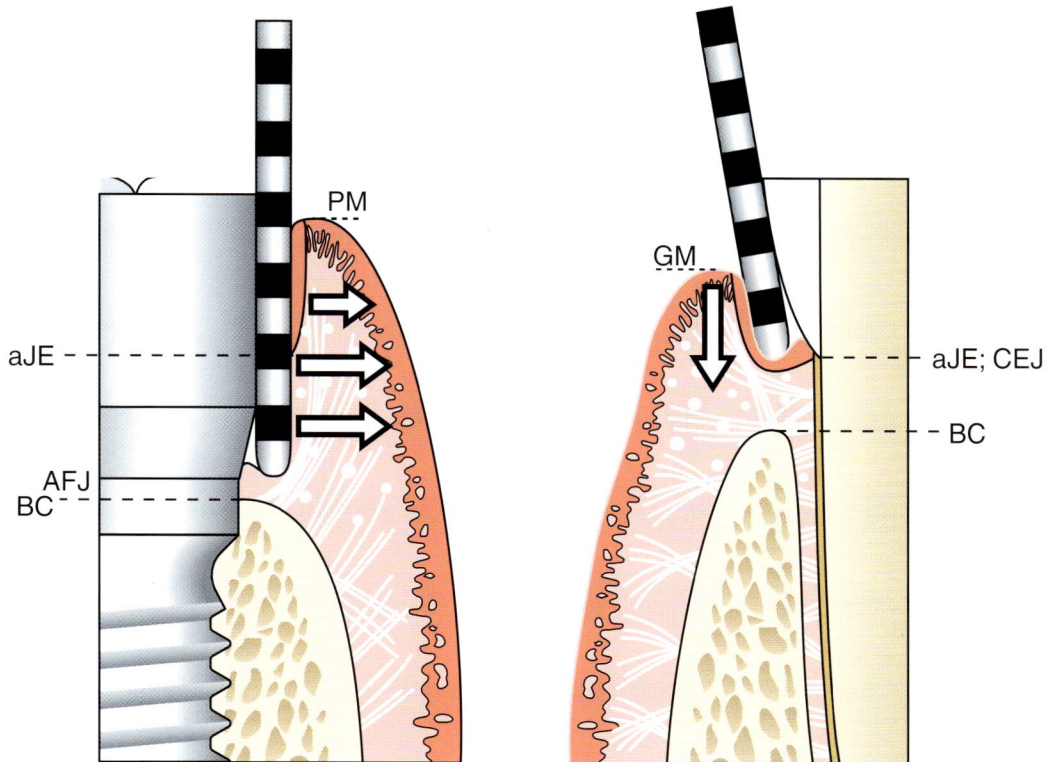

Fig 2-9 Results of probe penetration of Brånemark implants *(left)* and teeth *(right)*. PM indicates peri-implant soft tissue margin; aJE, apical termination of the junctional epithelium; AFJ, abutment-fixture junction; BC, marginal bone crest; GM, gingival margin; and CEJ, cementoenamel junction.

support the suggestion made by Buser et al (1992) that the peri-implant soft tissue may have impaired defense capacity against exogenous irritation, for example, bacterial plaque.

Ericsson and Lindhe (1993), using the beagle model, examined the resistance to mechanical probing of clinically healthy gingival tissue and peri-implant mucosa at titanium dental implants. The authors reported that the probe penetration was more advanced at implants than at teeth (approximately 2.0 mm and approximately 0.7 mm, respectively). Thus, at the implant sites the probe tip displaced the junctional epithelium as well as the connective tissue portion facing the abutment surface in the lateral direction and stopped close to the bone crest (Fig 2-9). The tip of the probe stopped within the supracrestal connective tissue portion, and the occasional rupture of some blood vessels resulted in bleeding. At the tooth sites, however, the tip of the probe consistently terminated coronally to the apical portion of the junctional epithelium, thus displacing the gingival margin apically and roughly identifying the bottom of the gingival pocket (see Fig 2-9). Bleeding on probing is an important tool in the analysis of the condition of the apical portion of periodontal soft tissue. In this study, however, bleeding on probing was sometimes observed at implants but very seldom at teeth. Based on current knowledge, the importance of such an observation at implants is doubtful.

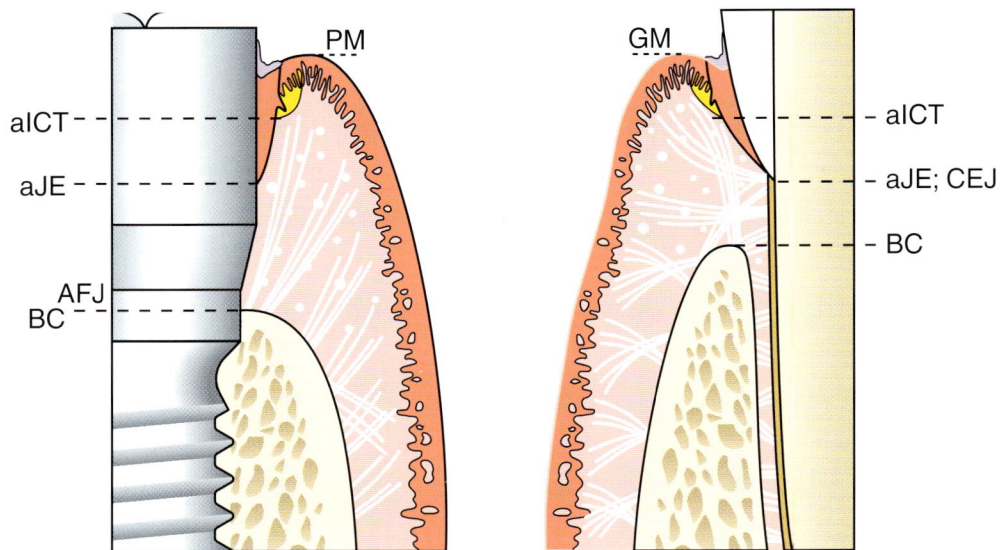

Fig 2-10 Anatomical landmarks of the peri-implant soft and hard tissue *(left)* and the periodontium *(right)* following de novo plaque formation. The violet area represents microbial plaque formation. PM indicates peri-implant soft tissue margin; aICT, apical termination of the infiltrated connective tissue; aJE, apical termination of the junctional epithelium; AFJ, abutment-fixture junction; BC, marginal bone crest; GM, gingival margin; and CEJ, cementoenamel junction.

Peri-implant Mucositis and Peri-implantitis

The effects of de novo (Berglundh et al 1992) and long-standing (Ericsson et al 1992) plaque formation on the gingiva and the peri-implant mucosa have been evaluated using the beagle model. Berglundh et al (1992) reported that both tissues responded to a 3-week plaque formation period with the development of an inflammatory lesion. Because of common features in size and composition of these two lesions (Fig 2-10), it can be observed that the gingiva and peri-implant mucosa had a similar host defense potential to de novo plaque formation. This observation is further supported by findings reported from a clinical trial by Pontoriero et al (1994). Twenty partially edentulous patients abstained from periodontal care following placement of implant-supported supraconstructions. The patients desisted from oral hygiene measures for 3 weeks following the connection of the fixed appliances. This resulted in gingivitis and peri-implant mucositis (reversible inflammation of the soft tissue surrounding implants in function) (Albrektsson and Isidor 1994). At the end of this 3-week period optimal oral hygiene was reinstituted. The authors concluded that "the period of no oral hygiene demonstrated a similar cause-effect relationship between the accumulation of bacterial plaque and the development of peri-implant mucositis as established for the gingival units by the experimental gingivitis model." In other words, it seems that "the need for supportive therapy at implant sites and tooth sites is of equal importance" (Pontoriero et al 1994).

Ericsson et al (1992) evaluated the response of gingival and peri-implant tissue to a 3-month

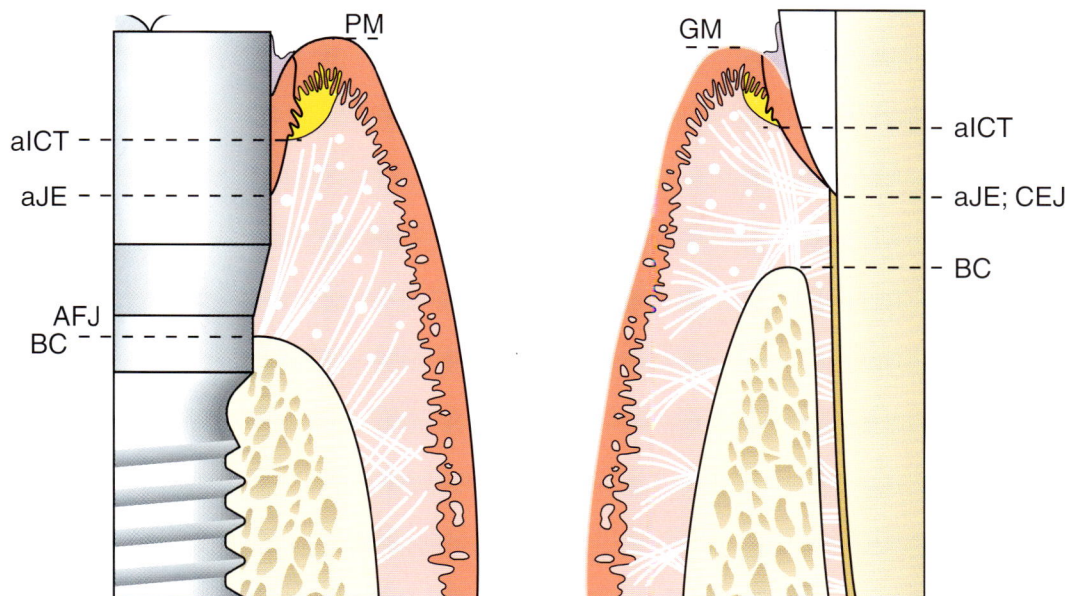

Fig 2-11 Anatomical landmarks of the peri-implant soft and hard tissue *(left)* and the periodontium *(right)* following long-standing plaque formation. The violet area represents microbial plaque formation. PM indicates peri-implant soft tissue margin; aICT, apical termination of the infiltrated connective tissue; aJE, apical termination of the junctional epithelium; AFJ, abutment-fixture junction; BC, marginal bone crest; GM, gingival margin; and CEJ, cementoenamel junction.

period of undisturbed plaque accumulation. Marginal soft tissue bleeding upon gentle touching was observed at both implants and teeth. The authors reported that the prolonged period of plaque accumulation resulted in the development of an inflammatory-cell infiltrate in the gingiva and the peri-implant mucosa. The two infiltrates had many features in common, but the apical extension was more pronounced in the peri-implant mucosa than in the corresponding lesion in the gingiva (Fig 2-11). The data indicate the following: *(1)* for teeth, 3 weeks to 3 months of undisturbed plaque accumulation resulted in no further extension of the inflammatory lesion; *(2)* at implants under identical experimental conditions, however, a further spread of the inflammatory-cell infiltrate in the apical direction was consistently observed. This finding implies that the defense mechanism of the gingiva may be more effective than that of the peri-implant mucosa in preventing further apical propagation of the pocket microbiota.

This hypothesis is further supported by Lindhe et al (1992) and Marinello et al (1995). Lindhe and coworkers (1992) induced the experimental breakdown of peri-implant and periodontal tissue in dogs by placing cotton-floss ligatures submarginally. They reported that 1 month after ligature removal, *"(1)* the resulting tissue destruction was more pronounced at implants than at teeth, *(2)* the size of the soft tissue lesion was larger at implants than at teeth, and *(3)* the lesion at implants but not at teeth frequently extended into the bone marrow" (Fig 2-12).

Using the same animal model, Marinello et al (1995) examined the "spontaneous" healing capacity of an advanced, experimentally induced, destructive peri-implantitis lesion (an inflammatory process affecting the tissues

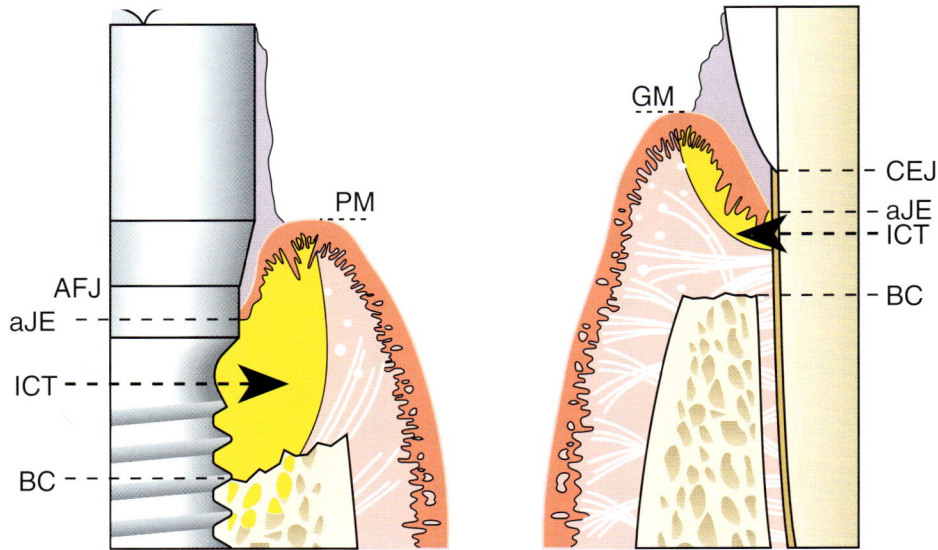

Fig 2-12 Anatomical landmarks of the peri-implant tissue *(left)* and the periodontal tissue *(right)* following experimental breakdown. The violet area represents microbial plaque formation. PM indicates peri-implant soft tissue margin; AFJ, abutment-fixture junction, ICT, infiltrated connective tissue; aJE, apical termination of the junctional epithelium; BC, marginal bone crest; GM, gingival margin; and CEJ, cementoenamel junction.

around an osseointegrated implant in function, resulting in loss of supporting bone) (Albrektsson and Isidor 1994). Marinello et al (1995) reported that the most common observation 3 months after ligature removal was that the soft and hard tissue lesion at most implant sites had converted to a resting and encapsulated lesion separated from the bone surface by a dense stroma of fibrous connective tissue. However, in one of the dogs monitored, three of four implants placed demonstrated a continuing loss of supporting bone, became unstable, and were consequently lost during the observation period (Fig 2-13).

Finally, it should be noted that microbial establishment and colonization on both healthy and diseased titanium implants in dogs follow essentially the same pattern as on teeth (Leonhardt et al 1992). This observation is further supported by Pontoriero et al (1994), who reported from their clinical trial that the

amount and composition of the bacterial plaque at implant sites and tooth sites were similar.

Conclusions

The attachment between the mucosa and the titanium implant surface consists of a junctional epithelium (approximately 2 mm high) and a connective tissue zone (approximately 1 mm high). This soft tissue seal protects the zone of osseointegration from the oral cavity, as well as from harmful substances produced by bacterial plaque. This soft tissue zone at implants shows some features in common with the corresponding zone at teeth but differs in regard to the composition of the connective tissue, the arrangement of the collagen fiber bundles,

3 Months

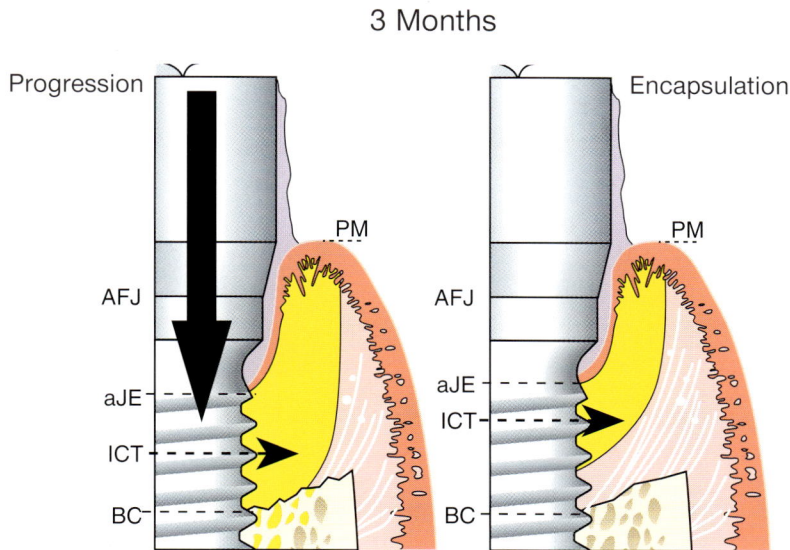

Fig 2-13 "Spontaneous" healing capacity (resolution) of peri-implantitis lesions during a 3-month period. The violet area represents microbial plaque formation. PM indicates peri-implant soft tissue margin; AFJ, abutment-fixture junction; aJE, apical termination of the junctional epithelium; ICT, infiltrated connective tissue; and BC, marginal bone crest.

and the vascular supply to the compartment apical to the junctional epithelium.

Based on the reported studies, it seems that the peri-implant mucosa has a lower capacity to encapsulate the plaque-associated lesion than does the gingiva and that peri-implantitis lesions involve bone tissue and may result in implant loss. According to clinical follow-up studies of dental implant treatment (for example, Adell et al 1981, 1990; van Steenberghe et al 1990; Lekholm et al 1994), peri-implantitis does not seem to be a frequent complication (for example, Esposito et al 1998a, 1998b; Mombelli and Lang 1998). However, consideration must be given to the possibility that peri-implant bone loss may occur as a result of occlusal overload (for example, Strub 1986; Rangert et al 1989; Quirynen et al 1992; Isidor 1996), submarginally located plaque formation (for example, Mombelli et al 1987; Nakou et al 1987; Sanz et al 1990; Rosenberg et al 1991; Leonhardt et al 1992, 1993; Mombelli and Lang 1998), or a combination of reasons.

Finally, periodontal and peri-implant soft tissue demonstrate many features in common but also some differences, such as the orientation of the collagen fibers and the fact that the peri-implant mucosa is characterized by a high collagen content and a low number of fibroblasts. The peri-implant mucosa has the characteristic of scar tissue, which will probably result in impaired defense against exogenous irritation such as plaque infection. This characteristic, in turn, underlines the importance of both the creation of a soft tissue anatomy around implants and proper superstructure design to facilitate a high standard of oral hygiene. Such measures will minimize the frequency of inflammatory conditions of the soft and hard tissue anchoring the implant.

References

Abrahamsson I, Berglundh T, Glantz PO, Lindhe J. The mucosal attachment at different abutments: An experimental study in dogs. J Clin Periodontol 1998;25:721–727.

Adell R, Eriksson B, Lekholm U, Brånemark P-I, Jemt T. A long-term follow-up study of osseointegrated implants in the treatment of totally edentulous jaws. Int J Oral Maxillofac Implants 1990;5:347–359.

Adell R, Lekholm U, Rockler B, Brånemark P-I. A 15-year study of osseointegrated implants in the treatment of the edentulous jaw. Int J Oral Surg 1981;6:387–416.

Adell R, Lekholm U, Rockler B, Brånemark P-I, Lindhe J, Eriksson B, et al. Marginal tissue reactions at osseointegrated titanium fixtures, I. A 3-year longitudinal prospective study. Int J Oral Maxillofac Surg 1986;15:39–52.

Akagawa Y, Takata T, Matsumoto T, Nikai H, Tsuru H. Correlation between clinical and histological evaluations of the peri-implant gingiva around single-crystal sapphire endosseous implant. J Oral Rehabil 1989;16:581–587.

Albrektsson T, Isidor F. Consensus report of session IV. In: Lang NP, Karring T (eds). Proceedings of the First European Workshop on Periodontology. London: Quintessence, 1994;365–369.

Berglundh T, Lindhe J. Dimension of the peri-implant mucosa: Biological width revisited. J Clin Periodontol 1996;23:971–973.

Berglundh T, Lindhe J, Ericsson I, Marinello CP, Liljenberg B, Thomsen P. The soft tissue barrier at implants and teeth. Clin Oral Implants Res 1991;2:81–90.

Berglundh T, Lindhe J, Jonsson K, Ericsson I. The topography of the vascular systems in the periodontal and peri-implant tissues in the dog. J Clin Periodontol 1994;21:189–193.

Berglundh T, Lindhe J, Marinello CP, Ericsson I, Liljenberg B. Soft tissue reactions to de novo plaque formation at implants and teeth: An experimental study in the dog. Clin Oral Implants Res 1992;3:1–8.

Brånemark P-I. Introduction to osseointegration. In: Brånemark P-I, Zarb GA, Albrektsson T (eds). Tissue-integrated Prostheses: Osseointegration in Clinical Dentistry. Chicago: Quintessence, 1985:11–76.

Buser D, Stich H, Krekeler G, Schroeder A. Faserstrukturen der periimplantären Mukosa bei Titanimplantaten: Eine experimentelle Studie am Beagle-Hund. Z Zahnärzttl Implantol 1989;5:15–23.

Buser D, Weber HP, Donath K, Fiorellini J, Paquette DW, Williams R. Soft tissue reactions to nonsubmerged unloaded titanium implants in beagle-dogs. J Periodontol 1992;63:226–236.

Carmichael RP, Apse P, Zarb GA, McCulloch CAG. Biological, microbiological and clinical aspects of the peri-implant mucosa. In: Albrektsson T, Zarb GA (eds). The Brånemark Osseointegrated Implant. Chicago: Quintessence, 1989:39–78.

Egelberg J. The blood vessels of the dento-gingival junction. J Periodontal Res 1966;1:163–179.

Ericsson I, Berglundh T, Marinello CP, Liljenberg B, Lindhe J. Long-standing plaque and gingivitis at implants and teeth in the dog. Clin Oral Implants Res 1992;3:99–103.

Ericsson I, Lindhe J. Probing at implants and teeth: An experimental study in the dog. J Clin Periodontol 1993;20:623–627.

Ericsson I, Nilner K, Klinge B, Glantz PO. Radiographical and histological characteristics of submerged and nonsubmerged titanium implants. An experimental study in the Labrador dog. Clin Oral Implants Res 1996;7:20–26.

Esposito M, Hirsch JM, Lekholm U, Thomsen P. Biological factors contributing to failures of osseointegrated oral implants, I. Success criteria and epidemiology. Eur J Oral Sci 1998a;106:527–551.

Esposito M, Hirsch JM, Lekholm U, Thomsen P. Biological factors contributing to failures of osseointegrated oral implants, II. Etiopathogenesis. Eur J Oral Sci 1998b;106:721–764.

Gould TRL. Clinical implications of the attachment of oral tissue to perimucosal implants. Excerpta Medica 1985;29:253–270.

Gould TRL, Brunette DM, Westbury L. The attachment mechanism of epithelial cells to titanium in vitro. J Periodontal Res 1981;16:611–616.

Hashimoto M, Akagawa Y, Nikai H, Tsuru H. Single-crystal sapphire endosseous dental implant loaded with functional stress: Clinical and histological evaluation of peri-implant tissues. J Oral Rehabil 1988;15:65–76.

Isidor F. Loss of osseointegration caused by occlusal load of oral implants: A clinical and radiographic study in monkeys. Clin Oral Implants Res 1996;7:143–152.

Jansen JA, de Wijn JR, Wolters-Lutgerhorst JML, van Mullem PJ. Ultrastructural study of epithelial cell attachment to implant material. J Dent Res 1985;64:891–896.

Lekholm U, Adell R, Lindhe J, Brånemark P-I, Eriksson B, Rockler B, et al. Marginal tissue reactions at osseointegrated titanium fixtures: A cross-sectional retrospective study. Int J Oral Maxillofac Surg 1986;15:53–61.

Lekholm U, Ericsson I, Adell R, Slots J. The condition of the soft tissues at tooth and fixture abutments supporting fixed bridges: A microbiological and histological study. J Clin Periodontol 1986;13: 558–562.

Lekholm U, van Steenberghe D, Herrman I, Bolender C, Folmer T, Gunne J, et al. Osseointegrated implants in the treatment of partially edentulous jaws: A prospective 5-year multicenter study. Int J Oral Maxillofac Implants 1994;9:627–635.

Leonhardt Å, Adolfsson B, Lekholm U, Wikström M, Dahlén G. A longitudinal microbiological study on osseointegrated titanium implants in partially edentulous patients. Clin Oral Implants Res 1993;4: 113–120.

Leonhardt Å, Berglundh T, Ericsson I, Dahlén G. Putative periodontal pathogens on titanium implants and teeth in experimental gingivitis and periodontitis in beagle-dogs. Clin Oral Implants Res 1992;3:112–119.

Lindhe J, Berglundh T, Ericsson I, Liljenberg B, Marinello CP. Experimental breakdown of peri-implant and periodontal tissues: A study in the beagle-dog. Clin Oral Implants Res 1992;3:9–16.

Listgarten MA, Buser D, Steinemann SG, Donath K, Lang NP, Weber HP. Light and transmission electron microscopy of the intact interfaces between nonsubmerged titanium-coated epoxy resin implants and bone or gingiva. J Dent Res 1992;71:364–371.

Marinello CP, Berglundh T, Ericsson I, Klinge B, Glantz PO, Lindhe J. Resolution of ligature induced peri-implantitis lesions in the dog. J Clin Periodontol 1995;22:475–480.

McKinney RV, Steflik DE, Koth DL. Evidence for junctional epithelial attachment to ceramic dental implants: A transmission electron microscope study. J Periodontol 1985;6:425–436.

Mombelli A, Lang NP. The diagnosis and treatment of peri-implantitis. Periodontol 2000 1998;17:63–76.

Mombelli A, van Osten MAC, Schürch E, Lang NP. The microbiota with successful or failing osseointegrated titanium implants. Oral Microbiol Immunol 1987;2:145–151.

Nakou M, Mikx FHM, Oosterwaal PJM, Kruijsen JCWM. Early microbial colonization of permucosal implants in edentulous patients. J Dent Res 1987;66: 1654–1657.

Pontoriero R, Tonetti MP, Carnevale G, Mombelli A, Nyman S, Lang NP. Experimentally induced peri-implant mucositis: A clinical study in humans. Clin Oral Implants Res 1994;5:254–259.

Quirynen M, Naert I, van Steenberghe D. Fixture design and overload influence marginal bone loss and fixture success in the Brånemark® system. Clin Oral Implants Res 1992;3:104–111.

Rangert B, Jemt T, Jörneus L. Forces and moments on Brånemark implants. Int J Oral Maxillofac Implants 1989;4:241–247.

Rosenberg ES, Torosian JP, Slots J. Microbial differences in 2 clinically distinct types of failures of osseointegrated implants. Clin Oral Implants Res 1991;2:135–144.

Sanz M, Newman MG, Nachnani S, Holt R, Stewart R, Flemmig T. Characterization of the subgingival microflora around endosteal sapphire dental implants in partially edentulous patients. Int Oral Maxillofac Implants 1990;5:247–253.

Schroeder A, van der Zypen E, Stich H, Sutter F. The reaction of bone, connective tissue and epithelium to endosteal implants with sprayed titanium surfaces. J Maxillofac Surg 1981;4:191–197.

Seymour GJ, Gemmel E, Lenz LJ, Henry P, Bower R, Yamazaki K. Immunohistologic analysis of the inflammatory infiltrates associated with osseointegrated implants. Int J Oral Maxillofac Implants 1989;4:191–197.

Strub JR. Langzeitprognose von enossalen oralen Implantaten unter spezieller Berücksichtigung von periimplantären, meterialkundlichen und okklusalen Gesichtspunkten [thesis]. Berlin: Quintessenz, 1986.

Ten Cate AR. The gingival junction. In: Brånemark P-I, Zarb GA, Albrektsson T (eds). Tissue-integrated Prostheses: Osseointegration in Clinical Dentistry. Chicago: Quintessence, 1985;145–153.

Van Drie HJY, Beertsen W, Grevers A. Healing of the gingiva following installment of Biotes® implants in beagle-dogs. Adv Biomater 1988;8: 485–490.

Van Steenberghe D, Lekholm U, Bolender C, Folmer T, Henry P, Herrmann I, et al. The applicability of osseointegrated oral implants in the rehabilitation of partial edentulism: A prospective multicenter study on 558 fixtures. Int J Oral Maxillofac Implants 1990;5:272–281.

Chapter 3

Practical Guidelines Based on Biomechanical Principles

Bo Rangert, Mech Eng, PhD, and Franck Renouard, DDS

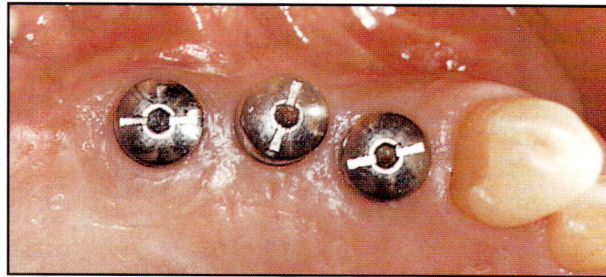

In implant dentistry biomechanics has long been used to explain many kinds of complications, and it has become evident that this discipline encompasses more than just screw loosening and prosthetic fit. In fact, implant treatment must be based on both biological tissue (bone) and mechanical components (the implant and the suprastructure). Consequently, many specialists—the radiologist, surgeon, prosthodontist, and technician, as well as the industry that provides the implant components and the specifications for their use—play a part in optimizing the patient's biomechanical condition.

In any structure subject to loading, overload and subsequent complications are possible. Overload in the biomechanical system encountered in implant dentistry can be defined as a condition in which functional or parafunctional forces exert loading that leads to implant failure, loss of bone support, component failure, or a combination of these conditions.

The various mechanical and biological parts or systems respond differently to overload. Loosening of components in an adverse situation may occur within a year's time, whereas component fractures usually occur only after an adverse situation of several years' duration (Rangert et al 1995). Interfacial bone seems to be sensitive to loading predominantly when it is healing and thereafter less often and only when damaged (Brunski 1999).

Consequently, implant failure is most likely during an early phase. The most important consideration, therefore seems to be control of the loading during the initial period so that the implant-bone interface has time to establish an equilibrium to be maintained over the implant's functional period. Only in extreme situations will bone lose its support capacity due to overload thereafter (Quirynen et al 1992; Rangert et al 1995). Mechanical complications, such as screw loosening, most often appear early and should be considered warning signs of excessive loading.

A clinical approach to analyzing these biomechanical factors in treatment planning is based on defining the load applied according to geometric load factors and occlusal load factors, as well as defining the support capacity according to bone/implant load capacity and technological factors (Rangert et al 1997; Renouard and Rangert 1999). This chapter will discuss the biomechanical risk factors, their effects on different types of complications, and a checklist for clinical examples.

Geometric Load Factors

Overload in the implant-supported biomechanical system is most often caused by excessive bending moments (Rangert et al 1997). An important consequence of the detrimental nature of bending is that a partially edentulous arch restoration is often more susceptible to overload than a full-arch restoration, because partially edentulous cases use a more in-line implant configuration.

The most comprehensive prospective long-term clinical study on implant treatment in partially edentulous patients is a prospective multicenter study with results at 3 years (Gunne et al 1994) and 5 years (Lekholm et al 1994). The authors reported a significantly lower failure rate for prostheses supported by three implants than those supported by two implants. From this study and a retrospective study on 732 consecutively placed implants in maxillae (Bahat 1993), it can be concluded that a sufficient number of implants is essential for minimizing complications because of the difference in bending versus axial loading (see "Transverse force, lever arm, and bending moment").

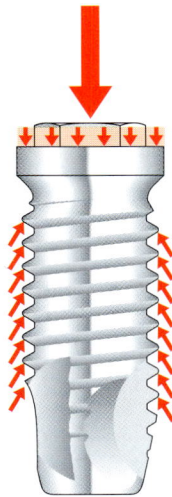

Fig 3-1 If a force is applied along the axis of an implant (axial force), the stress will be well distributed around the implant cross section and the implant threads.

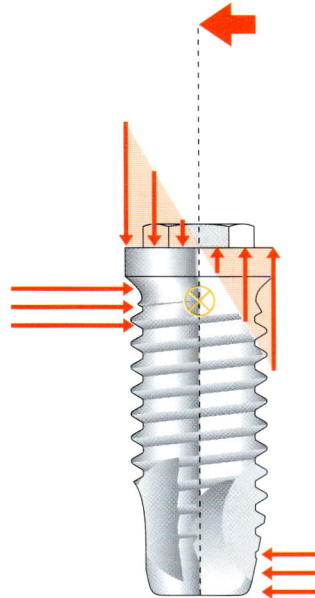

Fig 3-2 If a force is applied in a transverse direction relative to the implant axis, a bending moment is introduced. Only a small portion of the implant cross section and only a few threads will counteract the load, leading to higher stress levels in both implant and bone.

Transverse force, lever arm, and bending moment

When a force is applied along the axis of an implant (axial force), the stress will be well distributed around the implant cross section and the implant threads (Fig 3-1), and the implant and the supporting bone will have a high load-bearing capacity. If, however, the force or a component thereof is applied in a transverse direction relative to the implant axis, it will result in a bending moment on the implant (Fig 3-2). In bending, only a small portion of the cross section of the implant will counteract the load; the bone will be loaded mainly at the terminal portions of the implant, giving rise to higher stress levels in both implant and bone (Rangert et al 1989).

The bending moment is defined as the force times the lever arm (the orthogonal distance between the line-of-force direction and the cross-section axis) (see Fig 3-2). The larger this lever arm, the larger the bending moment and the greater the stress. Thus, although the acting force itself may be of reasonable magnitude, the forces needed to counteract the bending may be excessive because of the leverage effect. Therefore, axial loading is preferred.

The full-arch restoration is based on the use of multiple implants positioned on a curved line dictated by the residual jaw bone. This curved line imparts an inherent high capacity to compensate a transverse force with axial forces; any potential bending around a line combining any two implants will effectively be counteracted by axial forces of the implants that are offset relative to that line (Fig 3-3). In the restoration of posterior edentulous spaces in partially dentulous jaws, however, the implants often are placed in a more linear configuration, which does not provide the compensating nature of an offset implant (Fig 3-4); the straighter the alignment, the greater the potential bending of the implants. In a prosthesis supported by one or two implants, no compensating effect is available. Posterior implant-supported prostheses, therefore, are more frequently exposed to bending moments.

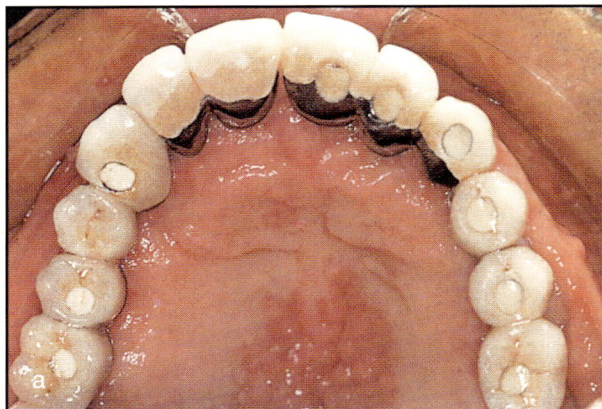

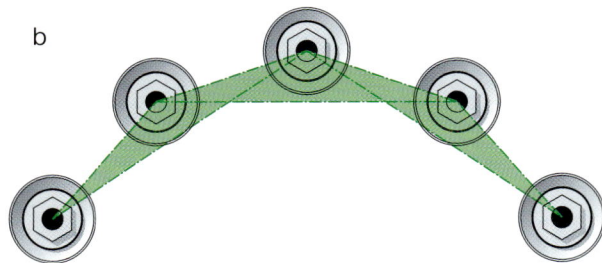

Fig 3-4 (a to c) In the restoration of posterior edentulous spaces in partially dentulous arches, implants often are placed in a linear configuration, which does not provide the compensating nature of an offset implant to counteract a transverse force.

Fig 3-3 (a and b) In the full-arch restoration, the implants are positioned on a curved line, and any potential bending around the line combining any two implants will effectively be counteracted by axial forces of the implants that are offset relative to that line.

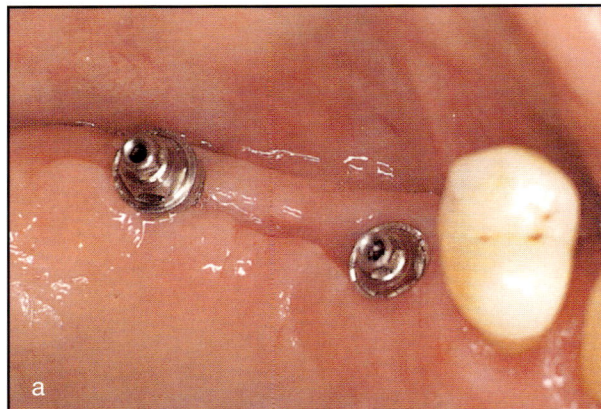

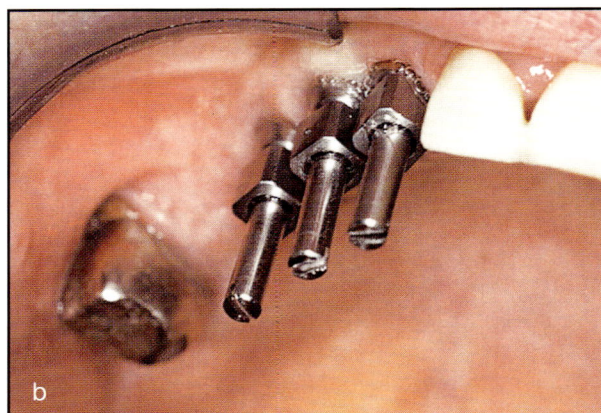

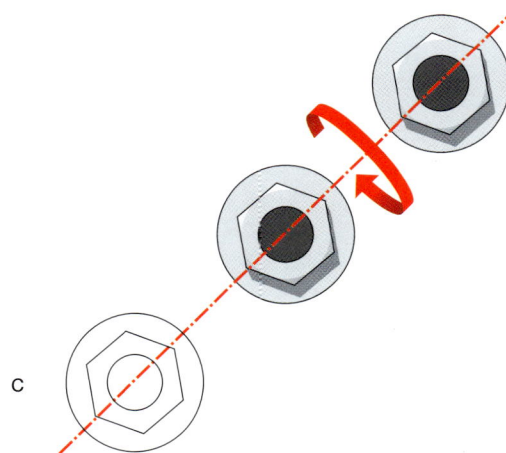

The leverage effect previously described can be caused by a variety of geometric conditions, including an extension beyond the implant support (Fig 3-5) or implants that are buccolingually offset relative to the prosthesis (Fig 3-6). In the single-implant molar replacement, the tooth crown is substantially larger than the diameter of the implant, leading to possible bending in all directions (Fig 3-7).

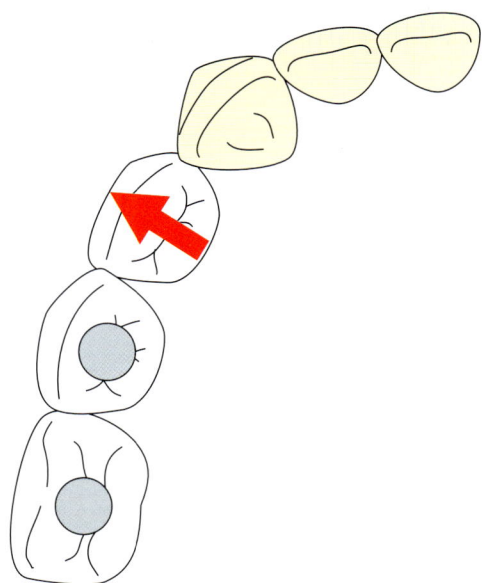

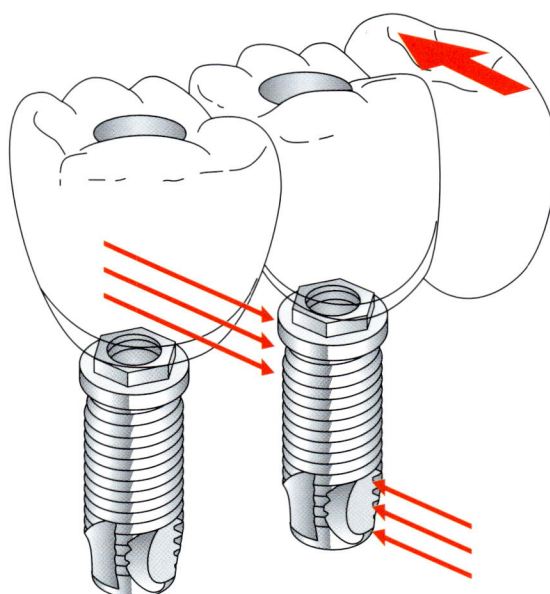

Fig 3-5 An extension beyond the implant support leads to an increased bending moment from a transverse force acting on the pontic.

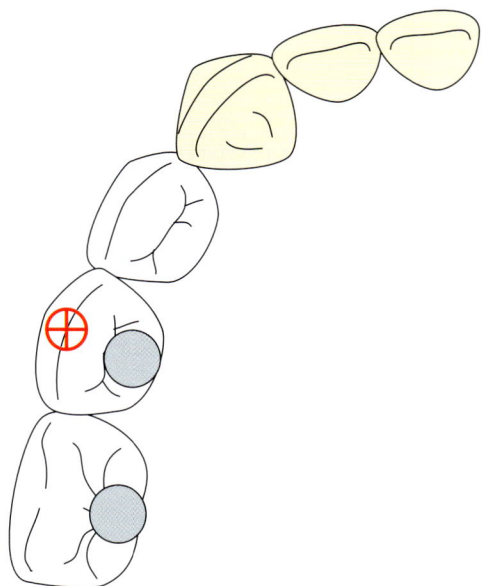

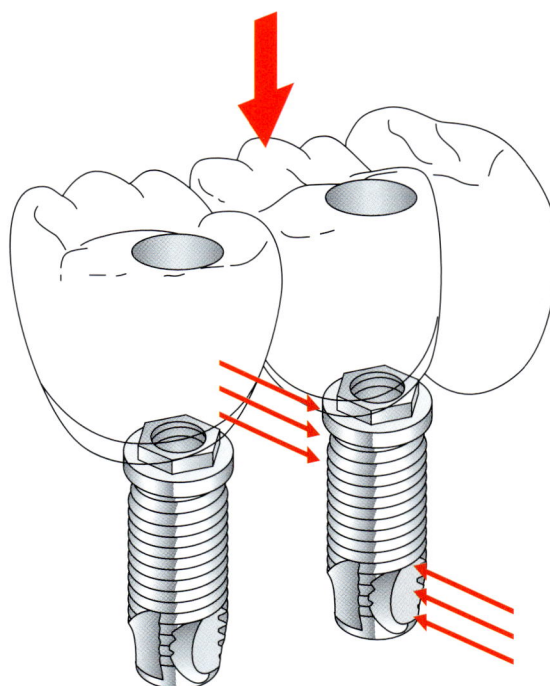

Fig 3-6 Implants that are buccolingually offset relative to a prosthesis may cause a bending moment from the axial force component's acting on the prosthesis.

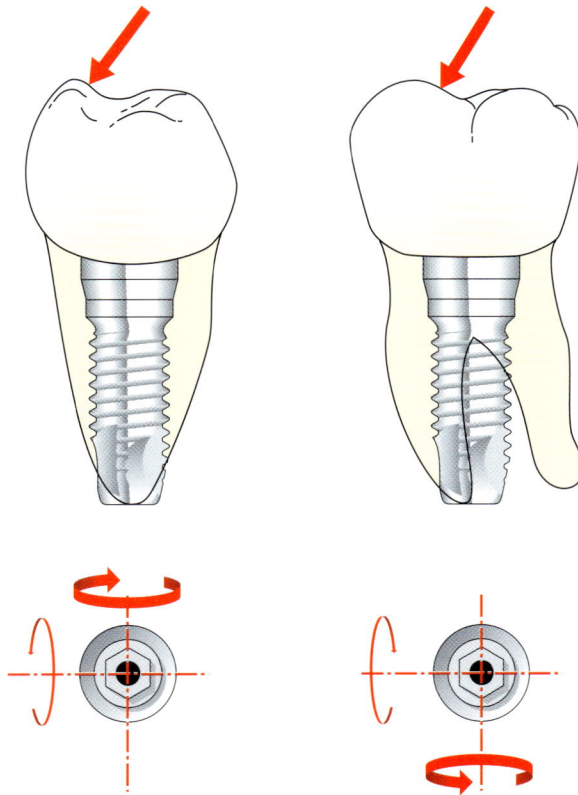

Fig 3-7 In a single-implant molar replacement, the tooth crown is substantially larger than the diameter of the implant, leading to possible bending in all directions.

Functional forces in individual cases are difficult to predict and control, as their intensity and direction vary from patient to patient. Furthermore, a rehabilitation phase in which the patient applies controlled force is not realistic in implant dentistry (as it is, for example, after orthopedic surgery). The only way to consider functional force is by estimation. Bruxism and parafunction are especially important to identify; such habits may contribute to bending overload as they increase both magnitude and frequency. Thus, observations of excessive occlusal wear, a history of fracturing natural teeth or veneering material, or both are indicators of increased loading. The implant reconstruction must be extra stable for patients with bruxism or parafunction, as the forces most often cannot be controlled. Other biomechanical risk factors should be avoided.

The effect of oral forces on the implants may differ depending on the occlusal condi-

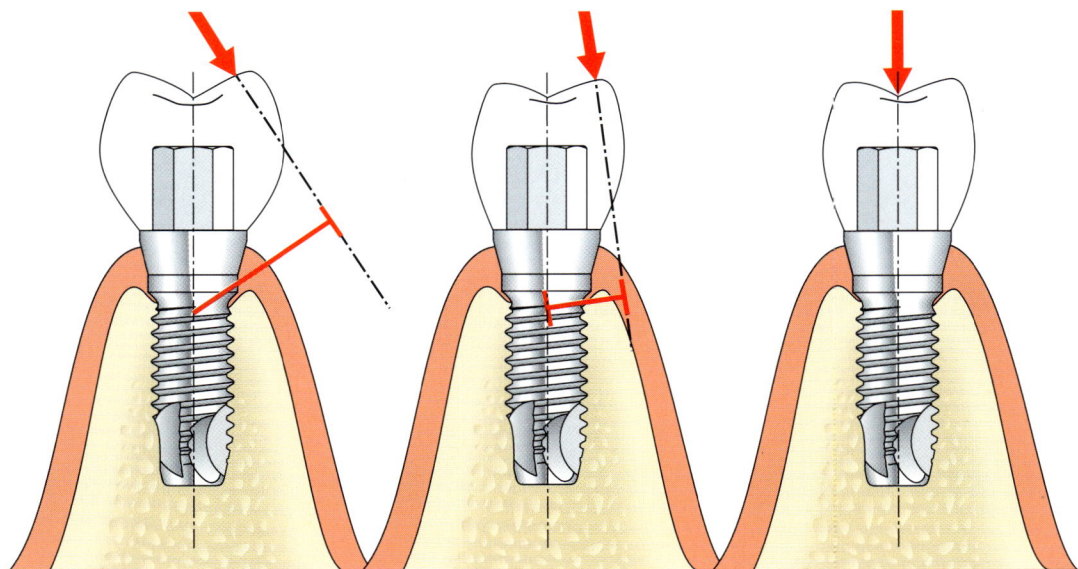

Fig 3-8 If cuspal contact is allowed, the cusp inclination and the position of the lateral excursive contact determine the leverage; the more lateral the contact and the larger the inclination, the greater the bending moment.

tions. If cuspal contact is allowed, higher cusp inclination leads to a higher magnitude of the transverse force components, and the more lateral the contact, the greater the leverage (Fig 3-8). However, centering the occlusal contact counteracts these effects. Careful consideration of the design of the occlusal surfaces and the contact pattern is therefore an important tool in limiting the bending forces on implant and bone. Because dental technicians create the basic design of the occlusal surfaces, it is important for them to be involved in the treatment planning.

Bone/Implant Load Capacity

Implant anchorage

Overall stability of implant anchorage is determined by bone quality and volume (Sennerby et al 1992; Ivanoff et al 1996). Cortical support (Fig 3-9) is important, as the engagement of the implant threads in strong, compact bone increases the load-carrying capacity

(Meredith et al 1997). Therefore, bicortical anchorage should be obtained where possible. Bicortical anchorage adds not only a greater amount of cortical bone support but also greater resistance to bending. A support at each end of the implant imparts an essentially greater capacity to withstand bending, as the stronger cortical bone will be present where the forces are greatest (see Fig 3-2).

Where not enough cortical bone is available for safe implant anchoring, new bone formation is needed to secure the implant. Ways to cope with this situation include allowing sufficient healing time, protecting the implant from full loading until the bone has proved its strength, or both. Dependence on newly formed bone in the absence of good initial mechanical fixation may be considered a risk factor.

According to empirical evidence, 3 months seems to be a sufficient healing period for implants in the anterior mandible, whereas 6 months is recommended for most maxillary implants (Adell et al 1985). Extended healing periods may be needed in posterior maxillae

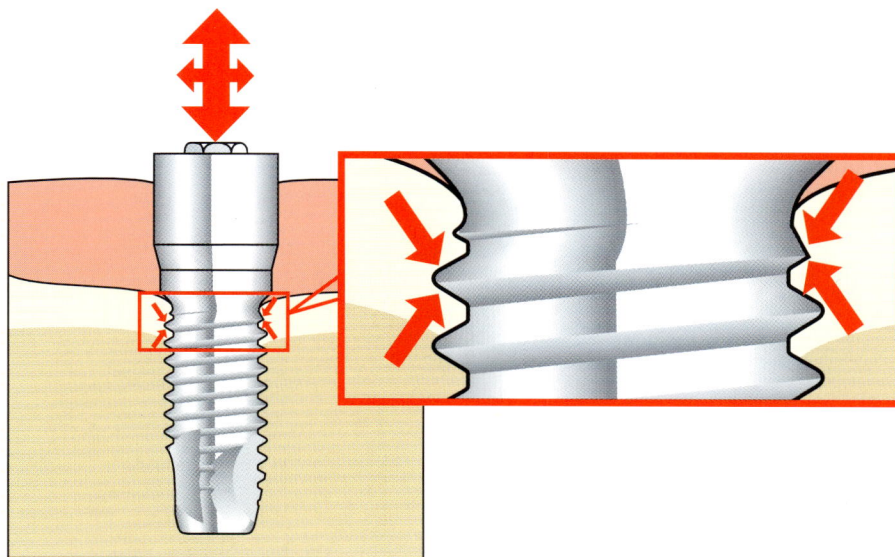

Fig 3-9 Implant thread interlocking in cortical bone, which is important for optimal load transfer.

(Bahat 1993). Recent research (Randow et al 1999) has demonstrated that the immediate function of Brånemark implants in the anterior part of the mandible is a viable concept. Ongoing research also indicates that immediate function with Brånemark implants may be possible in other clinical situations, provided the balance between applied load and initial bone anchorage is favorable (Malo et al 2000).

In addition to healing time, surgical technique is also important for the effective use of available bone. In maxillae, both bone com-pression by underpreparation and minimizing or eliminating countersinking are viable techniques to improve initial stability (Bahat 1993). In the posterior part of the mandible, where bicortical anchorage of the implant is usually not possible, countersinking must be minimized to avoid reducing the available bone support. Because dense mandibular bone in the posterior areas often has low vascularity, extra care with surgery in these areas is recommended, especially with wide-diameter implants (Polizzi et al, in press).

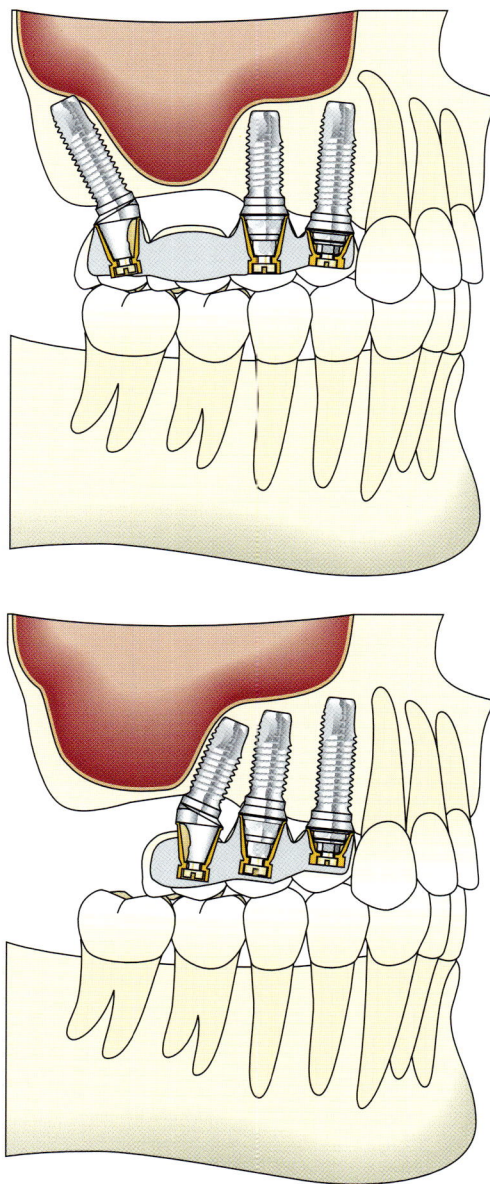

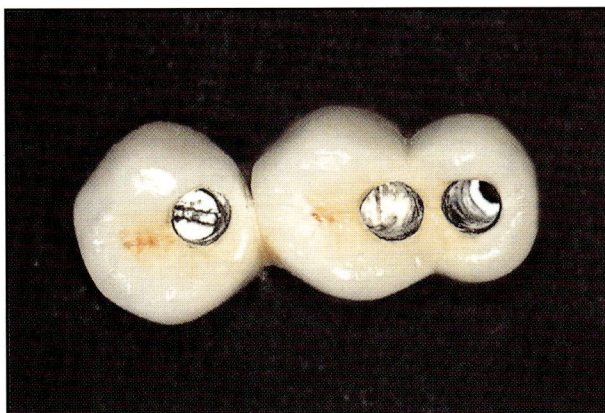

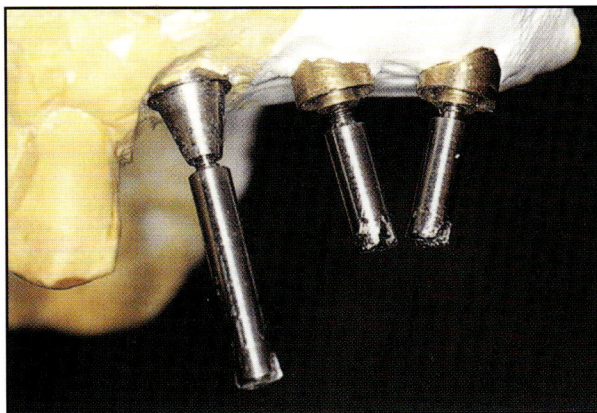

Fig 3-10 A mesiodistal inclination in a multiple-implant arrangement does not lead to increased loading, as a bending in the plane defined by the prosthesis's long axis and the implant direction will be counteracted by the suprastructure.

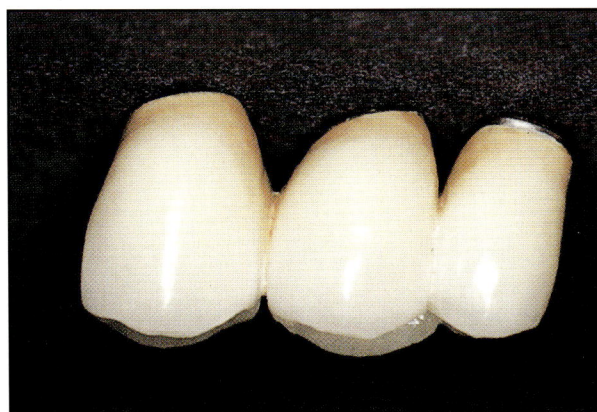

Implant inclination

Besides making optimal use of bone at the intended implant site, the anchorage sometimes can be improved by tilting (inclining) the implant (Fig 3-10). Dense bone structures remote from the intended implant position then may be utilized. In certain situations tilting the implant may also provide a better coronal position for the implant, thus improving the support of the prosthesis.

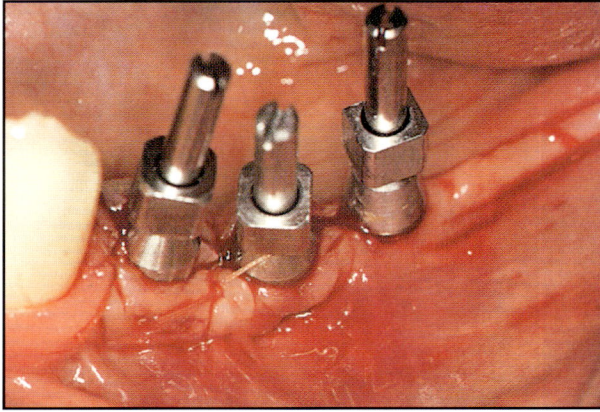

Fig 3-11 As long as the position of the implant head is unaltered, a limited inclination of the implant itself has minor influence on the load transfer to the implant. No additional bending of the implant is induced, and bone stress will be only slightly increased.

Limited inclination (15 to 30 degrees) of an implant is of minor importance in bone stress concentration (Fig 3-11). Furthermore, any potential bending of a mesiodistally tilted implant will be counteracted by the rigidity of the prosthesis (Krekmanov et al 2000). However, implant inclination in the buccolingual direction is a potential problem; if the prosthetic reconstruction becomes offset relative to the implant head, a bending moment is introduced on the implant (Fig 3-12).

The goal, then, should be to place the implant head as close as possible to the acting direction of the force, thus reducing the lever arm and bending moment. Using that selected position of the implant head, the implant may be tilted to improve its anchorage.

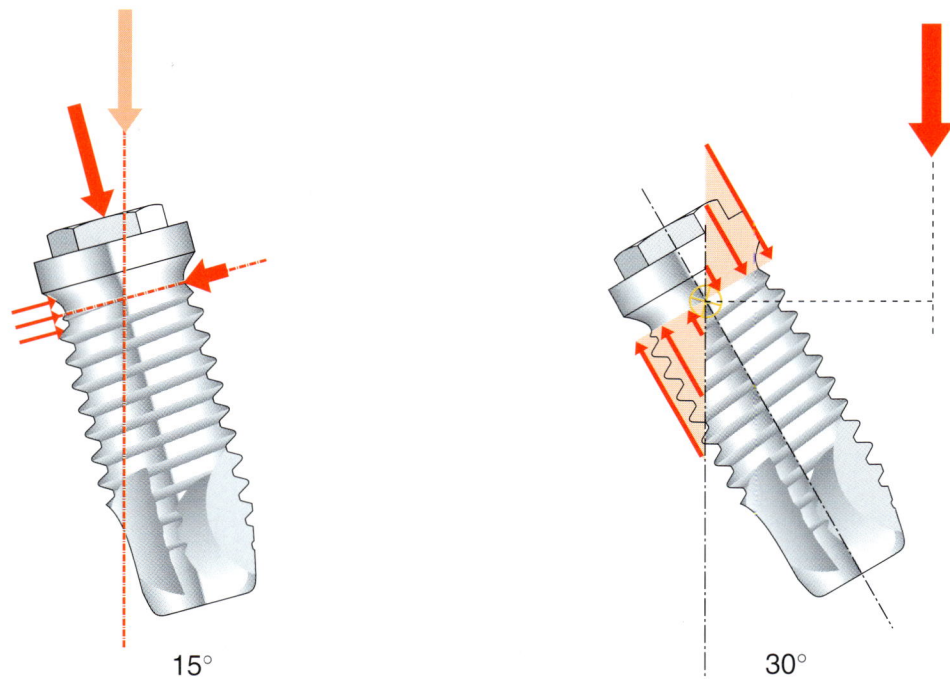

15°   30°

Fig 3-12 Implant inclination in the buccolingual direction may occur in situations where the prosthetic reconstruction is offset relative to the implant head, thus introducing a bending moment on the implant.

Technological Factors

The mechanical features of implant components, such as the precision of interfaces, screw joint preload, and fastening techniques, may influence the load capacity of the implant restoration. Technological factors are not always evident and may add to other factors without any apparent warning. The best way to eliminate component problems seems to be the establishment of a proven routine for component choice and handling.

Precision

A misfit between prostheses and implants generates static loads on the bone, and in vivo measurements indicate that prostheses considered clinically well fitting still may have implant loads corresponding to those found with open screw joints (Lindström et al, unpublished data) and that such misfits are not reduced over time (Jemt and Book 1996). A follow-up study after 5 years on 50 patients with complete-arch prostheses found that a substantial number of the patients had partially loose gold screws and misfit of the prostheses without any major clinical consequences (Kallus and Bessing 1994). Furthermore, it has been reported that no correlation exists between misfit and bone loss or other complications in complete-arch restorations followed for 5 years (Jemt and Book 1996).

Thus, misfit alone does not seem to be a major cause of complications for Brånemark system implants supporting complete-arch prostheses, probably because there is a certain degree of redundancy in situations with optimal spread of the implants. In short-span fixed partial dentures, however, where each implant has a strategic value, precision is of greater importance. If one out of two or three implants is not fully supportive because of lack of precision, the risk of the remaining implants being overloaded may increase dramatically.

Screw retention

The presence of screw joints that are not optimally tightened, as well as ill-fitting prostheses, leads to a higher risk of screw loosening and screw overload (Burguete et al 1994). It has been demonstrated that burnout casting of gold cylinders, as opposed to machining of cylinders, may reduce the screw preload significantly for the same torque and that screw joints that look alike may have large differences in preload (Carr et al 1996). Therefore, stable screw joints should be ensured by the selection of the proper components, the correct handling of the components, and use of optimal tightening torque.

Cementation

The cementation of prostheses to natural tooth abutments has a long clinical history, and its use with implant restorations may seem attractive in compensating for prosthetic misfit. A potential problem with definitive cementation of prostheses to implants, however, is the loss of retrievability. In the long-term follow-up of implant-supported restorations, adjustment or revision is sometimes required. The ability to unscrew a prosthesis is very useful in these situations.

The cementation of single-implant restorations on the optimized CeraOne screw joint (Jörnéus et al 1992) has a documented high clinical success rate (Henry et al 1996; Andersson et al 1998). This screw joint has been used in the development of the cement-over abutments now available (Brånemark system). However, it is recommended that cement-over solutions be used primarily in situations with limited load factors; if an overload should occur, the retrievable system is easier to deal with.

Treatment Planning Based on Biomechanical Risk Factors

The information previously discussed can be used to develop guidelines, mainly from a biomechanical point of view, for the design of implant-supported reconstructions. First, it is important to visualize the design of the final prosthetic reconstruction in terms of dimension, occlusal contacts, and function. Next, it is necessary to consider the anatomical limitations determined by the number and position of implants and how these limitations match the expected support needs. As early as the initial stage of treatment planning, there should be a balance between demand and possibilities.

During the design process it is possible to identify and evaluate different risk factors, each of which can be assigned a score. The sum of all the scores is the Biomechanical Risk Score for the specific clinical situation.

A score of 0 to 1 indicates no particular risk for the treatment plan. A score of 2 to 3 represents a moderate to major risk, whereas a score greater than 3 is a contraindication for the implant treatment plan, which should then be stopped. The score for each risk situation is based on an "average" clinical situation. These scores may be adjusted depending on the specific clinical situation. For example, the presence of a lateral incisor extension may give a score of 0.5, whereas a molar extension represents a score of 1. It is, however, always possible to modify the treatment plan, for example, by adding an extra implant or adjusting the prosthesis or occlusal scheme.

If a complication occurs after treatment, the biomechanical risk factors should be reviewed and the treatment adjusted accordingly to eliminate the cause of the problem. Five types of biomechanical risk factors may be defined:

1. **Geometric risk factors:** number of implants, their reative position, and prosthesis geometry (Table 3-1)
2. **Occlusal risk factors:** lateral contact in excursive jaw motions and parafunctional habits
3. **Bone/implant risk factors:** dependence on newly formed bone in the absence of good initial mechanical stability and implant diameter considerably smaller than what would be ideal
4. **Technological risk factors:** lack of prosthetic fit, nonoptimal screw joints, and cemented prostheses
5. **Warning signs:** indication of overload during clinical function

The presence of several of these factors indicates a risky situation for the implants, prosthesis, or both.

Table 3-1 Geometric Risk Factors

Risk Factors	Score
Number of implants < number of root supports (for N < 3)	1
Use of wide-platform implants (per implant)	–1
Implant connected to a natural tooth	0.5
Implants placed in tripod configuration	–1
Presence of a prosthetic extension (per pontic)	1
Implants placed offset to the center of the prosthesis	1
Excessive height of the restoration	0.5

Seven geometric risk factors

Number of implants less than number of root supports

The ideal number of implants in a given clinical situation depends not only on the number of teeth but also on the kind of teeth. For example, a canine represents one support, whereas a molar represents two supports. This evaluation is especially important for restorations based on one or two implants. For restorations based on three implants or more, it is possible to use fewer implants than lost supports without a substantial load increase.

One implant replacing a molar. A molar needs to be supported by two or three roots to avoid the crown's extending over the roots. Using one regular-platform implant for a molar restoration, therefore, leads to a geometric risk score of 2 (number of implants < number of root support + the presence of a prosthetic extension). The load risk score may be reduced by the use of a wide-platform (score, −1) or two regular-platform implants. (Narrow-platform implants are not recommended in the posterior area because of their low mechanical strength.)

Two implants supporting three roots or more. Replacing three or more roots with two regular-platform implants yields a geometric risk score of 1 (number of implants < number of root supports). The use of two wide-platform implants eliminates this risk factor.

Use of wide-platform implants

The wide-platform implant has increased mechanical strength and greater load support than the regular-platform implants. It should be noted, however, that with very dense (type 1) in the posterior mandible, the use of a wide implant may lead to marginal bone resorption before loading because of the low vascularity in the area.

Implants connected to natural teeth

Teeth are approximately 10 times more mobile than implants. Combining these two systems with very different resilience leads to a risk of unbalanced load sharing between the supports. However, it is important to note that this factor is often combined with other geometric factors, such as lack of bone support and extension. Furthermore, if two or more implants are connected to teeth, the rigidity of the implants causes the implants to take the major share of the load; the tooth connection will act more or less as a cantilevered pontic and should be assigned risk factors accordingly.

Implants placed in a tripod configuration

Placing implants along a straight line at a posterior restoration allows lateral forces to induce adverse bending of the implants. In contrast, when the implants are in a tripod configuration, these lateral forces, to a large extent, will be counteracted by the more favorable axial forces. In the full-arch restoration, straight-line placement leads to severe risk of overload. It is important to spread the implants along the alveolar ridge.

Presence of a prosthetic extension

In any clinical situation the presence of an extension considerably increases the load to the implants, and each pontic will add 1 to the score. Generally, the use of two regular-platform implants and an extension in the posterior region is not acceptable (geometric risk score of 2) if additional biomechanical risk factors are present.

Implants placed offset to the center of the prosthesis

If the implant axis is placed at a distance from the center of the prosthetic crown, occlusal contact may lead to screw loosening or component fracture because of the relationship of lever arm position to implant axis. However, as part of a tripod arrangement, such an offset is favorable.

Excessive height of the restoration

When the height of the abutment-crown complex is substantially increased above the implant head, the lever arm is increased as well. Lateral forces may cause screw loosening or component fracture.

Occlusal risk factors

The occlusal risk factors also must be considered. The first is a patient with bruxism, parafunction, or natural tooth fractures that are due to occlusal factors (risk score, 2). Knowledge of the etiology of tooth loss aids in the evaluation of the patient's occlusal state. Both force intensity and parafunctional habits can have a considerable negative effect on the stability of implant components. This risk is elevated if the forces are not transmitted through the implant axis. A patient with bruxism or tooth loss that is due to fracture should be considered at high risk, and the implant restoration should be reinforced by optimal support to compensate for the severe load.

The second occlusal risk factor is the presence of lateral occlusal contacts on the implant-supported prostheses only (risk score, 1). Natural teeth "suspended" by their periodontal ligaments have physiological mobility and the capacity for orthodontic movement. In contrast, implants are rigid and fixed, so they may take a larger part of the load than the teeth.

To compensate for this risk, the implant prosthesis ideally should be designed with occlusal contact at the central fossa, low inclination of the cusps, and reduced size of the occlusal table. It should be noted that most occlusal overload in the posterior regions is due to implant bending induced by lateral forces. Minimizing or eliminating lateral contacts will therefore significantly reduce the risk

of overload. Furthermore, the prosthesis should be designed and the implants positioned so that the occlusal forces act mainly along the implant axes.

The final occlusal risk factor is the elimination of lateral occlusal contact with the implant-supported prostheses (risk score −1), which represents a more favorable situation. The proprioreceptor capacity of the adjacent teeth may also help reduce the applied load, particularly during mandible excursive motions. In the design of the occlusal contact, the difference in mobility and fixation between implants and teeth must be considered. If the occlusal contact is eliminated completely and the antagonists are natural teeth, the opposing teeth may erupt and establish contact over time. Therefore, centric contact should be established in light occlusion, and lateral contact is acceptable in heavy occlusion.

Bone/implant risk factors

Bone/implant risk factors include dependence on newly formed bone in the absence of good initial mechanical stability (risk score, 1) and a smaller implant diameter than desired (risk score, 0.5). After surgery it is important to evaluate the initial stability of each individual implant to select early loading or define a proper healing time before loading the implants. If the primary stability of the implant is not satisfactory, the healing time should be prolonged and the implant protected from too much load during the first period of function. The absence of good primary implant stability should be considered a risk factor only during the first year of function.

Implants with smaller diameters have a lower capacity to support bending forces than do implants with wider diameters. In the posterior regions, therefore, implants with a 4-mm diameter are a recommended minimum. A narrow-platform implant used in the posterior region should be considered a major risk factor (risk score, 1). A regular-platform implant with a 3.75-mm diameter used in the posterior region in combination with a stronger gold alloy abutment screw (CeraOne, CerAdapt, TiAdapt) should be considered a moderate risk factor (risk score, 0.5).

Technological risk factors

Technological risk factors include lack of prosthetic fit (risk score, 0.5) and cemented prostheses (risk score, 0.5). Studies of complete-arch prostheses on implants have shown that most often there is considerable misfit between prosthesis and implant. This factor alone does not seem to lead to complications, as the number of implants is usually more than sufficient to support the prosthesis. For short-span prostheses in the posterior region, however, where each implant has a strategic value, the lack of prosthetic fit or proper screw tension may cause complications and should be considered a risk factor.

If a screw joint will be cemented over, it is important to have high and stable screw tension, such as that obtained with gold alloy screws (CeraOne, CerAdapt, TiAdapt, or AurAdapt) when using a torque controller. Otherwise, retightening is difficult to accomplish. A screw-retained prosthesis is preferable in a situation with elevated risk (risk score greater than or equal to 3). Warning signs are easier to detect, adjustments are easier to perform, and complications are easier to handle.

Note that the technological risk factors are often hard to detect. Therefore, to reduce their possible negative influence, the best solution is the use of proven and standardized protocols for prosthesis fabrication, premachined prosthetic components, and tightening instruments with stable and predefined tightening torque.

Warning signs

Brånemark system implants are designed to support prostheses in virtually any clinical situation, provided the previously discussed treatment planning recommendations are followed. Should an overload situation occur, warning signs usually appear before the complication leads to failure. Warning signs include repeated loosening of prosthetic or abutment screws (risk score, 1), repeated fracture of veneering material (risk score, 1), fracture of prosthetic or abutment screws (risk score, 2), and bone resorption below the first thread of the implant (risk score, 1).

These warning signs should not be neglected but rather trigger an analysis of their origin and the proper response. In case of screw loosening or screw fracture it is not enough to replace or retighten the components (or both); rather, the cause of the complication should be identified and the reasons for it eliminated, or the problem may continue and lead to implant failure. A warning sign should trigger a review of the biomechanical risk factors with the goal of modifying the situation and reducing or eliminating excessive risk factors (for example, reducing or eliminating cantilevers, modifying the occlusion, or inserting extra implants).

Clinical Examples

Three-unit prosthesis

In the case of a three-unit prosthesis, the ideal design from a biomechanical point of view is three implants placed in a slightly curved configuration, with the middle implant offset a minimum of 2 to 3 mm in the buccolingual direction (Fig 3-13). This tripod implant configuration allows a largely axial load response to bending forces, minimizing the stress level (Fig 3-14). It can be estimated that the stress will be reduced approximately 50% by the tripod configuration compared with a straight-line configuration with the same number of implants. The tripod placement should be determined by where the implant heads pierce the anchoring bone. A slight inclination of the implant may be useful in achieving such placement (Fig 3-15).

If only two implants can be placed, they are best used as end supports to eliminate extensions (Fig 3-16). A three-unit prosthesis with one cantilever pontic basically doubles the stress level at the implant closest to the extension (see Fig 3-5) in comparison with the design where the pontic is placed between the two implants. Two implants cannot prevent a possible bending moment (see Fig 3-4), so it is important to diagnose the patient's functional habits and, if needed, reduce the consequences of any parafunction. Centering the occlusion and eliminating lateral excursive contacts should be considered (see Fig 3-8). There could be as much difference in risk factor as 6 between the most adverse load situation (two implants with an extended pontic) and the most optimal situation (tripod placement) because of the implant support only (Fig 3-17). Consideration of the occlusal control possibilities would lead to an even larger difference between the worst and best situations.

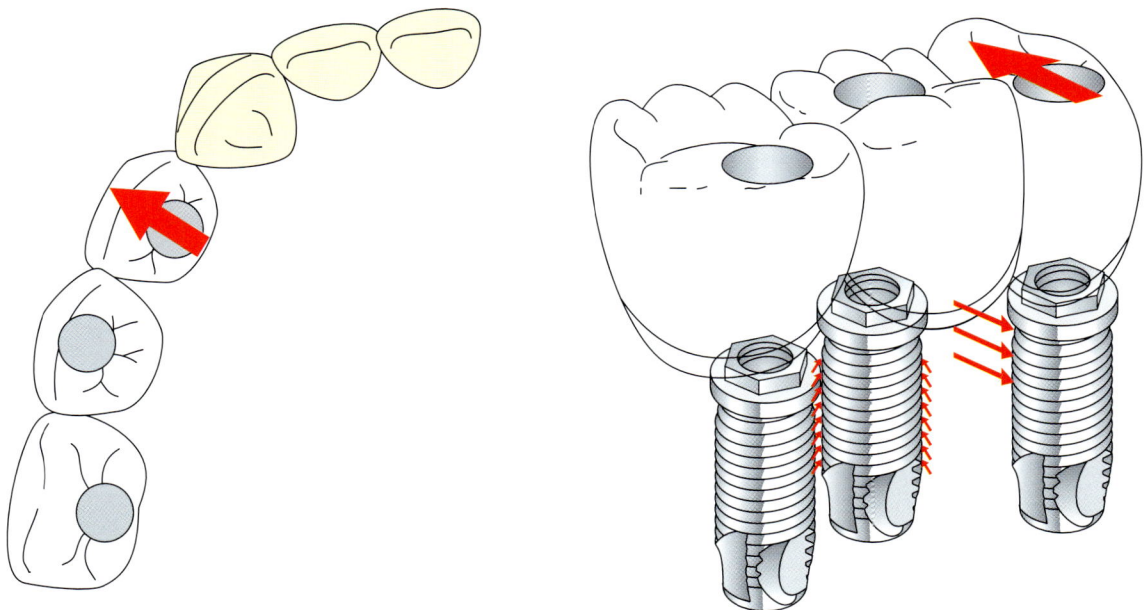

Fig 3-13 The ideal situation from a biomechanical point of view for a three-unit prosthesis is three implants in a slightly curved configuration, with the middle implant offset a minimum of 2 to 3 mm in the buccolingual direction.

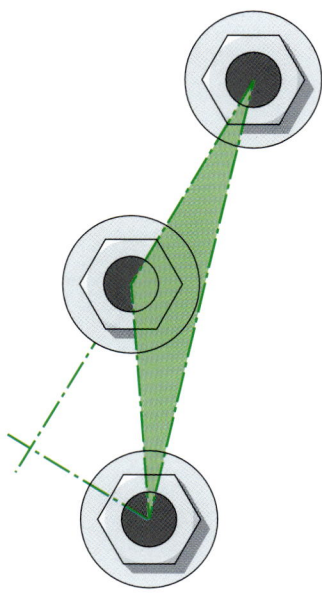

Fig 3-14 A tripod implant configuration allows the load response to bending forces to be predominantly axial, minimizing the stress level.

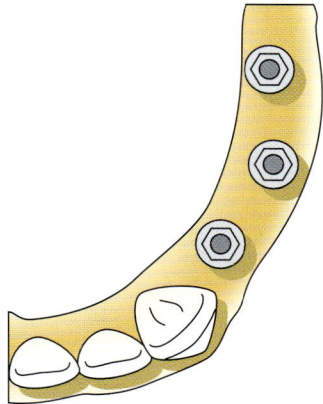

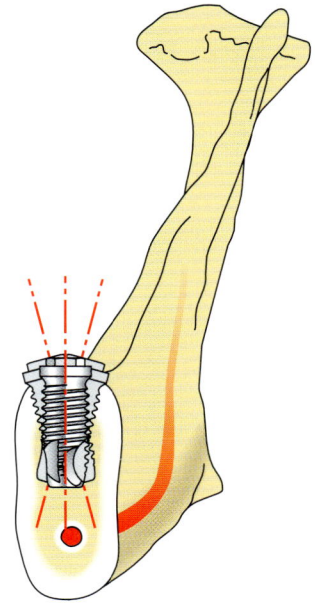

Fig 3-15 The implant head defines the position of the prosthesis support in the bone; a slight inclination of the implant may be useful for optimizing its location.

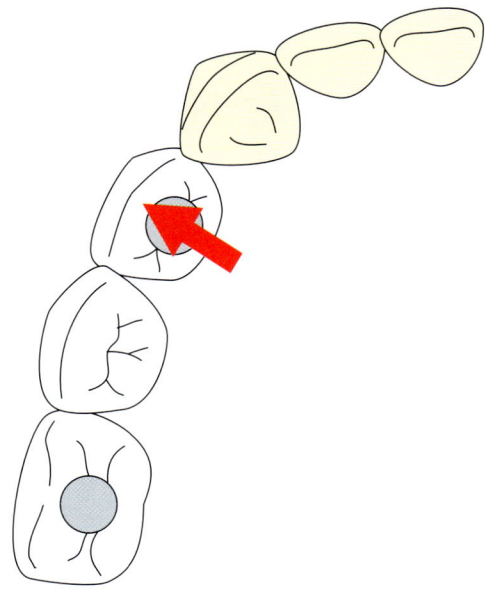

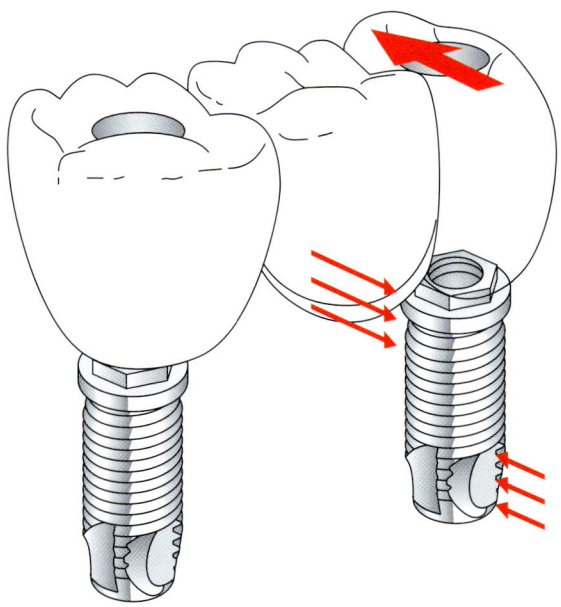

Fig 3-16 If only two implants can be placed, they should preferably be end supports to eliminate extensions.

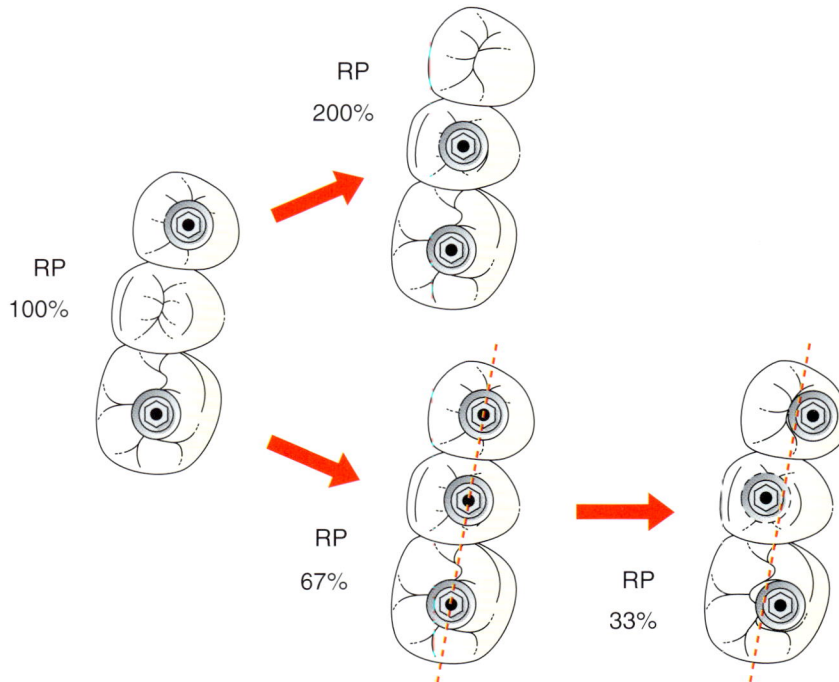

Fig 3-17 The same prosthetic situation is supported by different implant configurations. The configuration with two end supports *(left)* is arbitrarily chosen as a reference for the implant stress (100%). The stress levels for each of the other configurations are illustrated. There could be a difference in risk factor of 6 between the situation with most stress (two implants with an extended pontic) and the optimal situation (tripod placement). RP indicates regular platform.

Wide-platform implants

Although the Brånemark system wide-platform components yield considerable gains in mechanical strength, bone quality and bone quantity are still patient-dependent variables. It is therefore important to consider the ability of the bone to support the projected prosthetic load by striving for an adequate number and arrangement of implants. Increasing the relative strength of mechanical components does not, in and of itself, eliminate the risk of overload. In fact, in patients with minimal ridge width, the use of a wider implant may actually compromise available bone support.

The importance of bone anchorage can be seen in a comparison of the use of three regular-platform versus two wide-platform components for a three-unit restoration (Fig 3-18). In this example, the increased mechanical strength of the wide-platform components reduces the material stress to approximately 63% of the regular-platform with the same prosthetic forces applied. However, the increased surface area per se reduces the bone stress level to only approximately 77%, and the bone is the limiting factor. Therefore, the use of two wide-platform implants—placed by geometric definition in line—is less favorable than the use of three regular-platform implants in a staggered configuration.

This analysis demonstrates the importance of biomechanical treatment planning and shows that a stronger component per se will

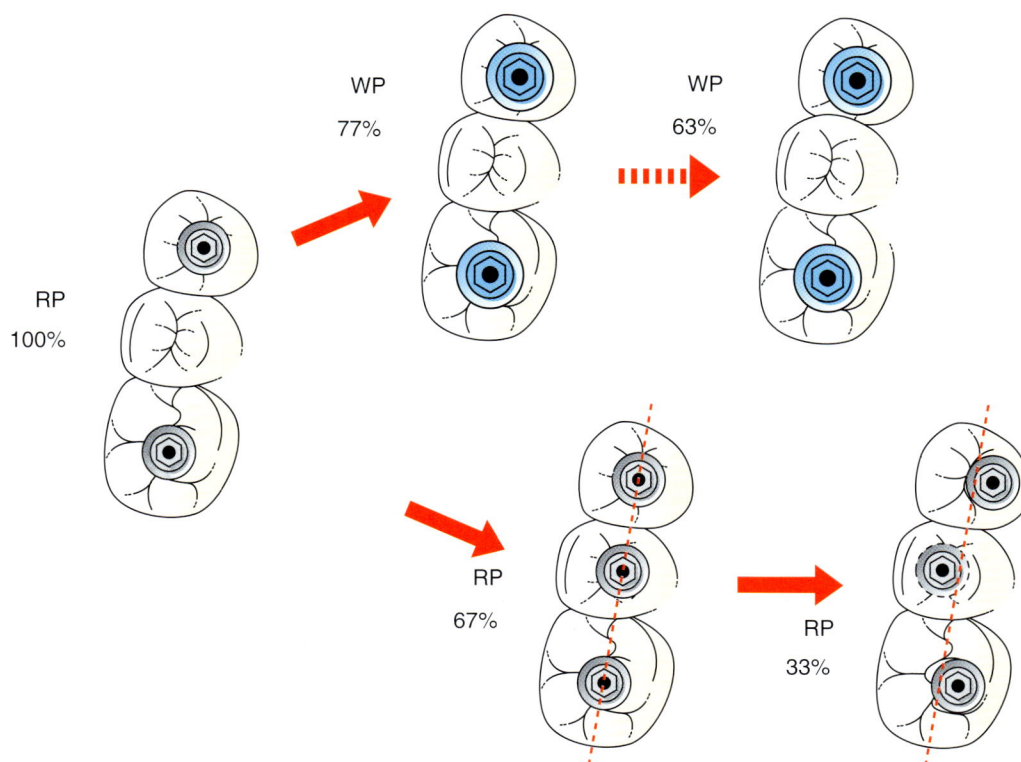

Fig 3-18 Two wide-platform (WP) implants used to support the prosthetic configuration illustrated in Fig 3-17. Because of the larger surface area, the bone stress may be reduced to approximately 77% that of two regular-platform (RP) implants. The mechanical stress, however, is reduced to approximately 63% as a consequence of the increased dimensions. Only if the wide implants allow improved cortical anchorage can the full benefit of the additional mechanical strength be realized (stress reduced to between 77% and 63%).

not necessarily eliminate overload. Finally, the choice between the platform options should be based on the surgeon's judgment of bone support and the healing capacity of the site, in addition to other factors. Especially in the posterior mandible, the vascularity of dense cortical bone may be compromised if a large implant is used without a matching width of bone cross section.

Narrow-platform implants

The narrow-platform implant has about 20% reduced mechanical strength relative to the regular-platform implant with a 3.75-mm diameter. However, with the increased fatigue strength (about 30% greater) of the commer-

cially pure titanium material used today, the implant strength is about the same as that of the previous regular-platform implant. Therefore, if needed in posterior situations with narrow ridges, the narrow-platform might be used as part of a restoration, especially with the more favorable staggered implant configuration (see Fig 3-17).

Single-implant molar replacement

The single-tooth molar replacement supported by a single implant has limited long-term clinical documentation at this time. This design is highly susceptible to bending overload, so the occlusion should be developed so that only centric contacts exist. Because of the potential high level of stress, implants with a diameter of 4 mm or more are recommended for single-implant molar replacements. It is virtually impossible to completely replace the lost root support of two or three natural molar roots with a single cylindrical pillar, so single-implant molar replacement, from a biomechanical viewpoint, should continue to be used with caution. Bruxism, clenching, and the periodontal condition of the adjacent teeth should be carefully evaluated, as they may be contraindications for single-implant molar restorations. In some situations two implants may be needed to sufficiently support a single molar. Even if the wide platform offers considerably increased strength, bone anchorage may still be a limiting factor.

Conclusions

Biomechanical considerations in implant dentistry to a large extent follow simple mechanical rules, based on the leverage principle and the implant's initial anchorage in dense bone. By ensuring good initial implant stability and a sufficient number of implants with strategic positions, considering the patient's functional behavior, limiting the extension of the prosthesis, and controlling the occlusal pattern and contacts, possible overload situations can be minimized. These requirements usually do not conflict with esthetic demands.

References

Adell R, Lekholm U, Brånemark PI. Surgical procedures. In: Brånemark P-I, Zarb G, Albrektsson T (eds). Tissue-integrated Prostheses: Osseointegration in Clinical Dentistry. Chicago: Quintessence, 1985:221–232.

Andersson B, Ödman P, Lindvall AM, Brånemark P-I. Cemented single crowns on osseointegrated implants after five years: Results from a prospective study on CeraOne. Int J Prosthodont 1998;11: 212–218.

Bahat O. Treatment planning and placement of implants in the posterior maxillae: Report of 732 consecutive Nobelpharma implants. Int J Oral Maxillofac Implants 1993;8:151–161.

Brunski J. In vivo bone response to biomechanical loading at the bone/dental implant interface. Adv Dent Res 1999;13:99–119.

Burguete R, Johns R, King T, Patterson E. Tightening characteristics for screwed joints in osseointegrated dental implants. J Prosthet Dent 1994;71:592–599.

Carr A, Brunski J, Hurley E. Effects of fabrication, finishing and polishing procedures on preload in prostheses using conventional "gold" and plastic cylinders. Int J Oral Maxillofac Implants 1996;11: 589–598.

Gunne J, Jemt T, Lindén B. Implant treatment in partially edentulous patients: A report on prostheses after 3 years. Int J Prosthodont 1994;7:143–148.

Henry PJ, Laney WR, Jemt T, Harris D, Krogh PHJ, Polizzi G, et al. Osseointegrated implants for single-tooth replacement: A prospective 5-year multicenter study. Int J Oral Maxillofac Implants 1996;11: 450–455.

Ivanoff C-J, Sennerby L, Lekholm U. Influence of mono- and bicortical anchorage on the integration of titanium implants: A study in the rabbit tibia. Int J Oral Maxillofac Surg 1996;25:229–235.

Jemt T, Book K. Prosthesis misfit and marginal bone loss in edentulous implant patients. Int J Oral Maxillofac Implants 1996;11:620–625.

Jörneus L, Jemt T, Carlsson L. Loads and design of screw joint for single crowns supported by osseointegrated implants. Int J Oral Maxillofac Implants 1992;7:353–359.

Kallus T, Bessing C. Loose gold screws frequently occur in complete-arch fixed prostheses supported by osseointegrated implants after 5 years. Int J Oral Maxillofac Implants 1994;9:169–178.

Krekmanov L, Kahn M, Rangert B, Lindström H. Tilting of posterior mandibular and maxillary implants for improved bridge support. Int J Oral Maxillofac Implants 2000;15:405–414.

Lekholm U, van Steenberghe D, Herrmann I, Bolender C, Folmer T, Gunne J, et al. Osseointegrated implants in the treatment of partially edentulous jaws. A prospective 5-year multicenter study. Int J Oral Maxillofac Implants 1994;9:627–635.

Maló P, Rangert B, Dvärsäter L. Immediate function of Brånemark implants in the esthetic zone: A retrospective clinical study with 6 months to 4 years of follow-up. Clin Implants Dent Res 2000;2:137–145.

Meredith N, Book K, Friberg B, Jemt T, Sennerby L. Resonance frequency measurements of implant stability in vivo: A cross-sectional and longitudinal study of resonance frequency measurements on implants in the edentulous and partially dentate maxilla. Clin Oral Implants Res 1997;8:226–233.

Polizzi G, Rangert B, Lekholm U, Gualini F, Lindström H. Brånemark system wide platform implants for single molar replacement: A clinical evaluation of prospective and retrospective materials. Clin Implants Dent Rel Res (in press).

Quirynen M, Naert I, van Steenberghe D. Fixture design and overload influence marginal bone loss and fixture success in the Brånemark system. Clin Oral Implants Res 1992:3;104–111.

Randow K, Ericsson I, Nilner K, Petersson A, Glantz P-O. Immediate functional loading of Brånemark dental implants: An 18-month clinical follow-up study. Clin Oral Implants Res 1999;10:8–15.

Rangert B, Jemt T, Jörneus L. Forces and moments on Brånemark implants. Int J Oral Maxillofac Implants 1989;4:241–247.

Rangert B, Krogh PHJ, Langer B, van Roekel N. Bending overload and implant fracture: A retrospective clinical analysis. Int J Oral Maxillofac Implants 1995;10:326–334.

Rangert B, Sullivan R, Jemt T. Load factor control for implants in the posterior partially edentulous segment. Int J Oral Maxillofac Implants 1997;12: 360–370.

Renouard F, Rangert B. Risk Factors in Implant Dentistry: Simplified Clinical Analysis for Predictable Treatment. Berlin: Quintessenz, 1999.

Sennerby L, Thomsen P, Ericsson L. A morphometric and biomechanic comparison of titanium implants inserted in rabbit cortical and cancellous bone. Int J Oral Maxillofac Implants 1992;7:62–71.

Chapter 4

Implant Placement Philosophy

Patrick Palacci, DDS, and Ingvar Ericsson, LDS, Odont Dr

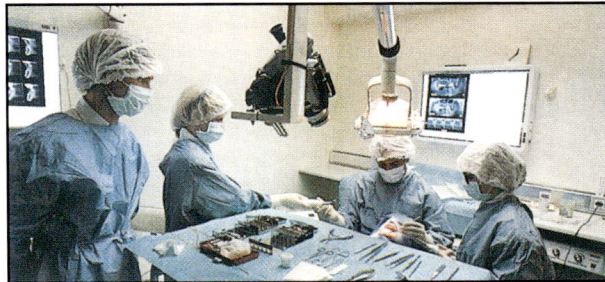

In occlusal rehabilitation using implants as anchors for reconstruction, the implant unit (titanium implant and abutment) must be considered a substitute for the tooth root. From a prosthodontic point of view, the implants replace the roots as support for the superstructure, so the implants must be placed so as to obtain the expected treatment outcome. The degree of bone resorption and other anatomical characteristics also must be considered. Furthermore, it is important to keep in mind that implant components are intended to support teeth of different sizes. Thus, the correct choice among a wide variety of prosthetic components, along with precision in implant placement, is needed to obtain the optimal treatment outcome.

Component Choice

Root and crown width vary greatly among different teeth. According to Wheeler and Ash (1984) (Table 4-1), the mesiodistal and buccolingual average extension of roots at the cementoenamel junction (CEJ) varies between 3.5 mm (mandibular central incisor) and 10.0 mm (maxillary molars). The mean width of the tooth crowns in the mesiodistal direction varies between 5.0 mm (mandibular central incisor) and 10.5 mm (mandibular molars). When considering only the incisors, canines, and premolars—the regions that are most important from an esthetic point of view—the corresponding figures still differ, but to a smaller degree. Thus, in the maxilla, the average width of the tooth crowns in the mesiodistal direction ranges from 6.5 mm (lateral incisor) to 8.5 mm (central incisor) and in the mandible ranges from 5.0 mm (central incisor) to 7.0 mm (canine and premolars). These values, which represent different tooth dimensions, must be compared with the design of the regular-platform implant components (Figs 4-1 and 4-2).

Table 4-1 Average Dimensions of Teeth*

Location of teeth	Mesiodistal crown diameter	Mesiodistal diameter at cervix	Buccolingual diameter at cervix
Maxillary teeth			
Central incisor	8.5	7.0	6.0
Lateral incisor	6.5	4.0	5.0
Canine	7.5	5.5	7.0
Premolars	7.0	5.0	8.0
Molars	10.0	8.0	10.0
Mandibular teeth			
Central incisor	5.0	3.5	5.5
Lateral incisor	5.5	4.0	5.5
Canine	7.0	5.5	7.0
Premolars	7.0	5.0	7.0
Molars	10.5	8.5	9.0

Dimensions in mm.
* Wheeler and Ash, 1984.

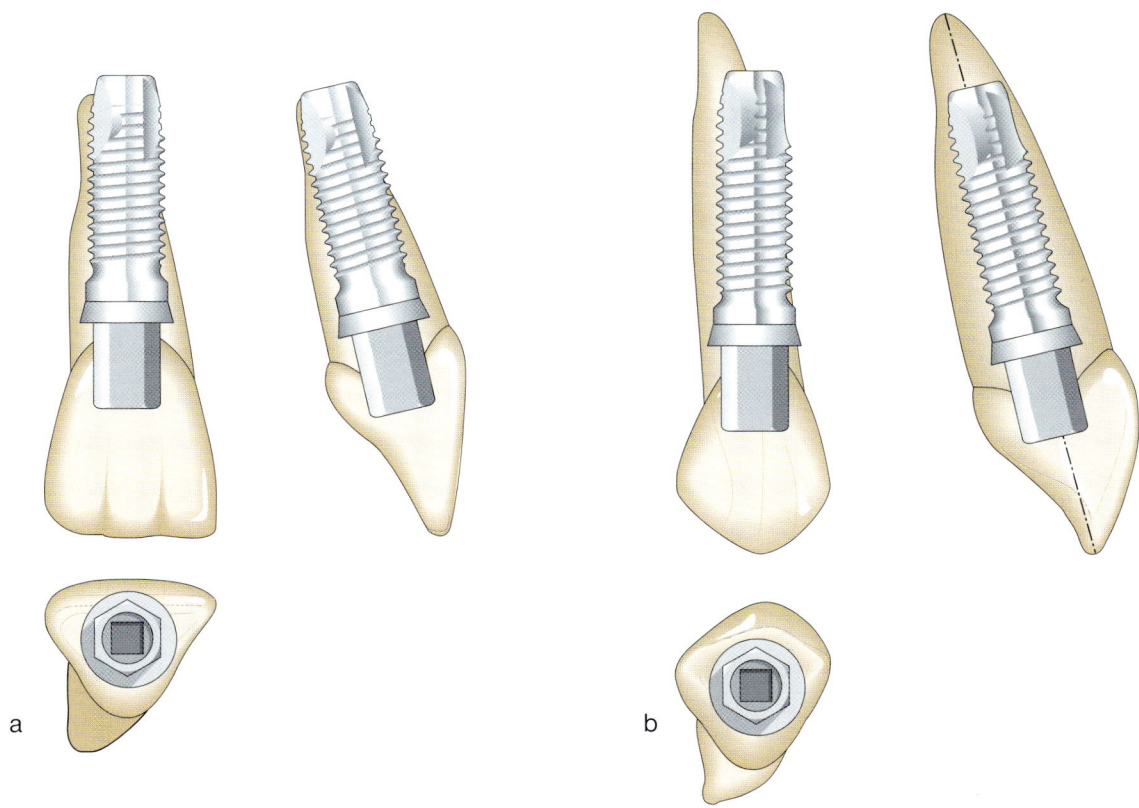

Fig 4-1 Relationship between the implant and the roots to be replaced. *(a)* Maxillary central incisor. *(b)* Maxillary canine.

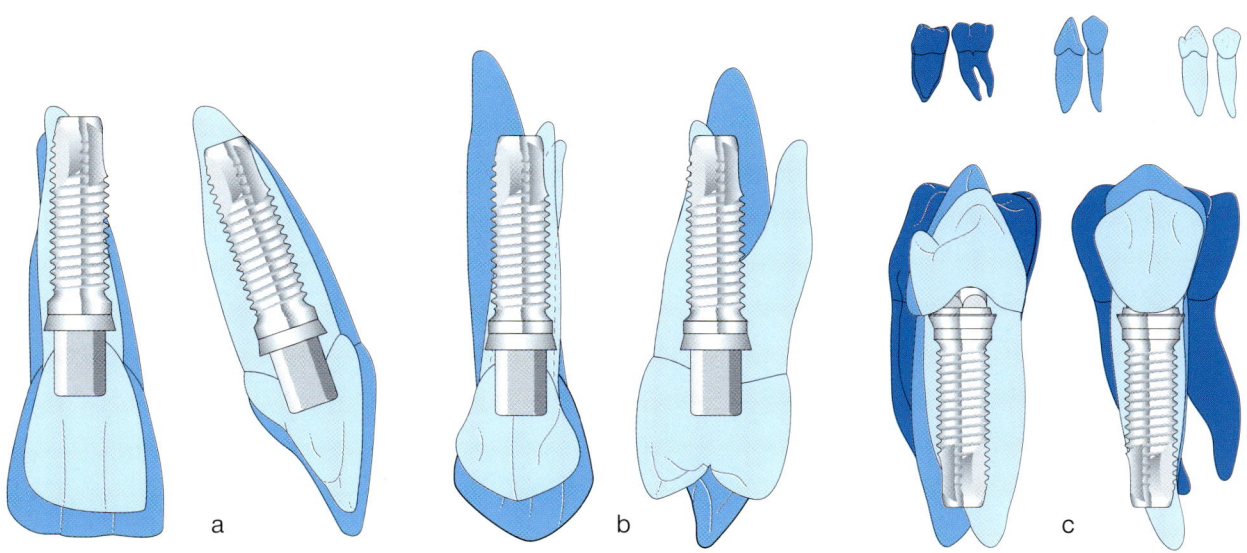

Fig 4-2 *(a to c)* Relationship between different tooth crowns and a regular-platform implant (implant supplied with a CeraOne abutment).

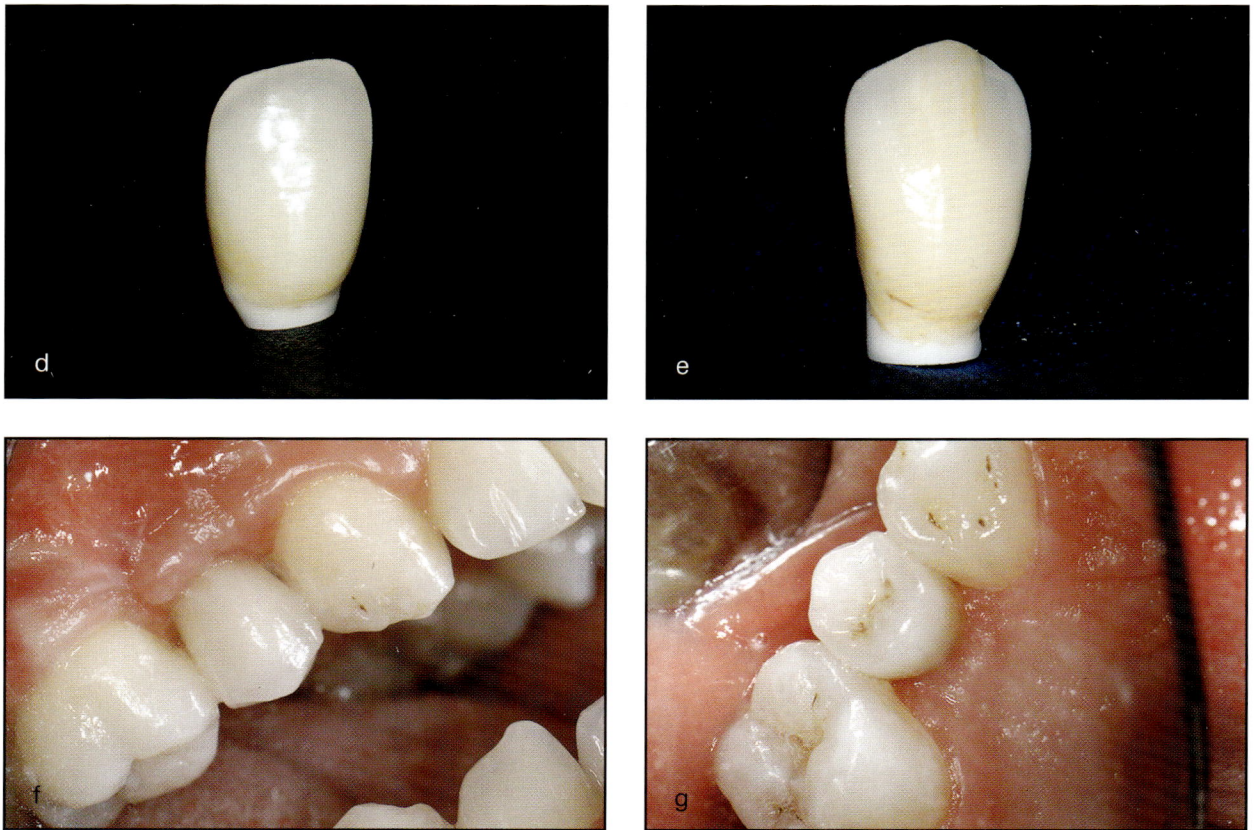

Fig 4-2 *(d and e)* Implant-supported maxillary lateral incisor, canine, and premolar illustrating the importance of optimal implant placement. Different teeth can be built on the same abutments. These two pictures illustrate the need for optimal implant placement, resulting in a better emergence profile. *(f and g)* Replacement of a maxillary premolar by an implant-supported restoration. Note the similarities in dimensions between the natural teeth and the prosthetic crown supported by a regular-platform implant.

The diameter of the threaded portion of the most frequently used implants is either 3.75 or 4 mm. At the implant head (that is, at the collar), the diameter is increased to 4.1 mm. The design of the standard, EsthetiCone, CeraOne, and MirusCone (Nobel Biocare, Göteborg, Sweden) abutments results in a further increase of the implant width, up to 4.8 mm (Fig 4-3).

Today implants of different diameters are available to better match the shape of the roots and crowns to be replaced (Fig 4-4). A wider implant (wide platform, diameter = 5.0 or 5.5 mm), as well as a narrow one (narrow platform, diameter = 3.3 mm), has been designed to be used mainly in the replacement of molars, and maxillary laterals and mandibular incisors, respectively. Furthermore, specific (preparable) abutments have been developed for even more precision in matching the anatomy of the different teeth to be replaced. Such abutments are particularly useful in the anterior maxilla, where esthetic demands are greater.

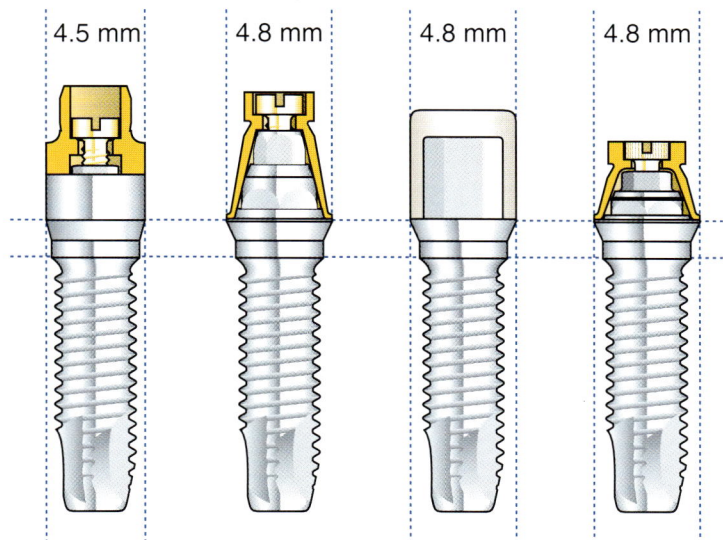

Fig 4-3 Widths of different types of prefabricated abutments for the Brånemark system (regular platform). *Left to right:* Standard abutment, EsthetiCone, CeraOne, and MirusCone.

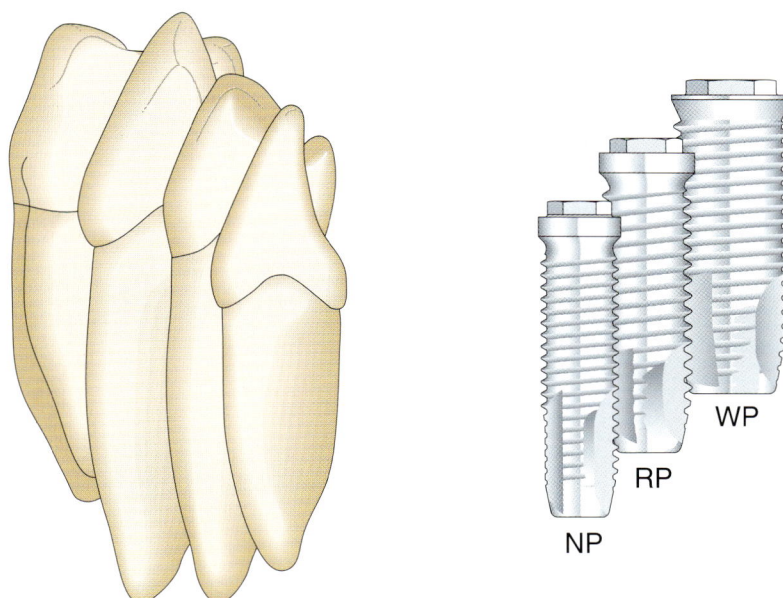

Fig 4-4 Evolution of Brånemark system implants with different widths to better match individual root anatomy. NP indicates narrow platform; RP, regular platform; and WP, wide platform.

For example, a maxillary central incisor may be replaced by a regular-platform implant with the abutment chosen to best match the shape of the tooth to be replaced (Fig 4-5). Different kinds of abutments, such as CeraOne, CerAdapt, and TiAdapt, can be evaluated.

The most common problems occur in the replacement of a maxillary lateral incisor. The diameter of a narrow- or regular-platform implant, combined with a CeraOne abutment, will yield a diameter of 4.8 mm at the crown-abutment junction level, which is approximately 0.5 to 1.0 mm wider than the "average" original root of a tooth at the CEJ level (Fig 4-6). When the space between the central incisor and the canine is limited, the best choice is a narrow-platform implant with a preparable abutment (TiAdapt) (Fig 4-7).

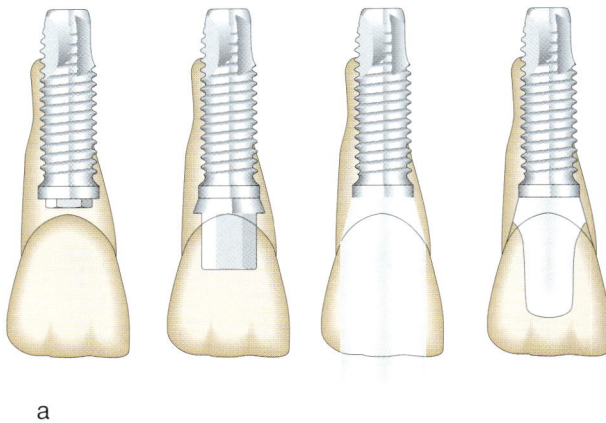

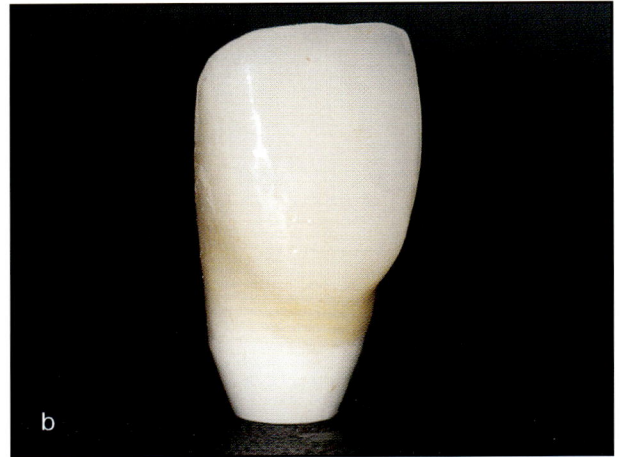

Fig 4-5 (a) Regular-platform implant replacing the root of a maxillary central incisor, supplied with both a CeraOne abutment and a CerAdapt/TiAdapt abutment. (b) The CerAdapt/TiAdapt abutment better matches the emergence profile of the tooth to be replaced than does the CeraOne abutment.

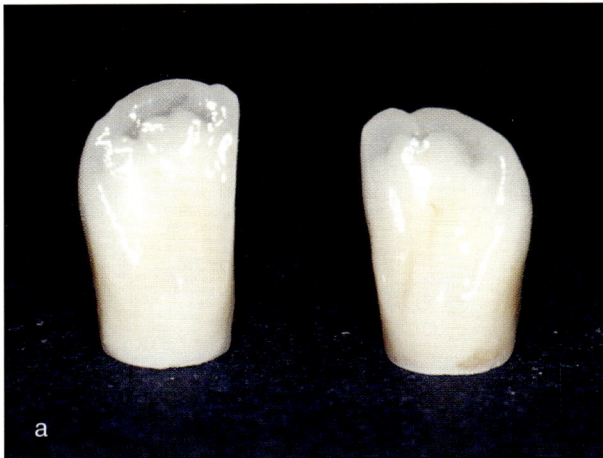

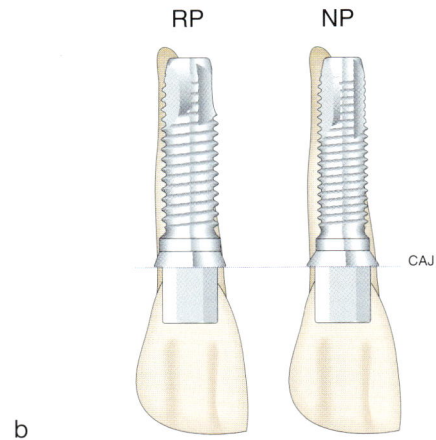

Fig 4-6 (a) Two lateral incisors which have been constructed on CeraOne abutments. It is obvious that a narrower abutment would have been indicated in this specific case. Narrow- and regular-platform implants replacing the root of a maxillary lateral incisor. (b) CeraOne abutments for both the regular- and narrow-platform implants have an identical prosthetic base (diameter = 4.8 mm). RP indicates regular platform; NP, narrow platform; and CAJ, crown-abutment junction.

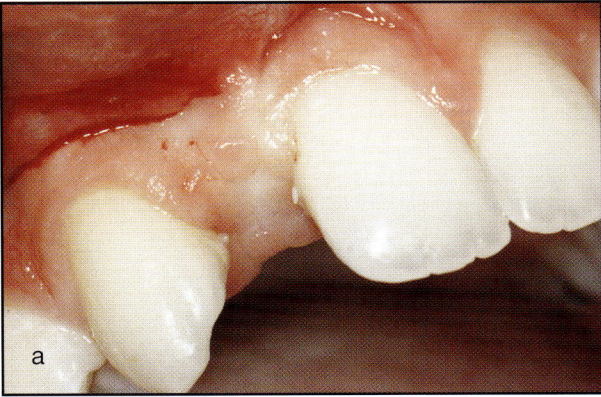

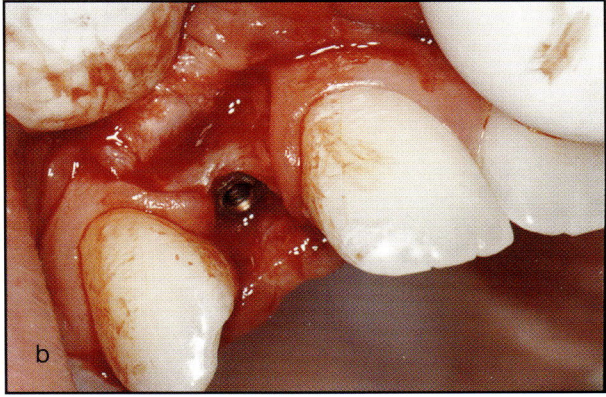

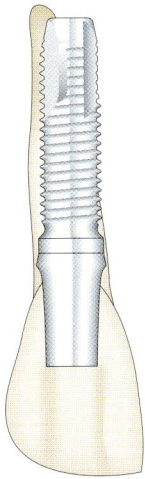

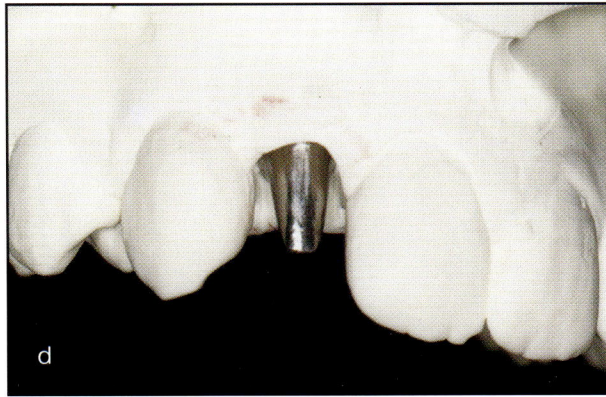

Fig 4-7 *(a to g)* Narrow-platform implant replacing the root of a maxillary lateral incisor and supplied with a TiAdapt abutment. This combination of implant and abutment matches the embrasure of the crown of the lateral incisor to be replaced.

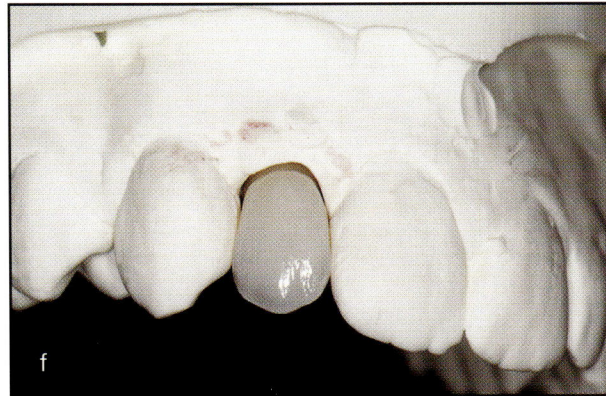

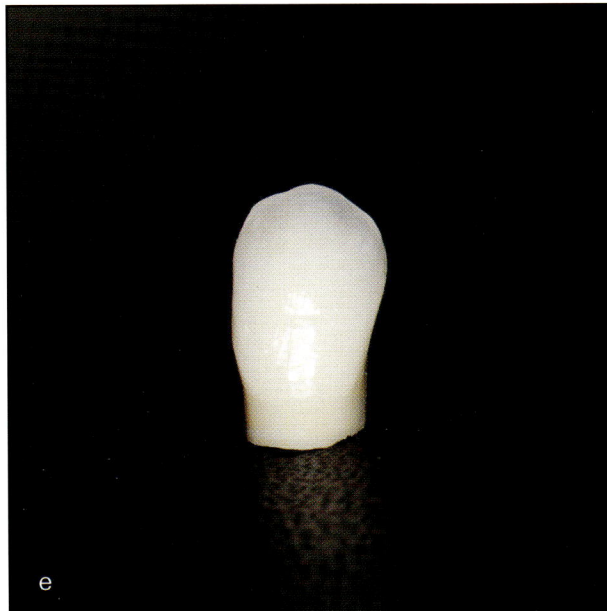

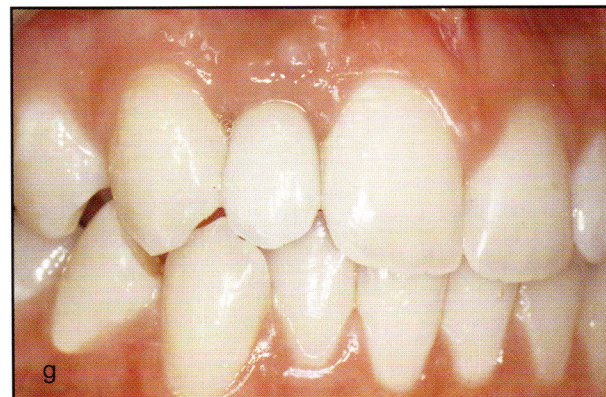

In the replacement of a single molar, a regular-platform implant can be used where the space between the adjacent teeth is limited (Figs 4-8a to 4-8c). A wide-platform implant, however, can also be used to create more favorable biomechanical conditions. The width of the wide-platform abutment will better match the anatomy of the original molar, thus allowing physiological embrasures (Fig 4-8d). According to Wheeler and Ash (1984) (see Table 4-1), the average mesiodistal diameter of a maxillary molar at the cervix is 8 mm. When using the wide platform, the base of the abutment will be about 6 mm, and only 1 mm needs to be added on each side to properly match the original anatomy. An ultimate pre-requisite for using the wide platform is sufficient bone width in the buccolingual/palatal direction. Where the ridge is thinner, either two regular-platform or two narrow-platform implants can be used if the space between the two adjacent teeth is sufficient (Fig 4-9). The crown restoration usually can be connected directly to the implants (without use of abutments) and designed as a "tunneled" molar.

Each tooth to be replaced represents a unique situation, so it is important for both surgeon and prosthodontist to be familiar with the dimensions of the prosthetic components in relation to the teeth to be replaced (Fig 4-10). As the implant system evolves, teeth can be replaced more effectively.

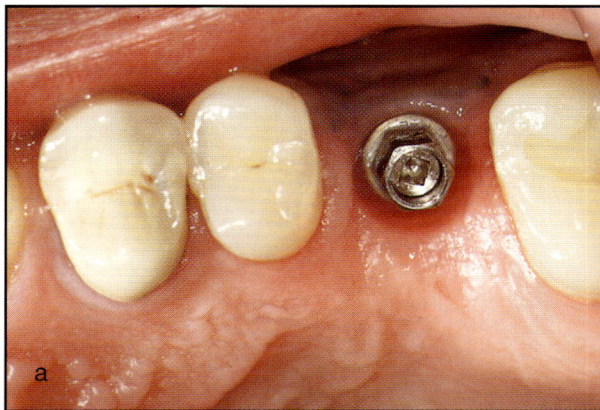

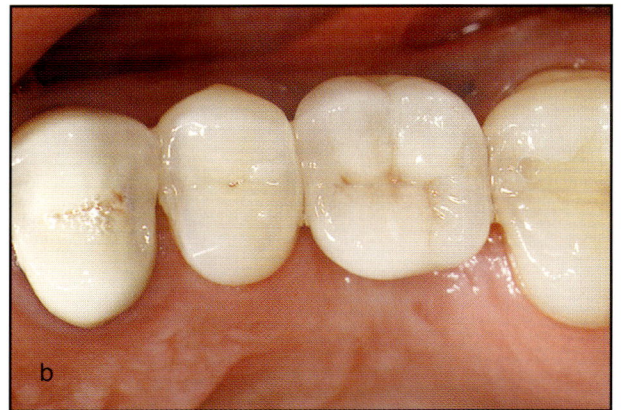

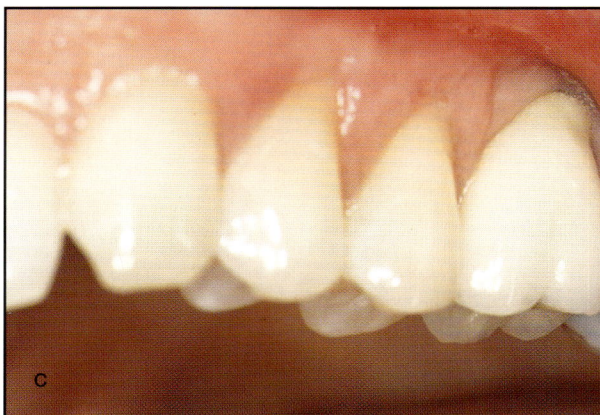

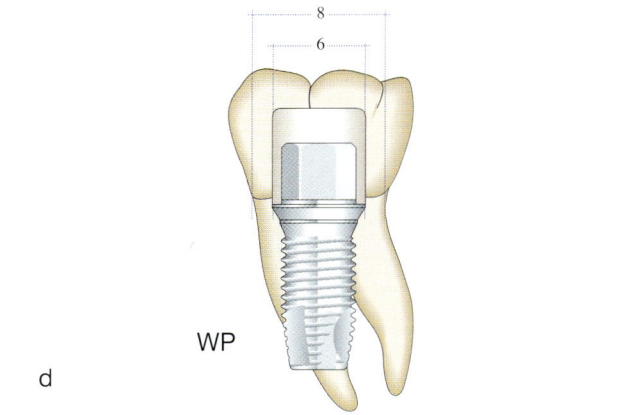

Fig 4-8 *(a to c)* Replacement of a maxillary first molar using a regular-platform fixture and a CeraOne abutment. Note that the mesiodistal space of the edentulous area is narrower than usual, thus allowing the use of a regular-platform implant. *(d)* Schematic drawing illustrating the relationship between a wide-platform (WP) implant supporting a CeraOne abutment and a mandibular molar.

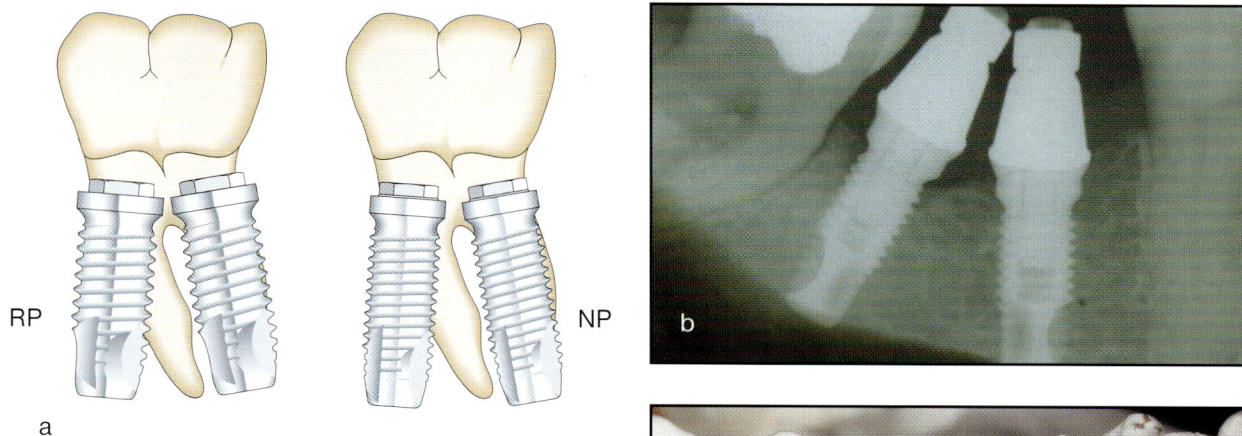

Fig 4-9 *(a)* Two regular- or narrow-platform implants (*left* and *right*, respectively) used to replace the roots of a molar. *(b and c)* In this treatment approach, the molar crown restoration has to be designed as a "tunneled molar" placed either with or without the use of abutments.

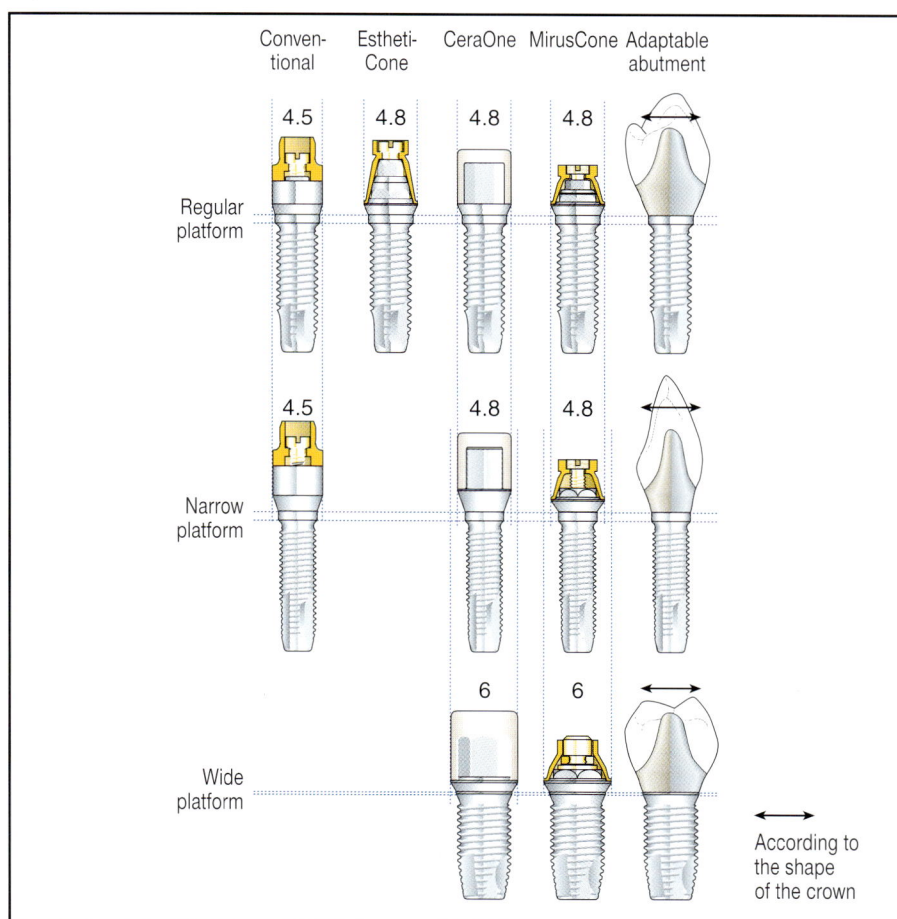

Fig 4-10 Dimensions (in mm) of various prosthetic components.

Implant Placement Considerations

The need for precision in implant placement varies according to the individual case. For example, in the edentulous mandible there is a need for precision only in the buccolingual direction. The need for precision increases in partially edentulous patients according to the jaw treated and the positions of the neighboring and opposing teeth. The most challenging situation is the single-tooth replacement, especially in the anterior maxilla, where a malposition of less than 1 mm and/or less than 10 degrees can jeopardize the overall treatment outcome (Fig 4-11).

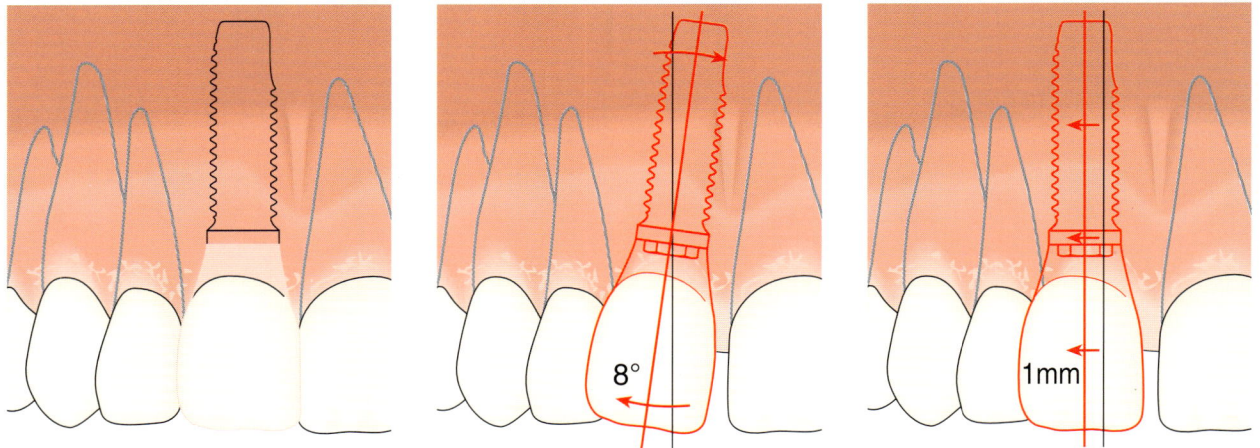

Fig 4-11 Ideal position and angulation of an implant to support a maxillary single-crown restoration are of utmost importance.

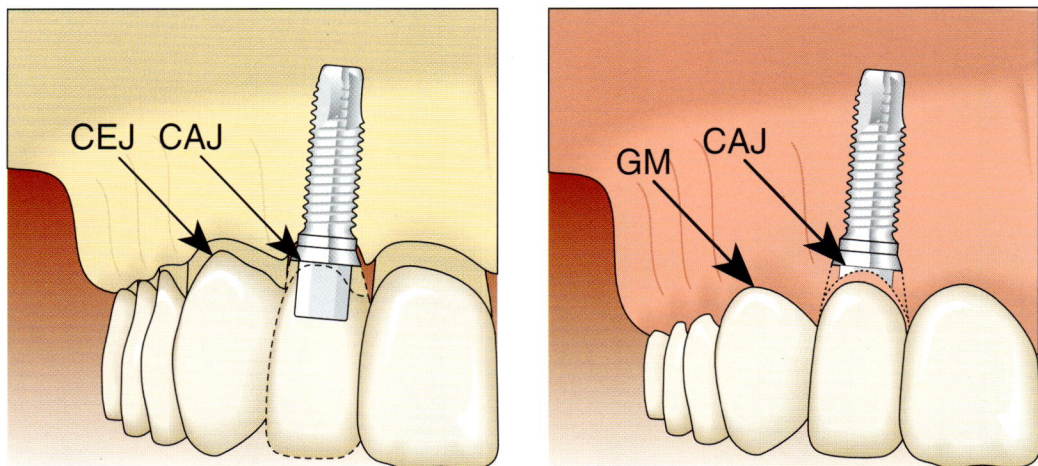

Fig 4-12 Ideal implant position where neighboring teeth demonstrate intact periodontal tissue support. The crown-abutment junction (CAJ) of the implant-supported restoration more or less coincides with the most apical extension of the cementoenamel junction (CEJ) of the neighboring teeth. GM indicates gingival margin.

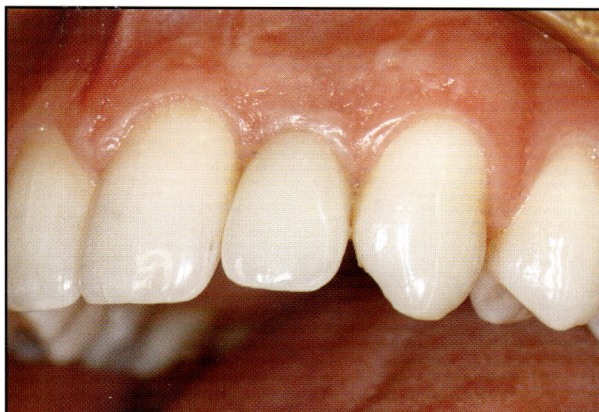

Fig 4-13 Replacement of a lateral incisor with an intact periodontal support.

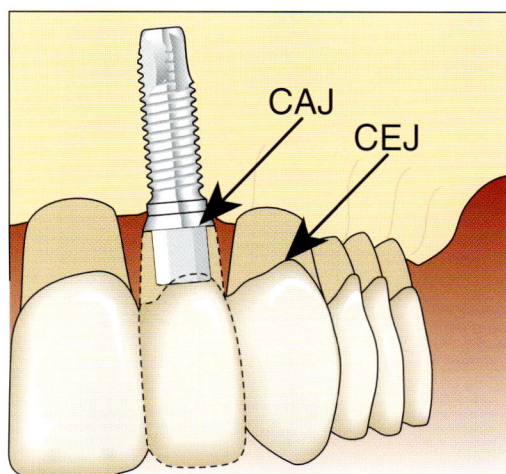

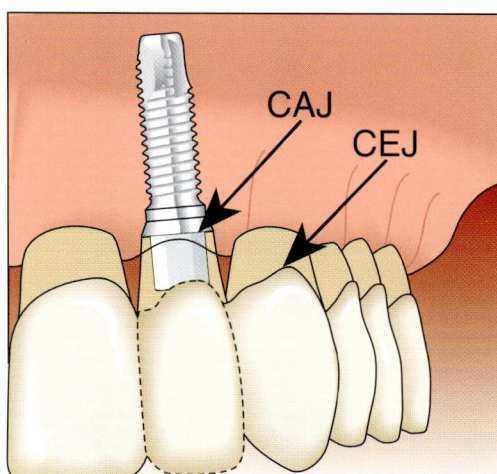

Fig 4-14 Ideal implant position where neighboring teeth demonstrate reduced periodontal tissue support. The crown-abutment junction is placed slightly submarginally. CAJ indicates crown-abutment junction; CEJ, cementoenamel junction.

A satisfactory esthetic treatment outcome in connecting the suprastructure to the implants depends on locating the most coronal extension of the crown-abutment junction approximately 0.5 to 3.0 mm submarginally. Thus, in partially edentulous patients in whom the neighboring teeth demonstrate intact periodontal tissue support, the crown-abutment junction must more or less coincide with the most apical extension of the CEJ of these teeth (Figs 4-12 and 4-13).

The crown-abutment junction must be placed more deeply (approximately 3 mm) when neighboring teeth demonstrate a pronounced difference in position of the CEJ at the buccolingual versus proximal sites. Consequently, in jaws with reduced periodontal tissue support and exposed root surfaces, the crown-abutment junction is most often placed more superficially than in periodontally intact situations, but still at a submarginal position (approximately 1 to 2 mm) (Figs 4-14 to 4-16).

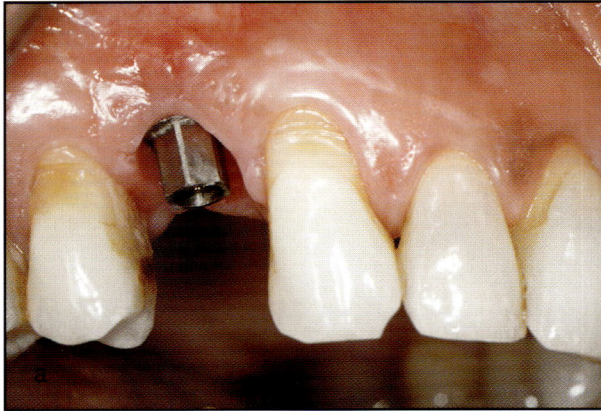

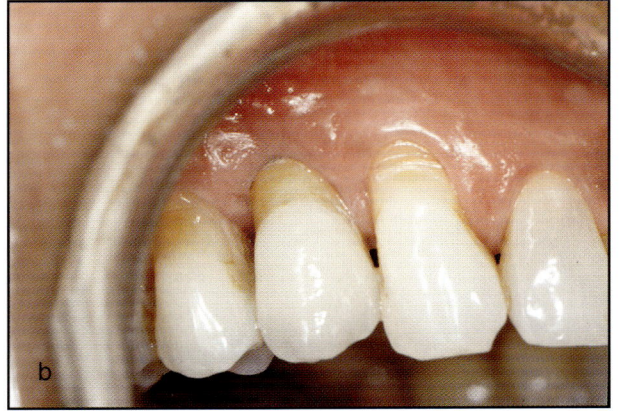

Fig 4-15 *(a and b)* Replacement of a first premolar and a lateral incisor with reduced periodontal support.

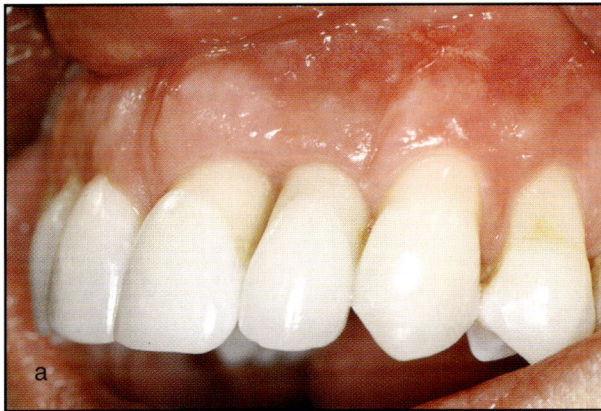

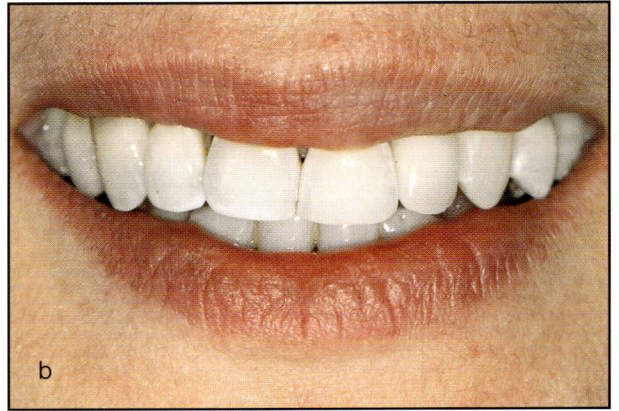

Fig 4-16 *(a and b)* Precision in implant placement permits the natural appearance of these teeth.

Implant placement to obtain this crown-abutment junction location will be discussed in detail in Chapter 6.

When replacing teeth in the anterior and premolar regions, except in the anterior mandibular region, the ideal distance in the mesiodistal direction between supporting implants usually is 7 to 12 mm (see Table 4-1). The shortest distance (7 mm) is used when each individual implant serves as an anchor for one crown; the longer distance is used when a pontic is placed between two implants; and a 9-mm distance is used in the molar regions (Figs 4-17 to 4-19). This concept can be applied in both totally and partially edentulous situations.

Ridge augmentation procedures allow more precise implant placement through more sophisticated soft tissue management in second-stage surgery. These procedures result in better prosthetic reconstruction in terms of emergence profile, function, biomechanics, phonetics, and esthetics.

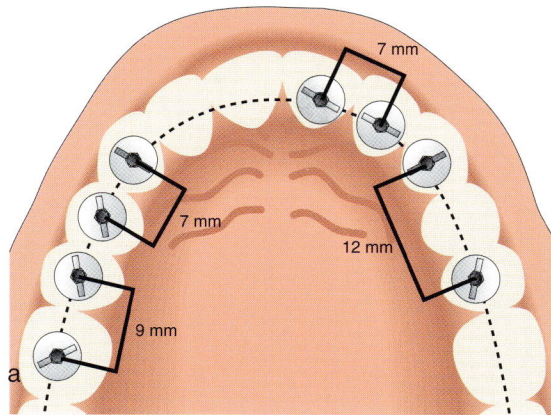

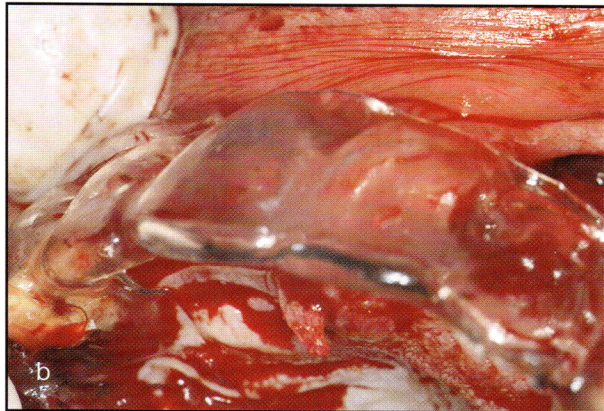

Fig 4-17 *(a)* Schematic drawing illustrating the proper distance between implants in different regions of the maxillary arch. *(b)* Surgical guide in place used for the treatment of an edentulous maxilla.

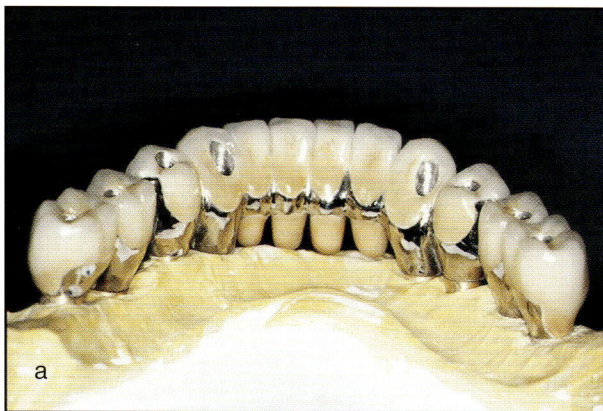

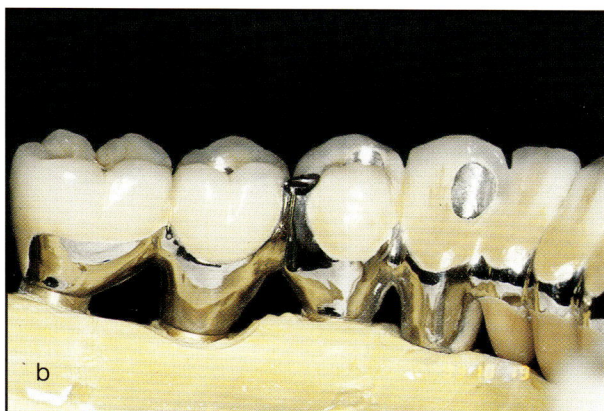

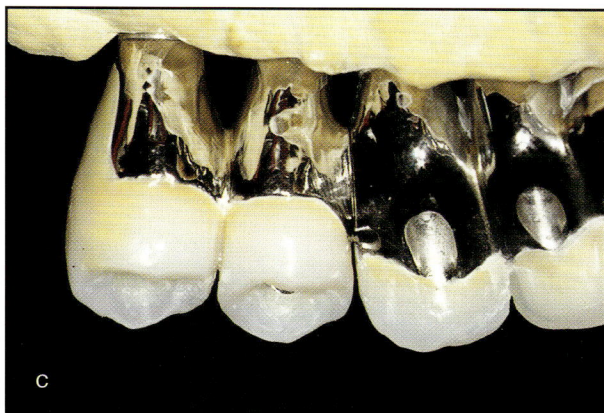

Fig 4-18 *(a to c)* Prosthetic reconstruction using the presented concept. Note the adequate space between implants as well as their correct angulation allowing physiologic embrasures and esthetic reconstruction.

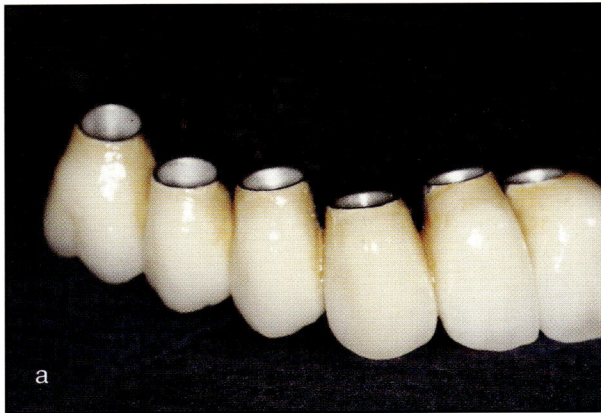

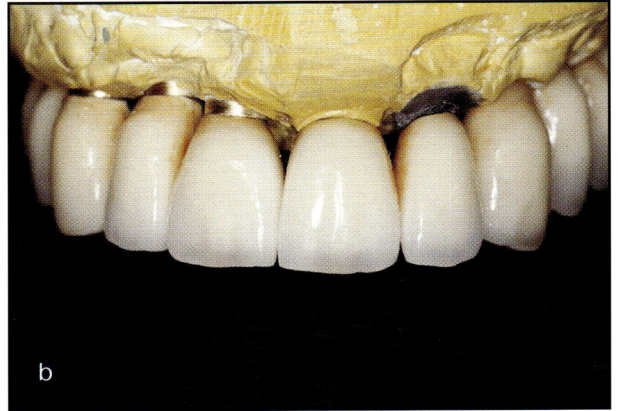

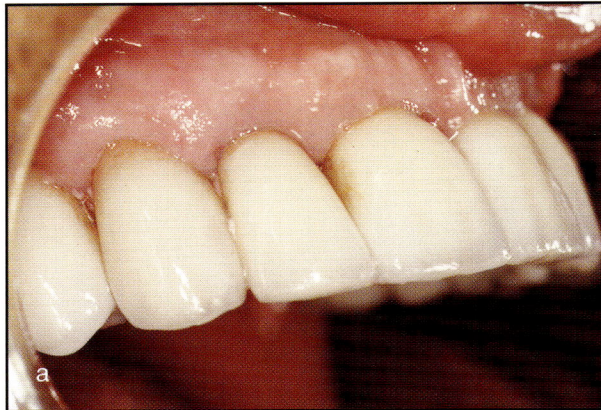

Fig 4-19 *(a to c)* Adequate angulation and placement (7 mm between fixture centers and 9 mm for molar region) permit the construction of a fixed partial denture with an optimal esthetic and functional result.

Spacing and angulation between implants

Even if the different implants and abutments match the anatomy of the various teeth, implant placement in bone is still based on individual anatomical dimensions that are due to the degree of bone resorption. This placement depends on two key factors: space and angulation between implants.

In an intact dentulous arch, the distance, from center to center, of incisors, canine, and premolars varies between 7 and 8.5 mm. The corresponding distance between premolar and molar and between molar and molar varies from 9 to 12 mm (see Fig 4-17).

A maxillary surgical guide stent is usually made according to the ideal positions of the teeth without consideration of the amount of horizontal bone resorption (Fig 4-20). In cases of pronounced resorption the circumference of the jaw is decreased, resulting in less favorable conditions for implant placement. Most often the proper clinical solution, at least from an esthetic point of view, is to decrease the number of abutments for the implant-supported fixed partial denture (Figs 4-21 and 4-22).

Fig 4-20 Schematic drawing illustrating a surgical guide stent with different levels of bridge resorption.

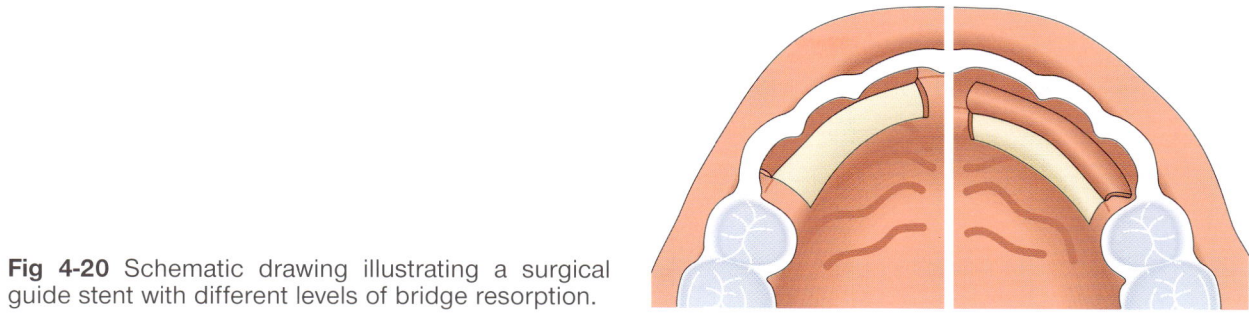

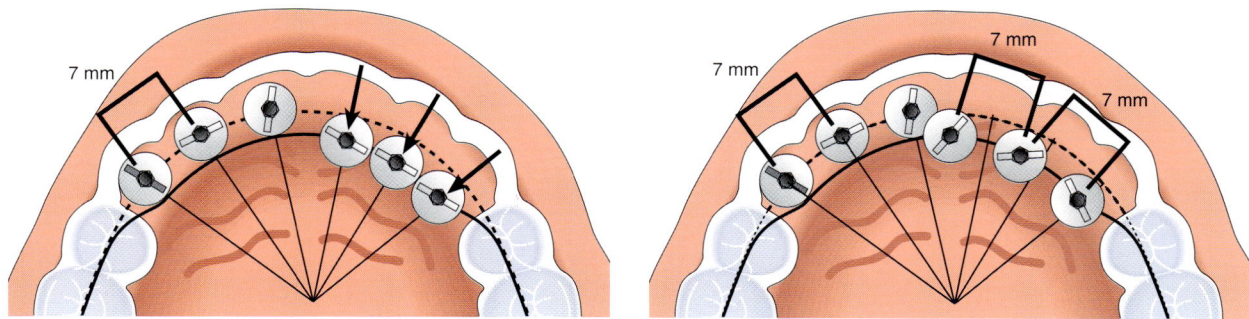

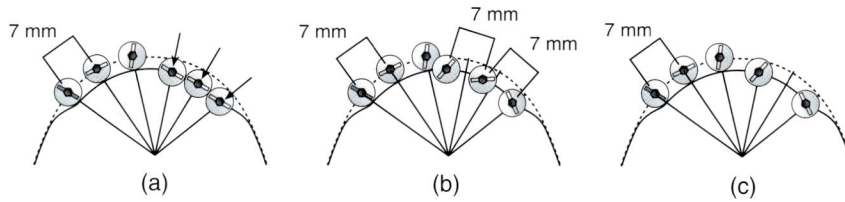

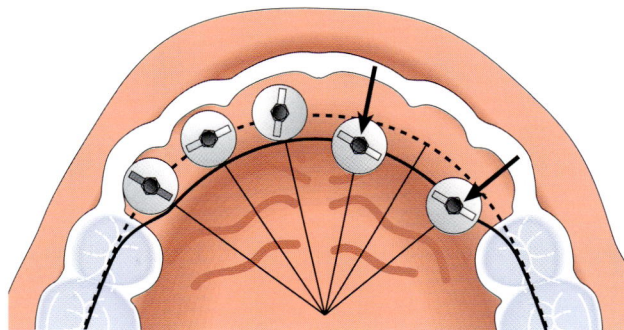

(a) (b) (c)

Fig 4-21 *(a to c)* Schematic drawings illustrating the situation following maxillary horizontal bone resorption and the subsequent problems faced for implant placement.

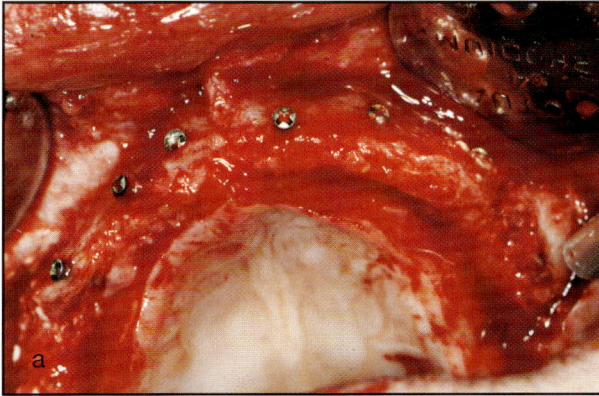

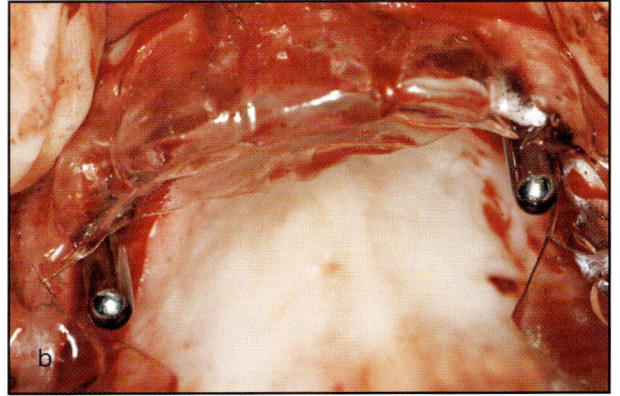

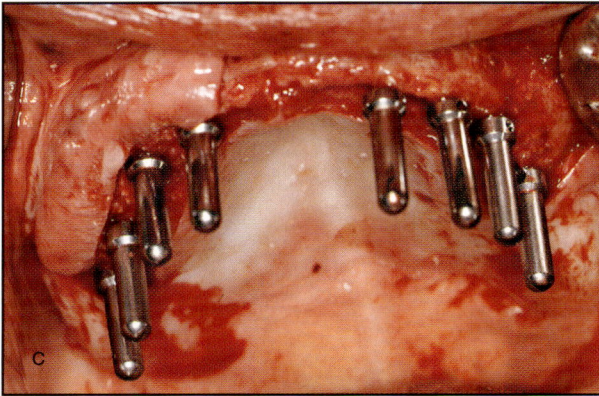

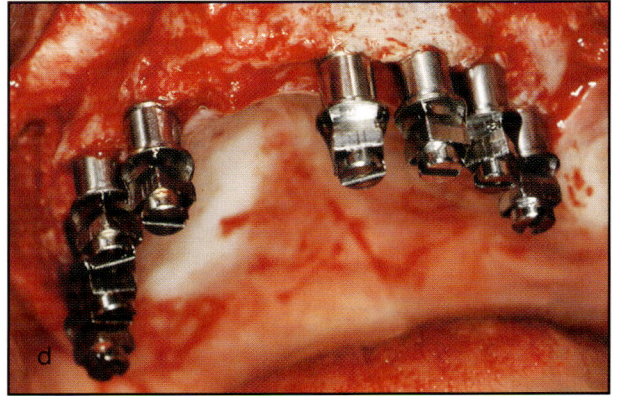

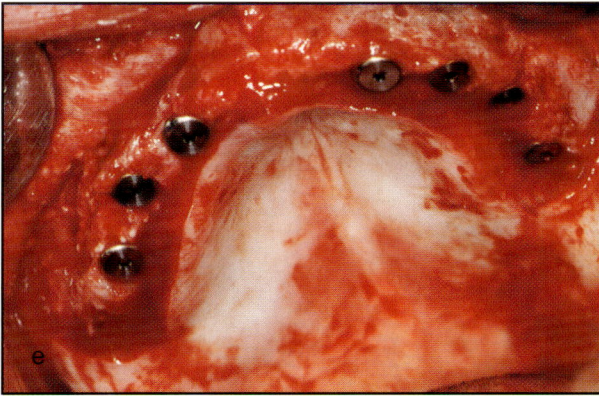

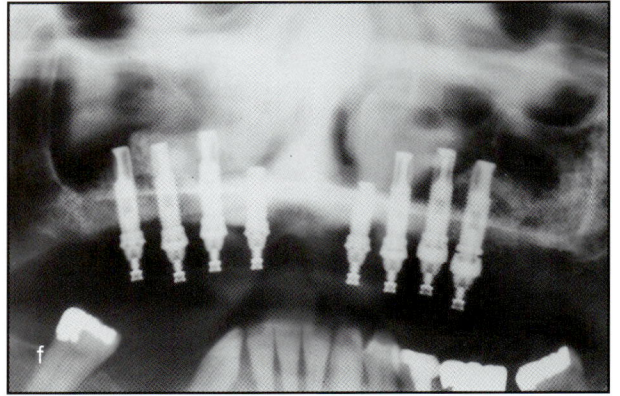

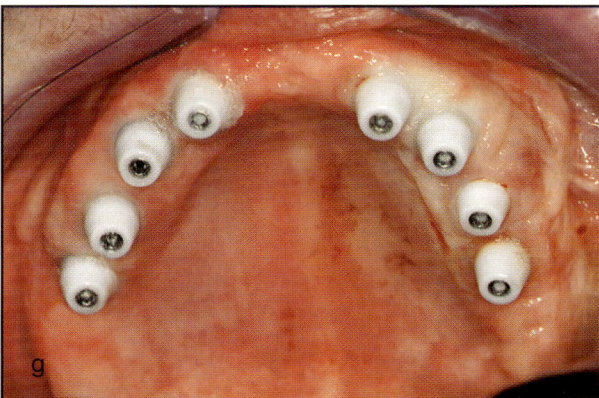

Fig 4-22 *(a to g)* A severely atrophic maxilla treated by bone grafting (onlay grafts plus sinus elevation). Implant placement will start at the canine area, then proceed to the lateral incisors, and continue with the premolars. The central region will be avoided, thus allowing more flexibility for the prosthetic restoration in terms of pontics, lip support, esthetics, and so on. (Bone grafting, P.K. Moy; implant placement, P. Palacci; second-stage surgery and prosthetic reconstruction, J-L. Vionnet).

Occlusion: Cusp-to-fossa relationship

Teeth normally occlude in a cusp-to-fossa relationship, resulting in more or less axial loading of the teeth. However, after implant treatment the jaw most frequently demonstrates both horizontal and vertical bone resorption, which results in a changed jaw relationship (Figs 4-23 and 4-24). As mentioned in previous chapters, axial loading of the implants is desired. At the time of implant placement, then, the opposing dentition should always be considered to obtain axial loading of the implants as much as possible. In the premolar and molar regions, attaining optimal axial loading of the implants will often result more or less in a crossbite (Fig 4-25).

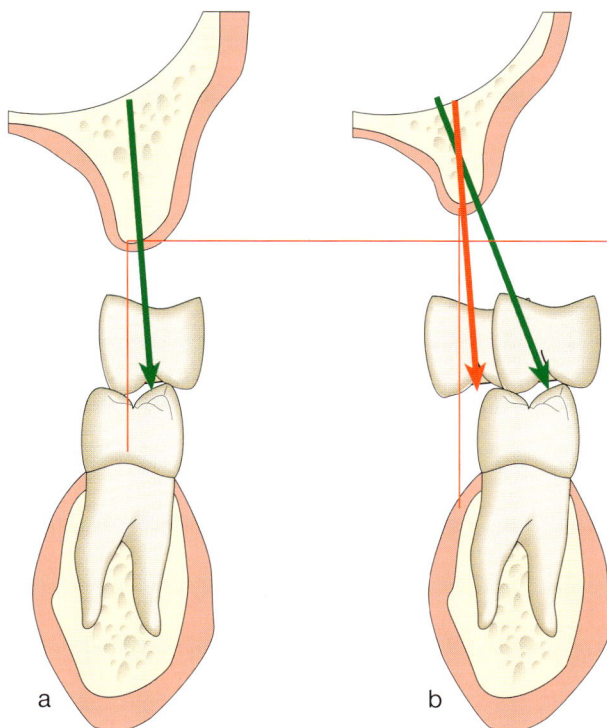

Anterior placement

The coordination of surgical and prosthetic treatment-planning procedures is certainly one of the most important factors in obtaining optimal esthetic and biomechanical results. In the anterior region, implants must be placed so that the screw-access holes are located lingual or palatal to the incisal edge of the crown restoration (Fig 4-26). Pronounced variances in implant angulation can jeopardize a good esthetic outcome (Fig 4-27). From an esthetic point of view, two or more implants should often be placed more or less parallel to each other. Thus, the position and angulation of the first implant placed will influence the placement of the following implants. These guidelines for implant placement also apply in the premolar and molar regions.

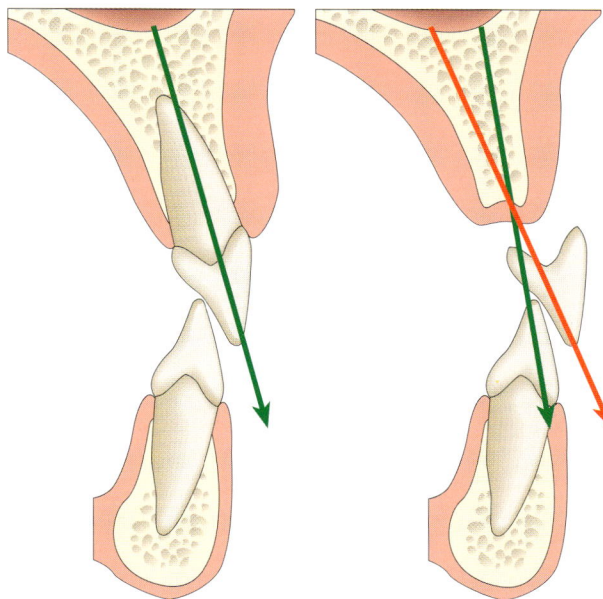

Fig 4-23 Schematic drawings illustrating proper jaw relationship and the compromised one following horizontal as well as vertical bone resorption in the anterior *(a)* and premolar/molar region *(b)*.

Fig 4-24 Schematic drawing illustrating the importance of the implant angulation for the location of the screw access hole in the anterior maxilla.

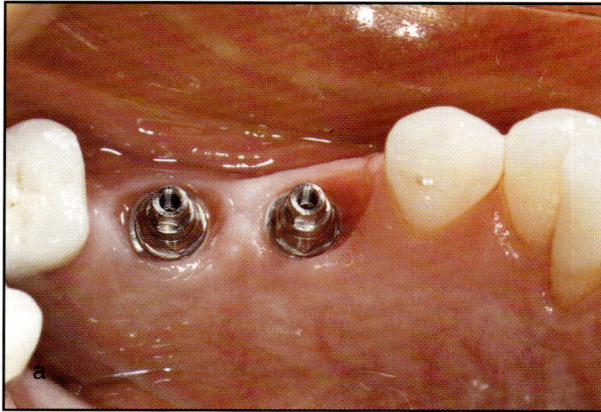

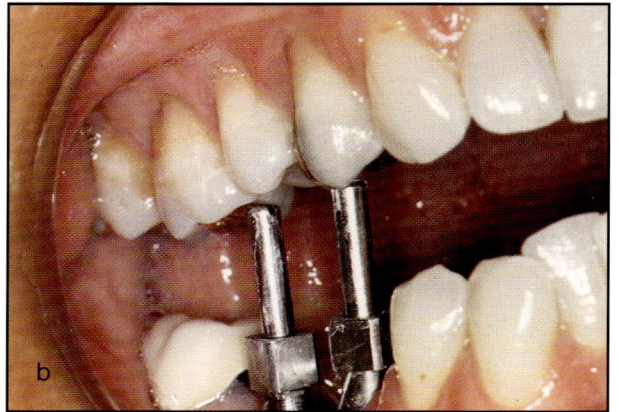

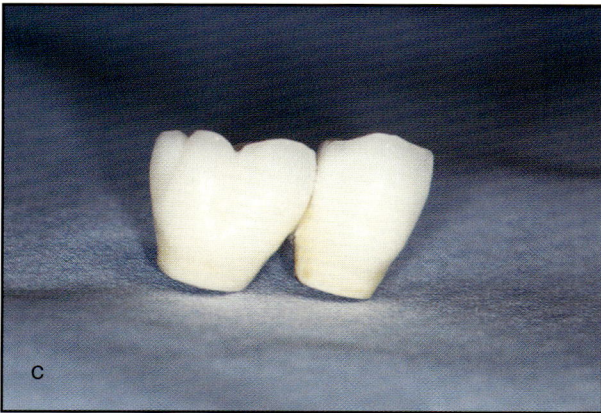

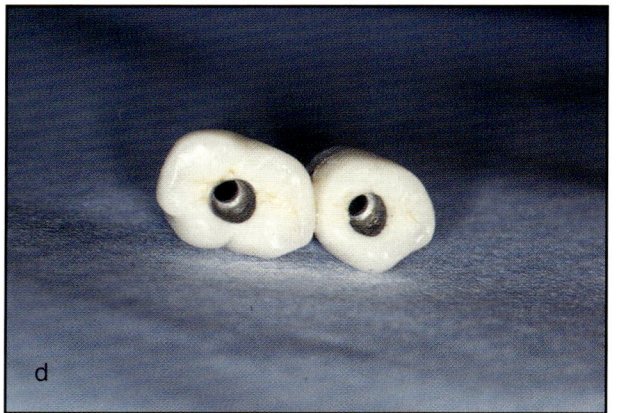

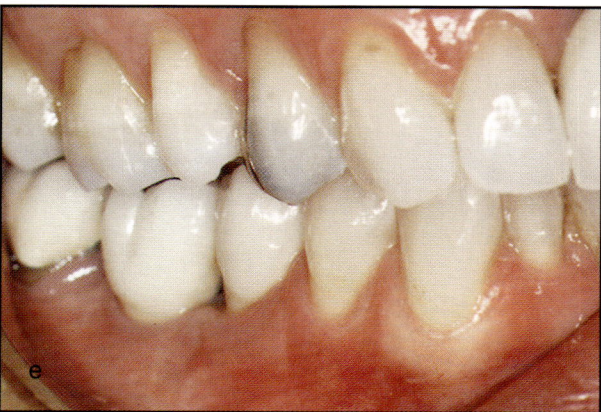

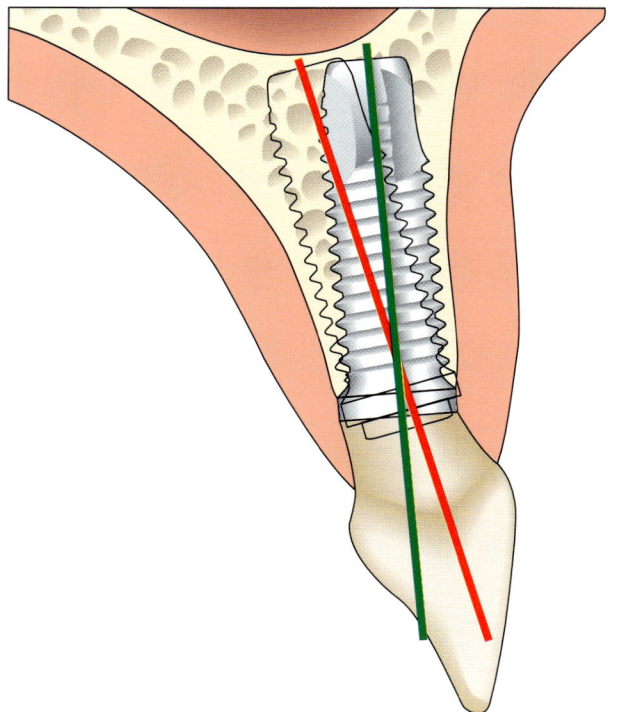

Fig 4-25 *(a to e)* Replacement of a mandibular pre-molar and molar. The space between these two implants from center to center is 9 mm. The clinical slide with the two impression copings in place illustrates the cusp-to-fossa relationship and the anatomy of the crowns due to proper implant position.

Fig 4-26 When dealing with the anterior maxilla, a slightly too labial angulation of the implant can jeopardize the whole treatment concept.

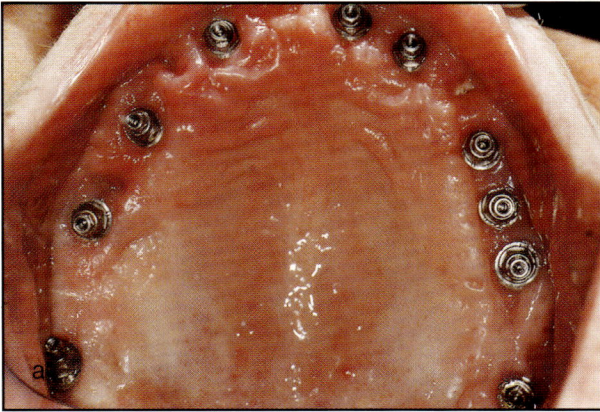

Fig 4-27 *(a to e)* The concept for optimal implant placement presented in this chapter is illustrated by these clinical cases. In both cases *(a)* and *(b to e)* implant placement has been optimized. Space between implants and angulation have been properly handled so that the emergence profile and teeth anatomy will be optimized.

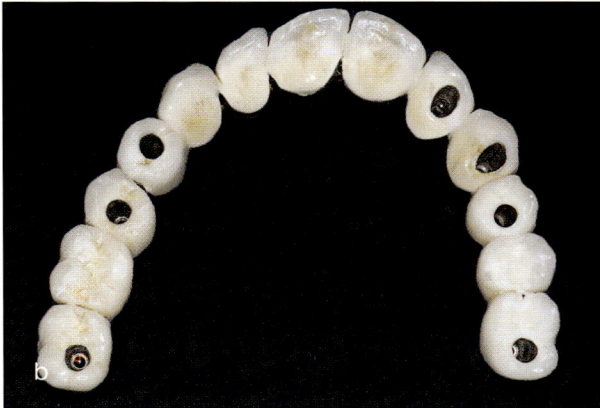

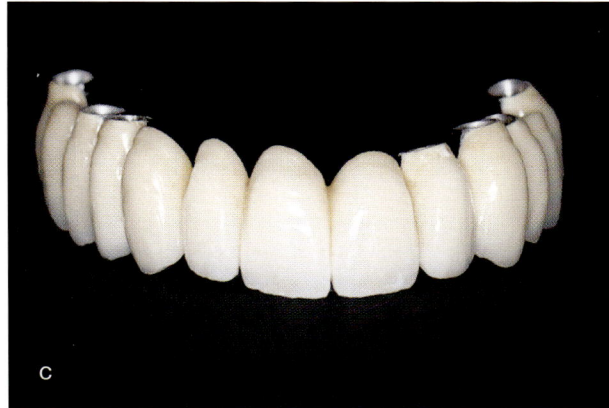

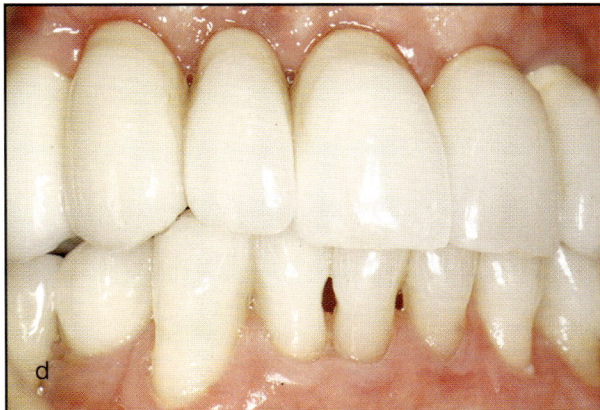

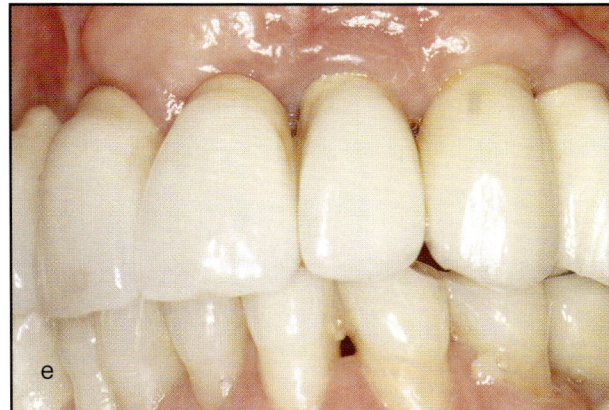

Conclusions

New components have been developed to facilitate optimal implant placement based on biological, biomechanical, and esthetic considerations while accommodating individual anatomical limitations. Descriptions of these components, as well their uses, are presented in Chapter 9.

Reference

Wheeler RC, Ash M (eds). Wheeler's Atlas of Tooth Form, ed 4. Philadelphia: Saunders, 1984.

Chapter 5

Anterior Maxilla Classification

Patrick Palacci, DDS, and Ingvar Ericsson, LDS, Odont Dr

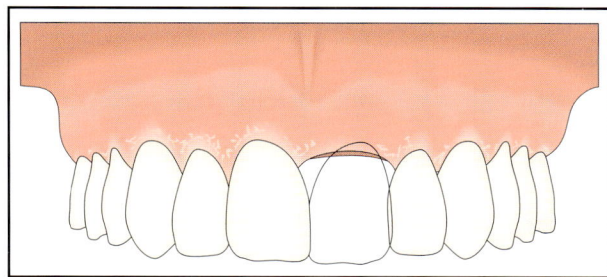

In 1985, Lekholm and Zarb presented a classification of the jaw bone, based on shape and quality, to be used to analyze implant anchorage. They described five groups of mandibular and maxillary cross-sectional shapes (Fig 5-1):

A. Most of the alveolar ridge is present.
B. Moderate residual ridge resorption has occurred.
C. Advanced residual ridge resorption has occurred (only basal bone remains).
D. Some resorption of the basal bone has started.
E. Extreme resorption of the basal bone has occurred.

The authors also described four groups of bone quality:

1 Almost the entire jaw bone is composed of homogenous compact bone.
2. A thick layer of cortical bone surrounds dense trabecular bone.
3. A thin layer of cortical bone surrounds a core of dense trabecular bone.
4. A thin layer of cortical bone surrounds a core of low-density trabecular bone.

In addition to this classification, the thickness of the ridge mucosa also has to be considered.

The classification of Lekholm and Zarb helps to clarify the relationship between the surgical technique to be used and jaw bone shape and quality. However, in the anterior maxilla, the position of the lip line (high or low), as well as the lip mobility, has to be considered. The architecture of the lip line, in combination with the mobility of the lip, determines the need for additional surgical procedures for an optimal esthetic outcome.

According to Seibert (1983), ridge defects in edentulous regions can be divided into three classes (Fig 5-2):

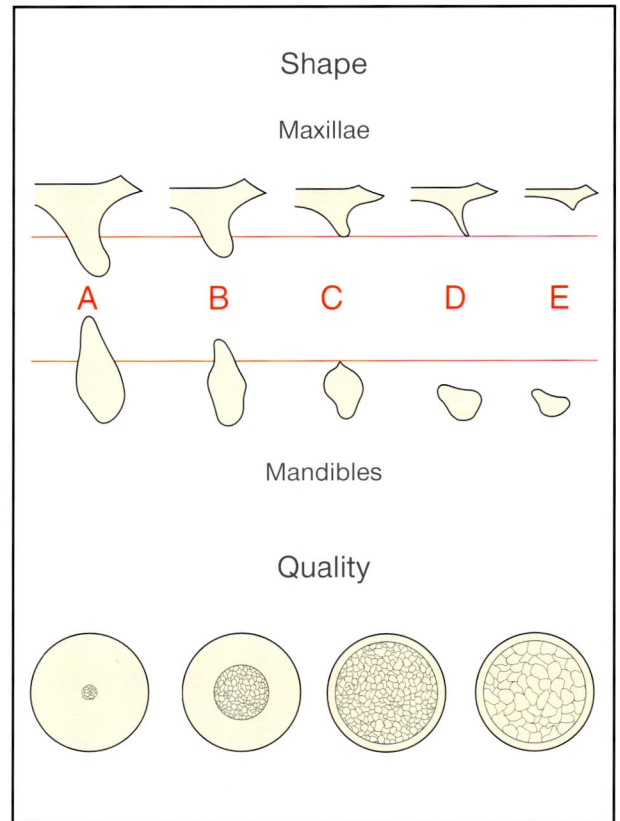

Fig 5-1 Bone shape and bone quality classification according to Lekholm and Zarb (1985).

1. Class I: loss of tissue in the buccolingual direction with normal height in the apical-coronal direction
2. Class II: loss of tissue in the apical-coronal direction, with normal width in the buccolingual direction
3. Class III: a combination of Class I and Class II (loss of both height and width)

The interdental papilla is the part of the periodontal soft tissue between two teeth and coronal to the cementoenamel junction (CEJ) (Fig 5-3). Its shape is defined by *(1)* the contact relationship between the teeth, *(2)* the width of the proximal tooth surfaces, and *(3)* the course of the CEJs. Thus, in the anterior

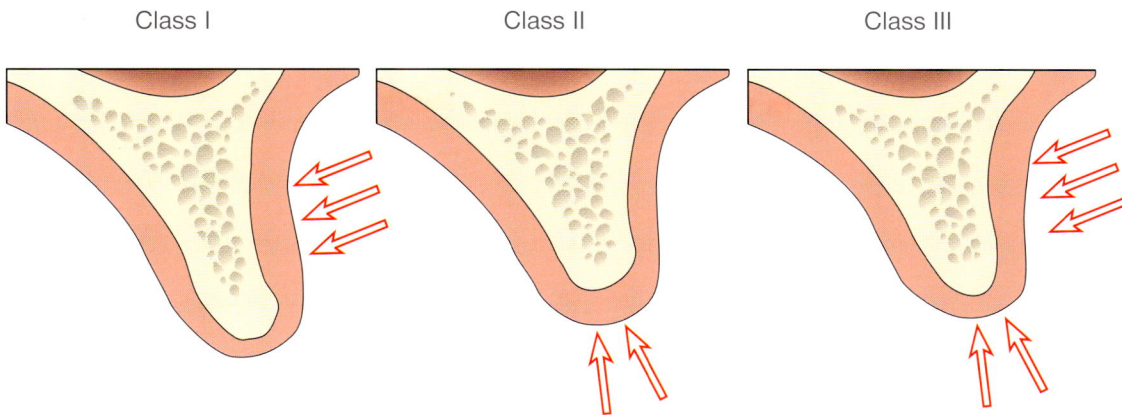

Fig 5-2 Ridge defect classification according to Seibert (1983).

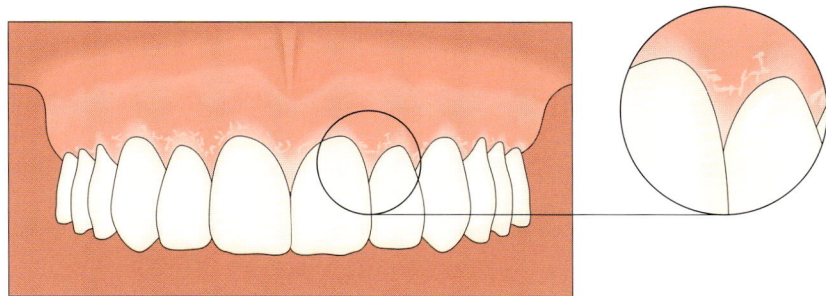

Fig 5-3 The interdental papilla.

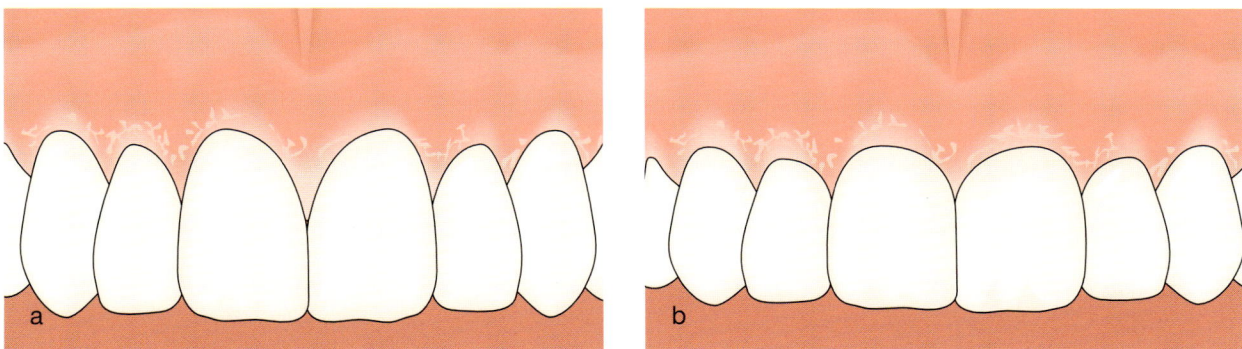

Fig 5-4 *(a)* "Scalloped-thin" gingival architecture. *(b)* "Flat-thick" gingival architecture.

regions of the dentition, the interdental papilla assumes a pyramidal or conical shape.

Two major types of gingival architecture have been described in the literature (for example, Olsson and Lindhe 1991; Olsson et al 1993; and Seibert and Lindhe 1997), namely the "scalloped-thin" and the "flat-thick" gingival architecture (Fig 5-4). The gingival architecture is mainly determined by the anatomy of the teeth and the position and size of the contact surfaces of the teeth.

Figs 5-5 to 5-8 Classifications of vertical dimension of soft and hard tissue.

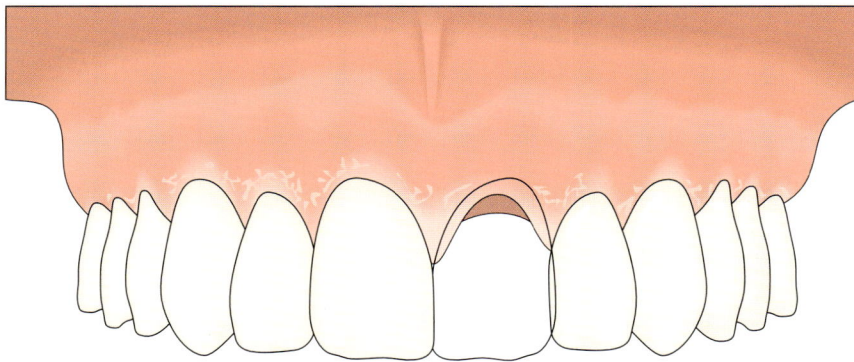

Fig 5-5 Class I.

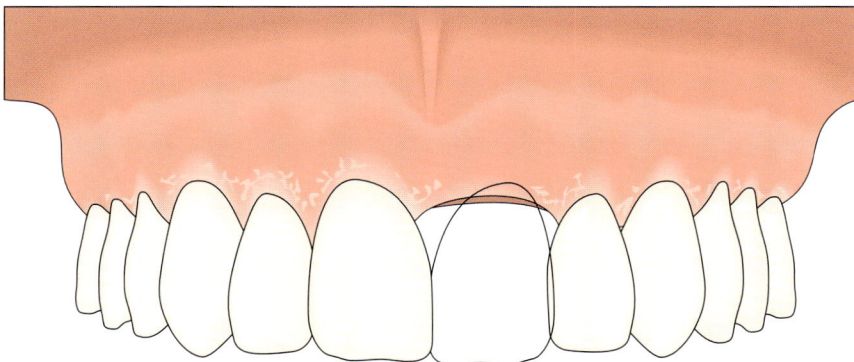

Fig 5-6 Class II.

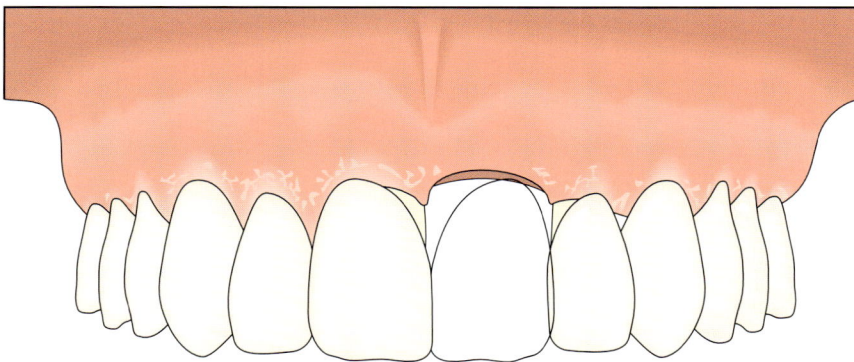

Fig 5-7 Class III.

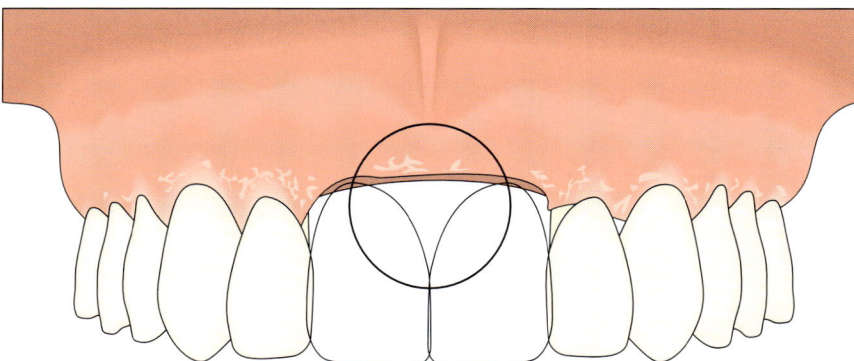

Fig 5-8 Class IV.

Figs 5-9 to 5-12 Classifications of horizontal dimension of soft and hard tissue.

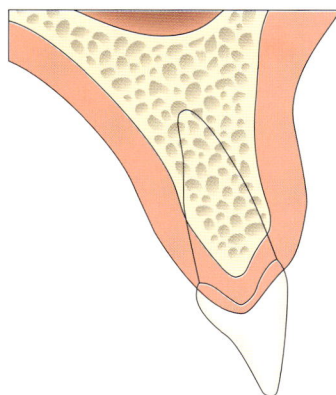

Fig 5-9
Class A.

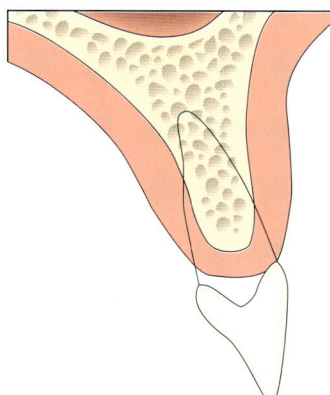

Fig 5-10
Class B.

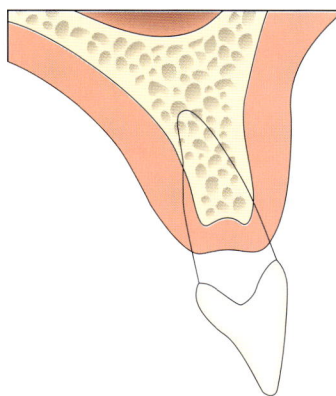

Fig 5-11
Class C.

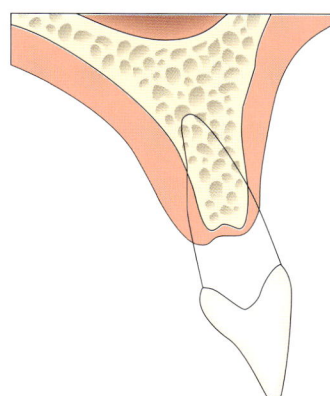

Fig 5-12
Class D.

Anterior Maxilla Classification for Optimal Esthetic Outcome

The use of a classification of the overall shape of the anterior maxilla (including the soft tissues) will help the practitioner evaluate the anatomical conditions in implant treatment. This classification is based on the amount of vertical and horizontal loss of soft tissue, hard tissue, or both. It is divided into four classes according to the vertical dimension and into four classes according to the horizontal dimension.

Based on vertical loss, Class I has intact or slightly reduced papillae (Fig 5-5). Class II has limited loss of the papillae (Fig 5-6). Class III has severe loss of the papillae (Fig 5-7), and

Class IV represents absence of the papillae (Fig 5-8).

Based on horizontal loss, Class A shows intact or slightly reduced buccal tissue (Fig 5-9). Class B has limited loss of buccal tissue (Fig 5-10). Class C has severe loss of buccal tissue (Fig 5-11). Finally, Class D has extreme loss of buccal tissue, often in combination with a limited amount of attached mucosa (Fig 5-12). Of course, many combinations of the different classes occur, and each patient must be viewed as unique.

A good final outcome depends on the clinician's understanding of the complexity of the overall treatment. The anterior maxilla classification should be used to document the anatomical condition before treatment and will guide the clinician in choosing proper

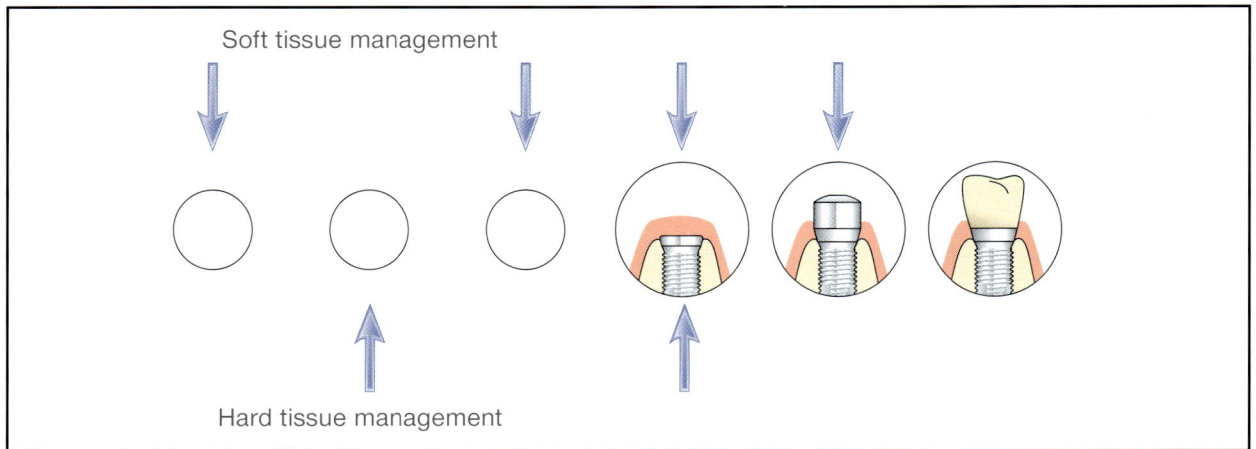

Fig 5-13 Different steps in the sequence of treatment.

treatment options to reach the expected final result. Some treatments (for example, Class IA) normally require only proper implant placement and minimal soft tissue handling at stage 2 surgery. Acceptable results in Class IVD, in contrast, may require additional hard and soft tissue surgical procedures prior to, at the time of, or after implant placement.

No scientific evidence for the absolute need for attached mucosa, from a functional or survival point of view, has been presented (Wennström et al 1994). However, from an esthetic and oral hygiene point of view, an adequate zone of attached peri-implant mucosa may be preferable.

Thus, the final esthetic and functional outcome is related to three main factors: the jaw bone, the soft tissue, and the design of the prosthetic reconstruction. The replacement of missing teeth is only one part of the treatment, especially in the anterior maxilla. Another part is the replacement of the lost portion of the alveolar process, the covering soft tissue, or both. The re-creation of a normal alveolar contour is an important key to esthetic success.

The understanding of the anterior maxilla classification will guide the therapist to find

adequate solutions to obtain consistent and predictable treatment results from a functional and esthetic point of view.

Treatment Philosophy

Success in implant dentistry involves four areas:

1. Pre-implant augmentative surgery
2. Precision in implant placement
3. Peri-implant soft tissue management
4. Quality of the prosthetic restoration

Augmentation of soft tissue is sometimes necessary to predict the final esthetic outcome of the treatment, for example, to obtain enough soft tissue to re-create the papillae. Depending on the loss of the alveolar ridge, the quality and quantity of available soft tissue and the needs for future ridge augmentation, soft tissue augmentation procedures can be performed prior to, after, or together with hard tissue augmentation, as well as at stage 1 and/or stage 2 surgery (Fig 5-13).

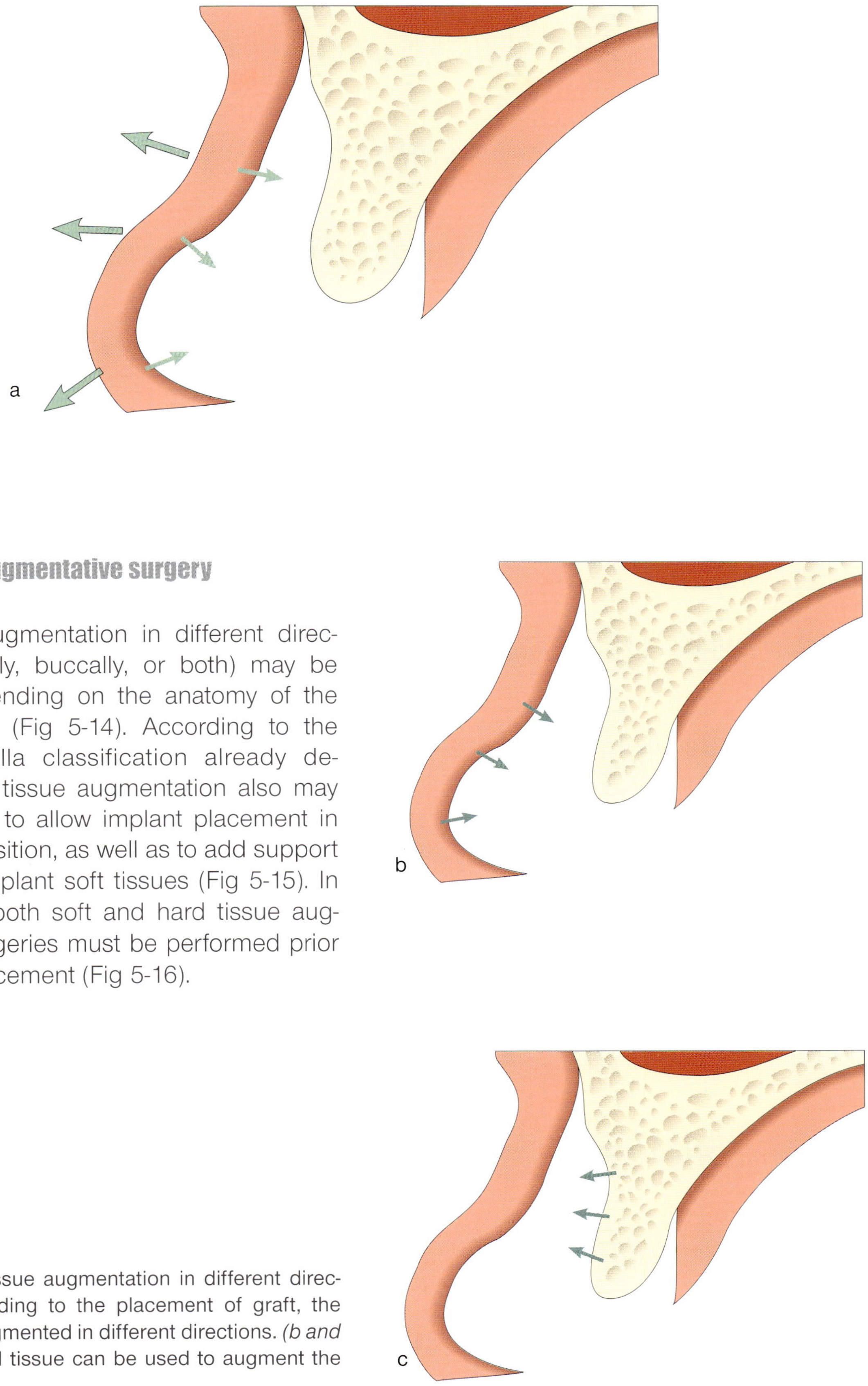

Pre-implant augmentative surgery

Soft tissue augmentation in different directions (coronally, buccally, or both) may be needed, depending on the anatomy of the alveolar ridge (Fig 5-14). According to the anterior maxilla classification already described, hard tissue augmentation also may be necessary to allow implant placement in an optimal position, as well as to add support for the peri-implant soft tissues (Fig 5-15). In some cases both soft and hard tissue augmentative surgeries must be performed prior to implant placement (Fig 5-16).

Fig 5-14 Soft tissue augmentation in different directions. *(a)* According to the placement of graft, the ridge can be augmented in different directions. *(b and c)* Soft and hard tissue can be used to augment the alveolar ridge.

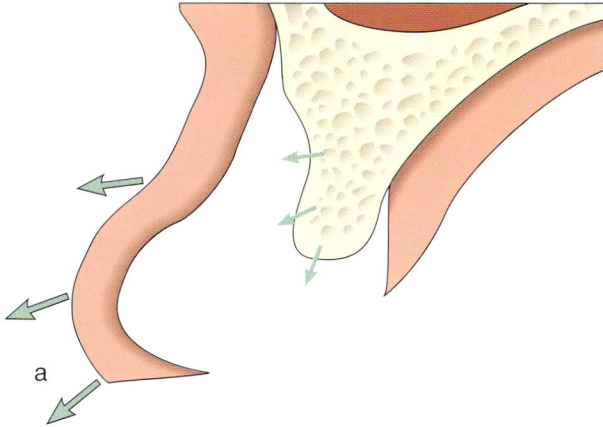

Precision in implant placement

A straightforward implant placement can be performed without any additional surgeries. However, at the time of implant placement, minor hard tissue augmentation may be needed to add support to the peri-implant mucosa. In other situations, soft tissue must be added to enhance the final result and thus facilitate soft tissue handling at stage 2 surgery (see Fig 5-16).

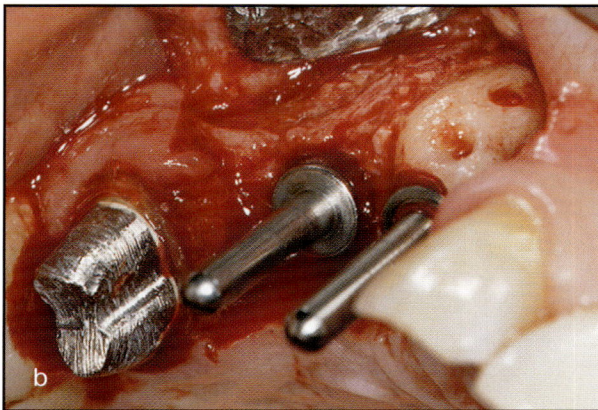

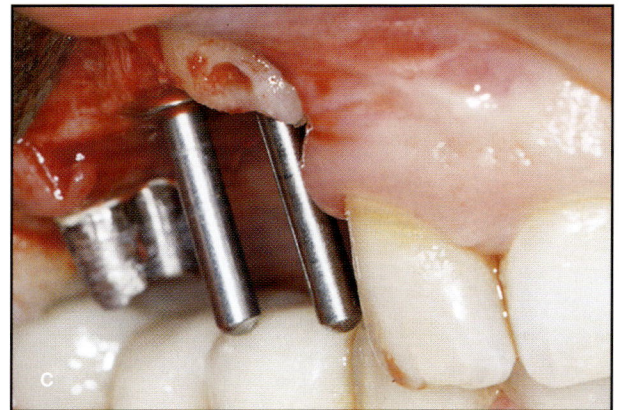

Fig 5-15 *(a)* Hard tissue augmentation in different directions. *(b and c)* In a case of bone loss in the maxillary canine region, a hard tissue graft will allow optimal implant placement, as well as adequate support for the covering soft tissues.

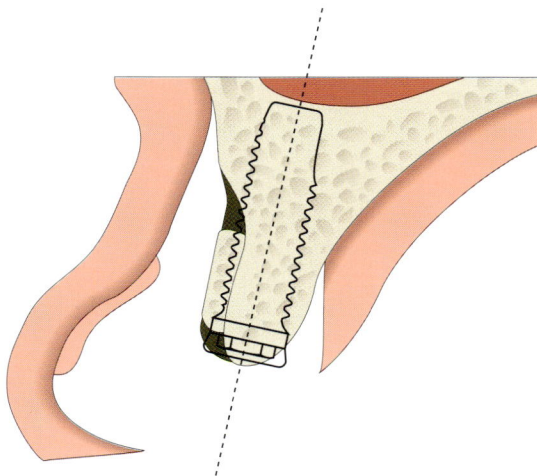

Fig 5-16 Pre-implant hard and soft tissue augmentation allowing ridge contour as well as optimal implant placement.

Peri-implant soft tissue management

If previous surgeries have created a favorable clinical situation, different surgical alternatives are possible. Sometimes a straightforward technique can be applied. In other situations the papilla regeneration technique, alone or in combination with additional soft tissue augmentation, must be performed.

Quality of the prosthetic restoration

The final esthetic result is related to the previously considered procedures. Optimal precision in implant placement will simplify the pros-thetic reconstruction and allow a favorable emergence profile, healthy peri-implant mucosa, facilitation of oral hygiene procedures, good phonetic conditions, and accordance with biomechanical principles (Fig 5-17).

The overall need for precision increases in the anterior maxillary arch. For example, when treating the edentulous mandible, a few millimeters of displacement or a few degrees of disangulation of one or several implants, probably will not affect the final result. In the anterior maxilla, in contrast, 1 mm of displacement and/or 10 degrees of disangulation of an implant may be more than enough to jeopardize the entire treatment.

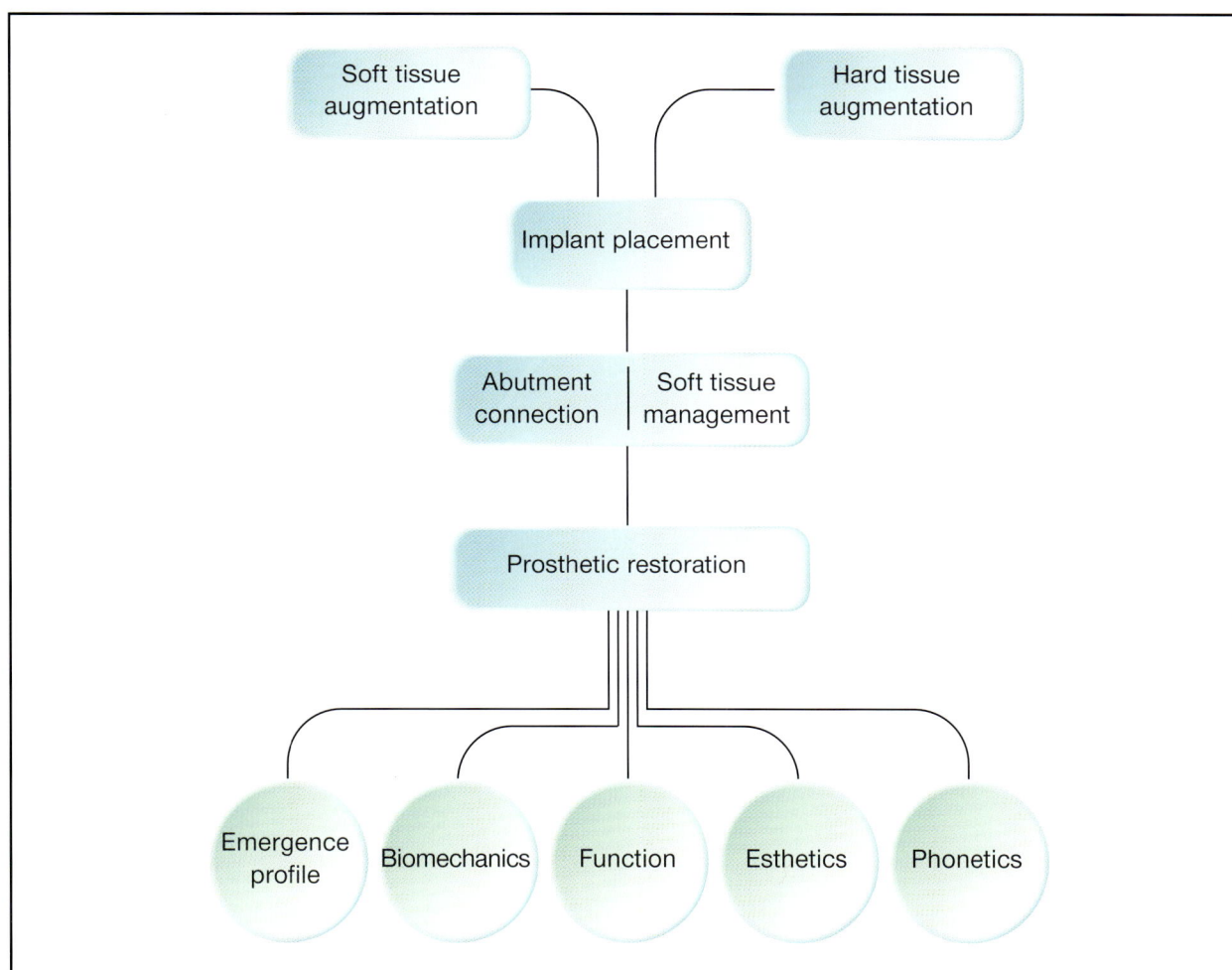

Fig 5-17 Steps in treatment and their implications.

Possible Treatment Sequences

The limitations of each procedure must be determined and explained to the patient. The complexity and number of surgeries are closely related to the amount of alveolar bone available. Depending on the lip line, the lip mobility, and the needs and expectations of the patient, more advanced surgery may be needed to attain an acceptable end result. The implant treatment will be simple in cases of minor or no tissue loss.

The following are possible treatment sequences based on the anterior maxilla classification:

- Class IA: no additional surgery
- Class IIB: at stage 1, soft tissue augmentation; at stage 2, papilla regeneration technique
- Class IIIC: possible pre-implant augmentative surgery: at stage 1, hard tissue augmentation, soft tissue augmentation, or both; at stage 2, papilla regeneration technique and, if needed, soft tissue augmentation
- Class IVD: pre-implant augmentative surgery, including hard tissue augmentation and, if needed, soft tissue augmentation: at stage 1, hard tissue augmentation, soft tissue augmentation, or both; at stage 2, papilla regeneration technique, soft tissue augmentation, or both

Each additional surgery adds an increased risk of failure. In other words, the simplest treatment approach applicable for a case is preferred.

The surgeon must respect the biological capacity of the hard and soft tissue involved; for example, it is not possible to go directly from Class IVD to IA. Each surgical procedure will allow, at most, a jump of one step (for example, IIIC to IIB). The goal of these augmentative procedures is to be as close as pos-

sible to Class IA at stage 2 surgery. Furthermore, it must be stressed that these surgical procedures apply in the edentulous patient only to a limited extent.

The treatment philosophy described in this chapter is illustrated by a case presentation (Fig 5-18).

Conclusion

A careful evaluation of the clinical situation has to be done before any implant treatment. The presented classification will help the practioner to evaluate this situation more precisely in the anterior maxilla and be a useful guide for the overall treatment in respect to the biological parameter.

References

Lekholm U, Zarb GA. Patient selection and preparation. In: Brånemark P-I, Zarb G, Albrektsson T (eds). Tissue Integrated Prosthesis: Osseointegration in Clinical Dentistry. Chicago: Quintessence, 1985: 199–210.

Olsson M, Lindhe J. Periodontal characteristics in individuals with varying form of the upper central incisors. J Clin Periodontol 1991;18:78–82.

Olsson M, Lindhe J, Marinello CP. On the relationship between crown form and clinical features in the gingiva in adolescents. J Clin Periodontol 1993;20: 570–577.

Seibert J. Reconstruction of deformed, partially edentulous ridges, using full thickness onlay grafts, II. Prosthetic/periodontal interrelationships. Compend Contin Educ Dent 1983;4:549–562.

Seibert J, Lindhe J. Esthetic in periodontal therapy. In: Lindhe J, Karring T, Lang NP (eds). Clinical Periodontology and Implant Dentistry, ed 3. Copenhagen: Munksgaard, 1997:647–681.

Wennström JL, Bengazi F, Lekholm U. The influence of the masticatory mucosa on the peri-implant soft tissue condition. Clin Oral Implants Res 1994;5:1–8.

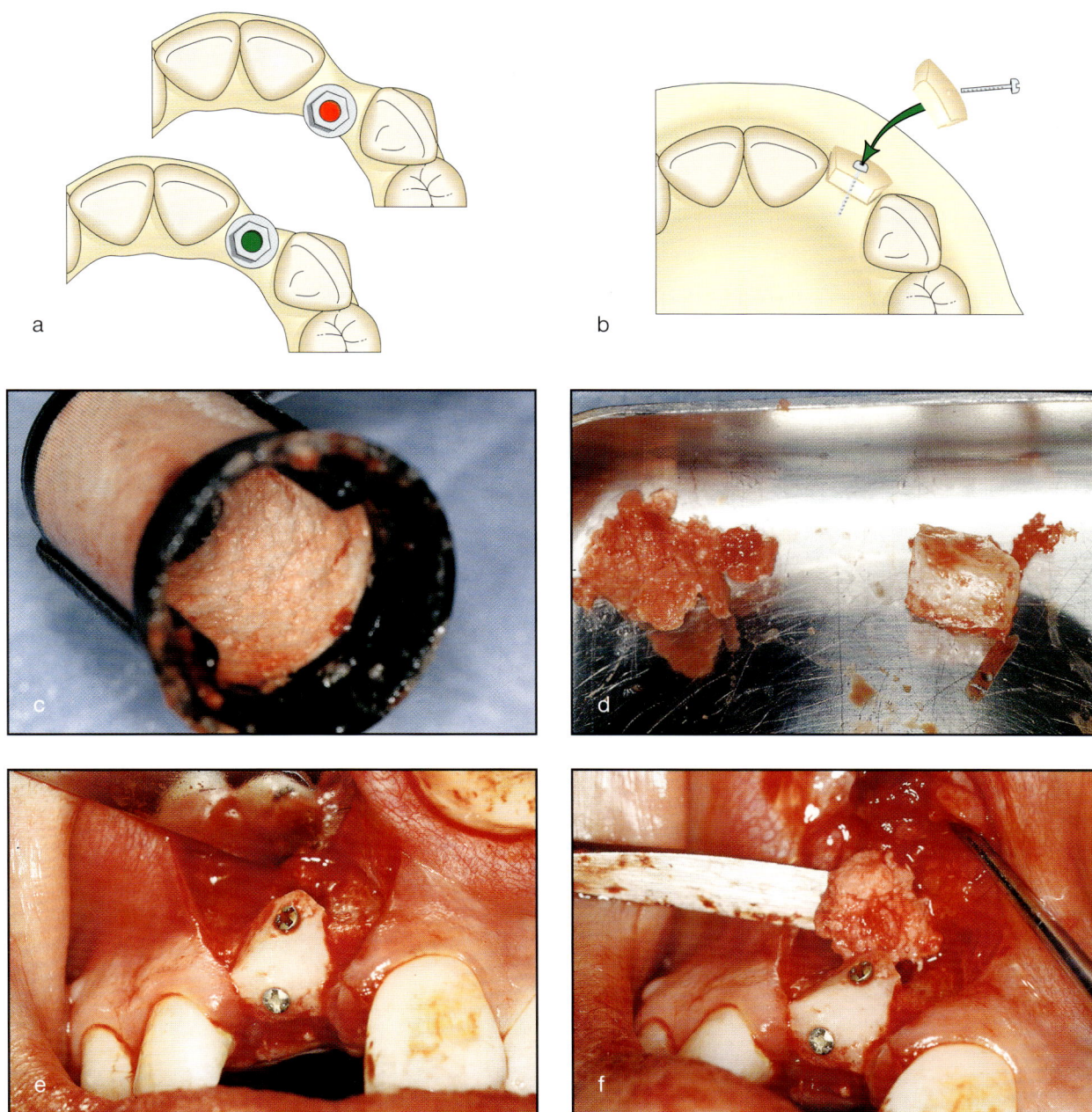

Fig 5-18 *(a)* Choices of implant placement when dealing with labial bone resorption. The green implant is optimally placed according to the adjacent teeth but the labial osseous wall is missing, jeopardizing the overall treatment. *(b)* To place this implant in an adequate position, a bone graft has to be placed labially to recreate an adequate ridge. *(c)* When drilling, a significant quantity of bone can be collected using a bone collector. *(d)* A block of cortical bone harvested from the chin area can be used to re-create an adequate ridge anatomy. Note the quantity of bone collected using the bone collector. *(e)* With a deficient alveolar ridge, the positioning of a block of reshaped cortical bone will be maintained with the use of fixation screws. *(f and g)* With the graft being stabilized, the collected bone, used as a space filler, is compacted in the graft area. *(h)* Occlusal view 4 months later. The ridge anatomy has been corrected. *(i to l)* With the flap elevated, a significant gain of hard tissue is visible. Optimal implant placement is now possible as presented in the schematic drawing. *(m and n)* Six months later, second-stage surgery using the papilla regeneration technique is performed.

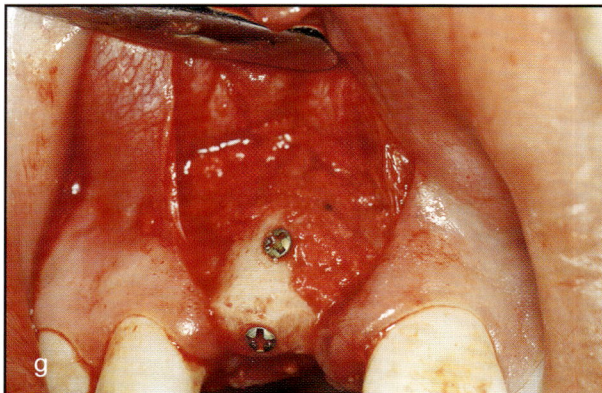

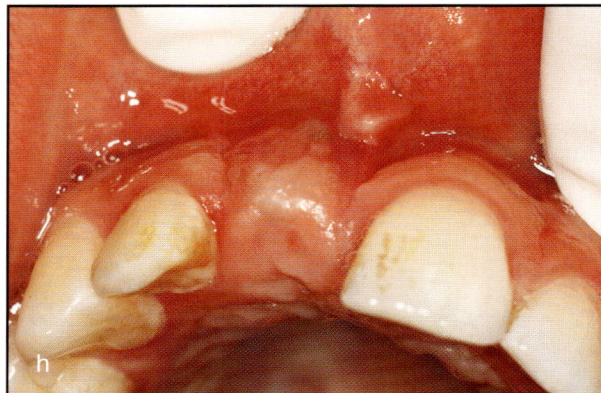

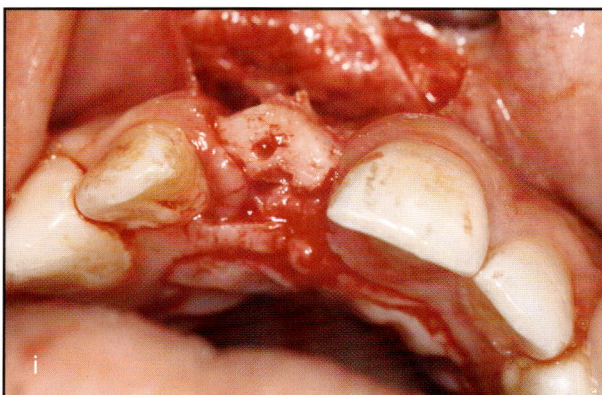

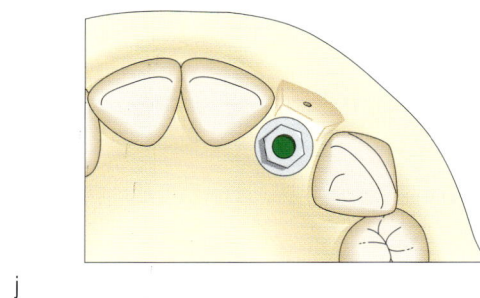

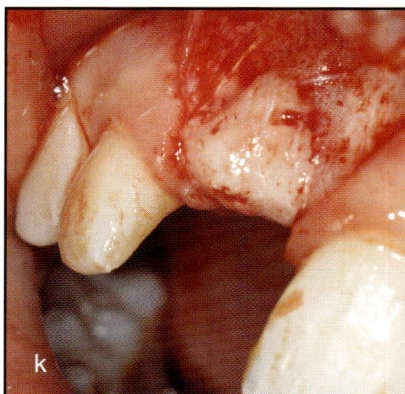

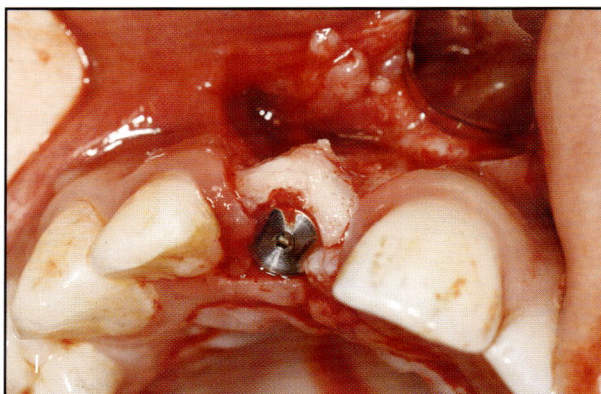

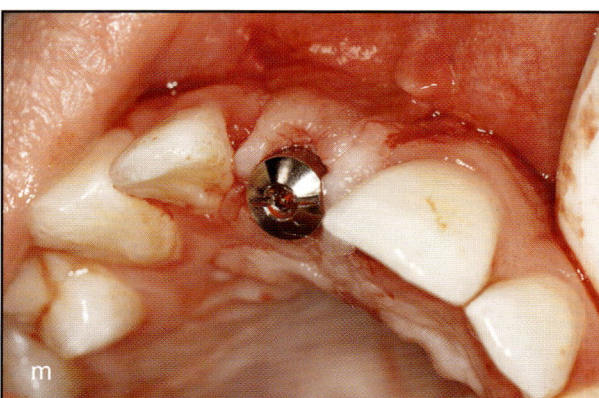

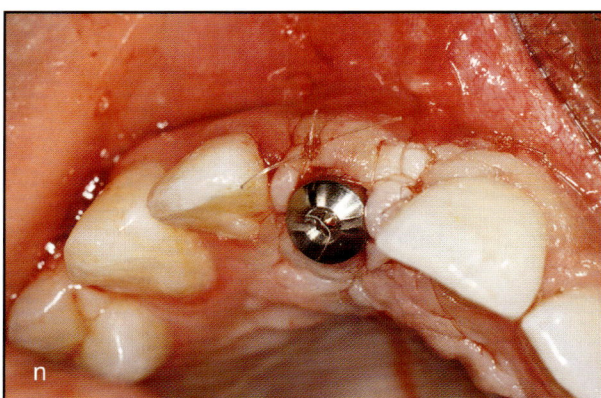

Chapter 6

Optimal Implant Positioning

Patrick Palacci, DDS

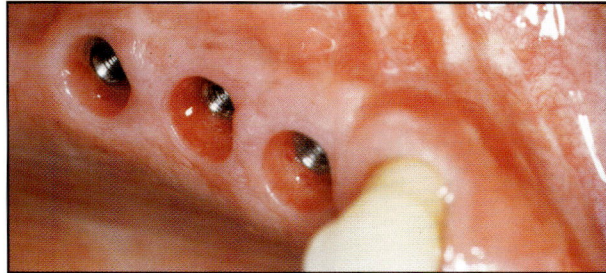

Proper implant treatment planning is important in obtaining an acceptable final result. A complete treatment plan includes both surgical and prosthetic aspects. From a surgical point of view, careful analysis of future implant positioning is essential. By tradition, surgeons have relied mainly on the use of a guide stent in combination with direction indicators. However, even when using these tools it is still difficult to visualize the final restorative result. Therefore, the author and Nobel Biocare designed presurgical and surgical components to enhance presurgical evaluation and subsequent implant placement. These tools simplify and facilitate implant placement according to biological, biomechanical, and esthetic considerations.

Previous chapters concluded the following:

1. A certain amount of space is needed between implants. A minimum of 7 mm from center to center results in a distance of 3 mm between the implants and 2 mm between the abutments.
2. The space varies according to the type of platforms used (narrow, regular, or wide platform) and the placement of the fixtures (pontic or not).
3. Ideally, each crown will be a continuation of a virtual cylinder emerging from the implant pillar.
4. Advanced bone resorption in the horizontal direction will influence the number of implants needed to support a fixed reconstruction. There is no relationship between the number of teeth to be replaced and the number of implants placed with the use of any surgical stent.
5. Platform selection is based on the position in the arch and the space between the adjacent teeth.

Presurgical planning is usually based on empirical evaluation of the patient. Casts of the maxilla and mandible are mounted in an articular, and waxups are made according to the ideal position of the teeth within the arch. In other words, the surgical guide stent mirrors an ideal situation without any consideration given to the anatomy of the future implant site. Thus, there is no correlation between the real placement of the implant and the surgical guide stent. Presurgical positioning guides are tools to increase the correlation between the presurgical evaluation and the surgery itself.

Presurgical Positioning Guides

When planning restorative treatment, clinicians frequently face problems related to the number and diameter of the implants to be placed. Presurgical positioning guides have been designed to help solve these problems. The guides can be used (1) intraorally before surgery to visual the future implant-supported restoration; (2) on the master cast to facilitate the fabrication of the stent to be used at the radiographic examinations, as well as the proper design of the surgical stent; and (3) during implant placement to facilitate optimal implant positioning. Figure 6-1 illustrates various presurgical positioning guides. Figures 6-1a to 6-1d show guides used in planning multiple-implant restorations. The guides shown in Figs 6-1e to 6-1g are used for single-implant restorations supported by narrow-, regular-, or wide-platform implants.

Multi-unit and single-tooth restoration guides

The guide shown in Fig 6-2 is designed to indicate when the mesiodistal space is sufficient to install a two-unit fixed partial denture supported by two regular-platform implants. Figure 6-3 shows a guide designed to indicate when the mesiodistal space is sufficient to install a two-unit fixed partial denture supported by two wide-platform implants. Fig 6-4 shows one wide- and one regular-platform guide together to illustrate the difference in

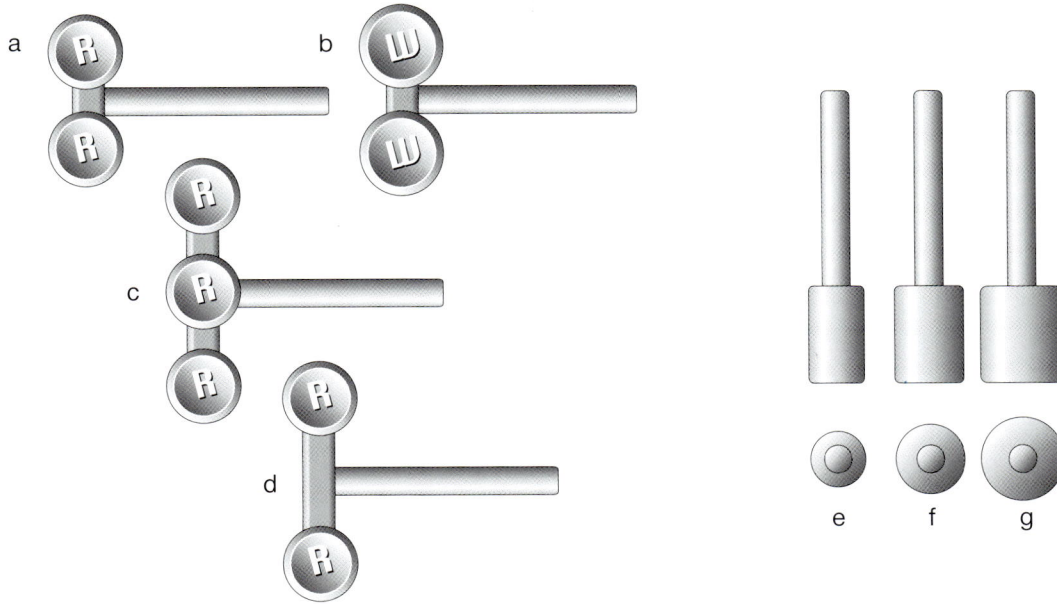

Fig 6-1 *(a and b)* Presurgical positioning guides used for implant restorations supported by two regular-platform or two wide-platform implants. *(c and d)* Guides used to determine the adequate number of regular-platform implants: three or two implants supporting a three-unit fixed partial denture. *(e to g)* Guides used for single-implant restorations supported by narrow-, regular- or wide-platform implants.

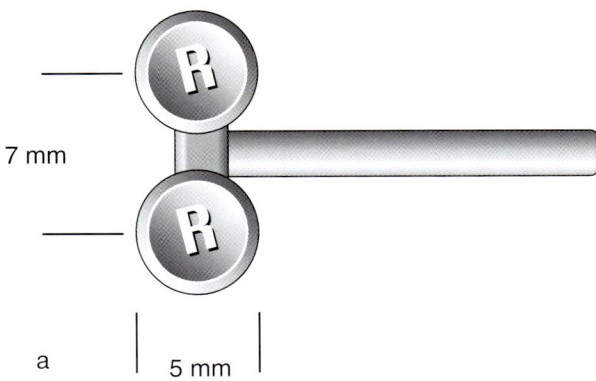

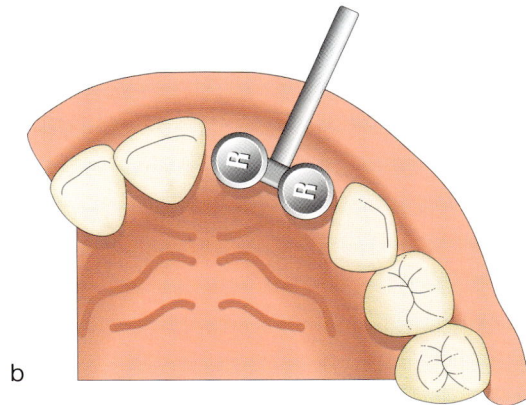

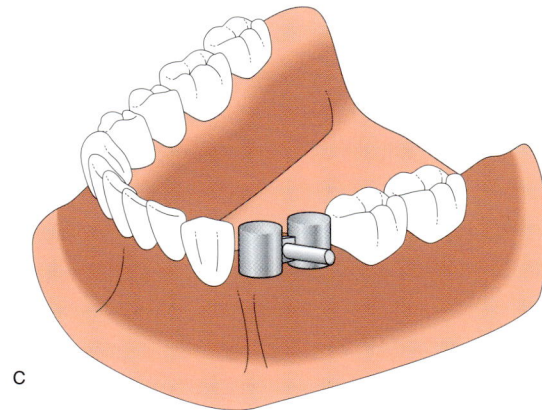

Fig 6-2 *(a)* Presurgical positioning guides made of two 5-mm-diameter cylinders. The distance is 7 mm from center to center, the minimum space recommended between regular-platform implants and the space occupied by the prosthetic abutment. *(b and c)* Guides in place between two teeth, showing the possibility of placing implants.

Fig 6-3 *(a)* Presurgical positioning guides made of two 6-mm-diameter cylinders. The distance is 8 mm from center to center, the space used when placing two consecutive wide-platform implants. *(b and c)* Guides in place between two teeth illustrating the possibility of placing two crowns on wide-platform implants.

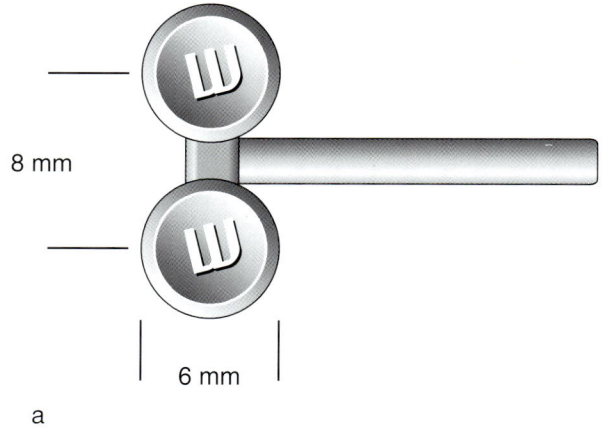

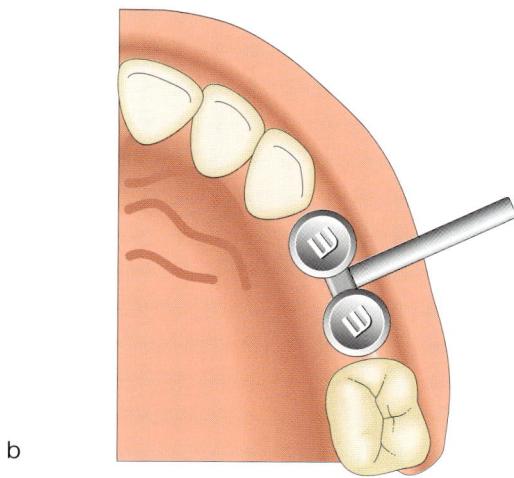

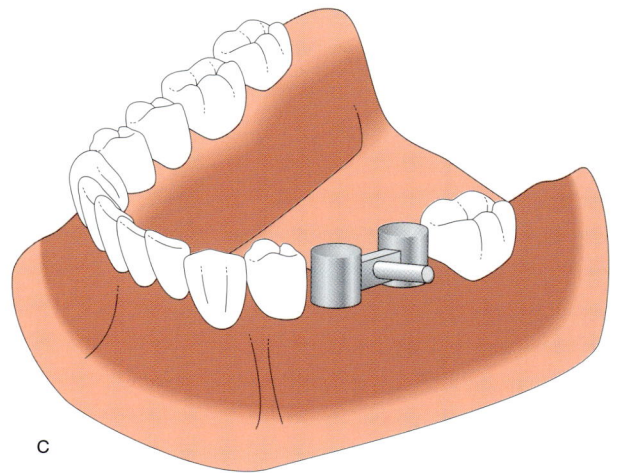

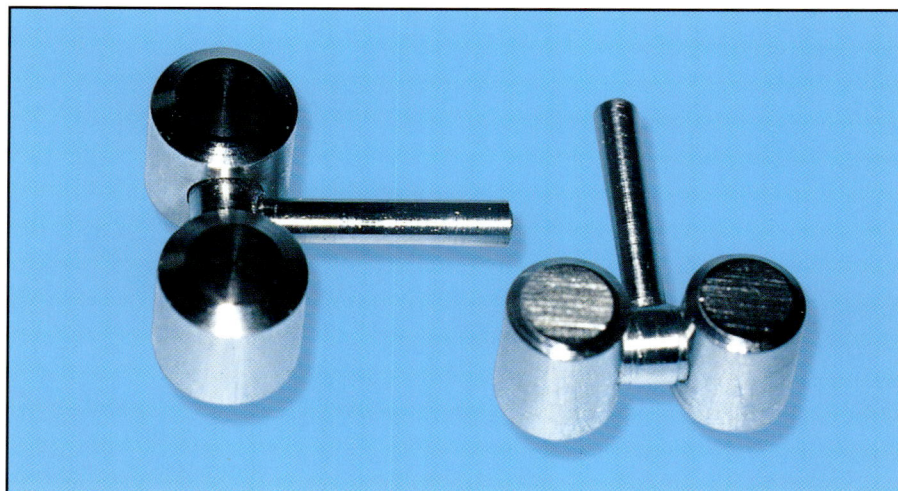

8 mm

6 mm

a

b

c

Fig 6-4 Regular- and wide-platform presurgical positioning guides.

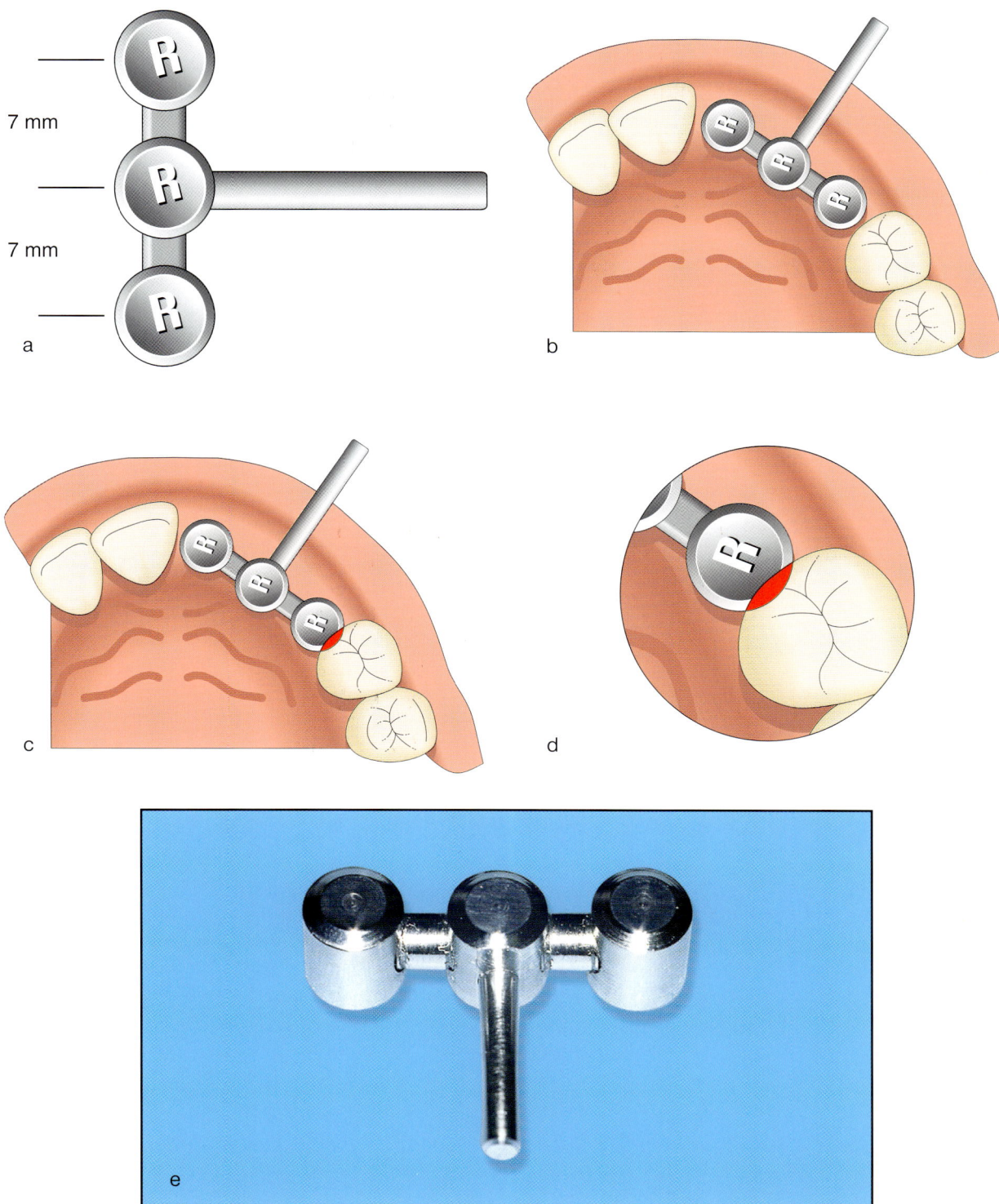

Fig 6-5 *(a)* Presurgical positioning guides made of three 5-mm-diameter cylinders used to determine the possibility of placing three consecutive regular-platform implants. *(b to d)* Due to the ridge resorption in the maxilla, it is not always possible to replace three lost teeth with a prosthetic restoration supported by three implants. In the clinical situation presented there is not enough space to place three regular-platform implants. *(e)* Presurgical positioning guide used for a three-unit fixed partial denture supported by three regular-platform implants.

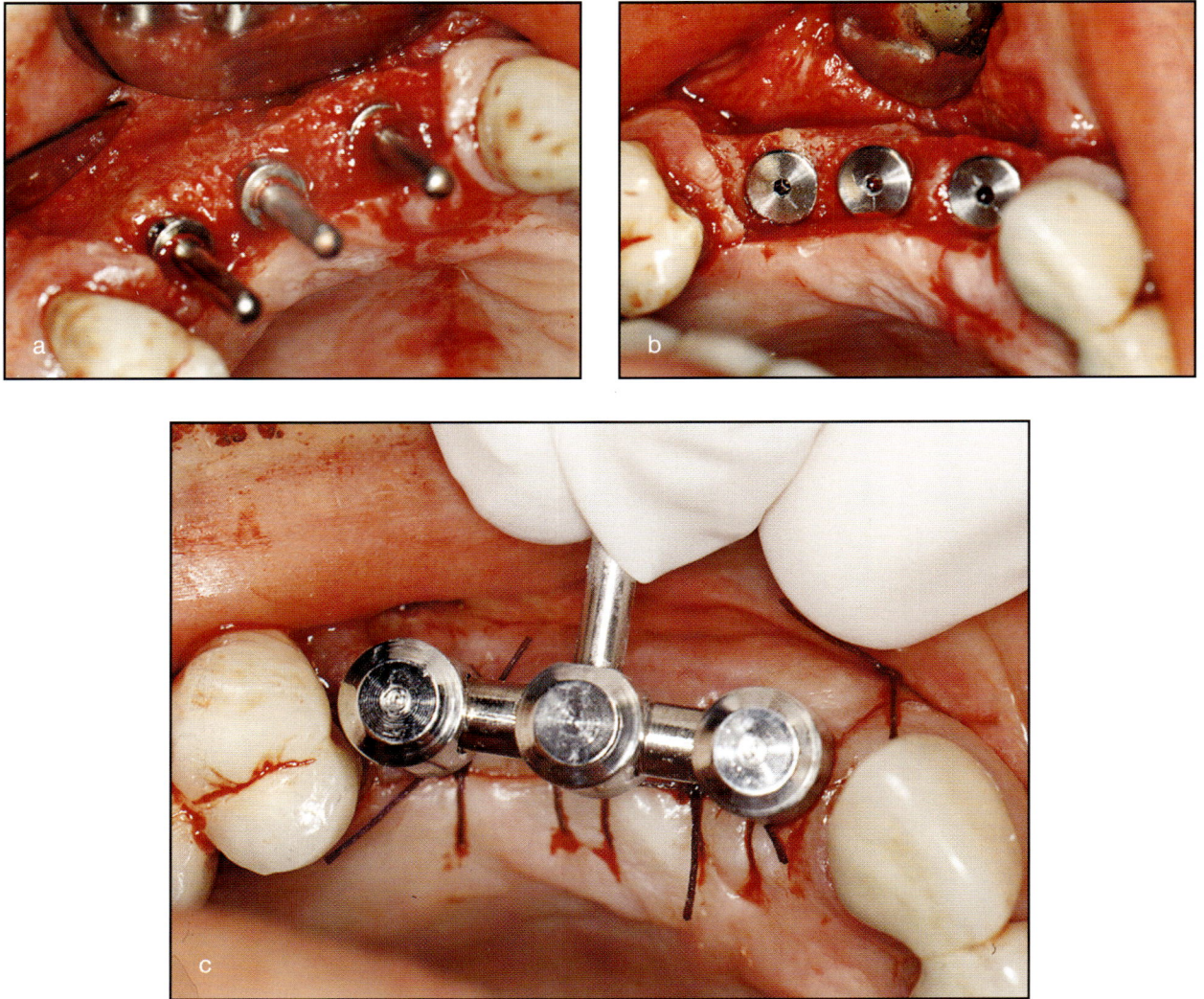

Fig 6-6 *(a to c)* Correlation between the presurgical positioning guide and implant positioning guide illustrated by the optimal placement of three implants to support a three-unit fixed partial denture. The use of the three-unit presurgical positioning guide intraorally as well as on the cast has demonstrated the possibility of placing the implants with sufficient mesiodistal space between the adjacent teeth. The implant positioning guides allow optimal precision in positioning in correlation with presurgical positioning guide measurements.

size between these components. The guide in Figs 6-5 and 6-6 is used to determine whether the mesiodistal space is sufficient to install a three-unit fixed partial denture supported by three regular-platform implants. Figure 6-7 shows a guide designed to indicate when the mesiodistal space is sufficient to install a three-unit fixed partial denture supported by two regular-platform implants.

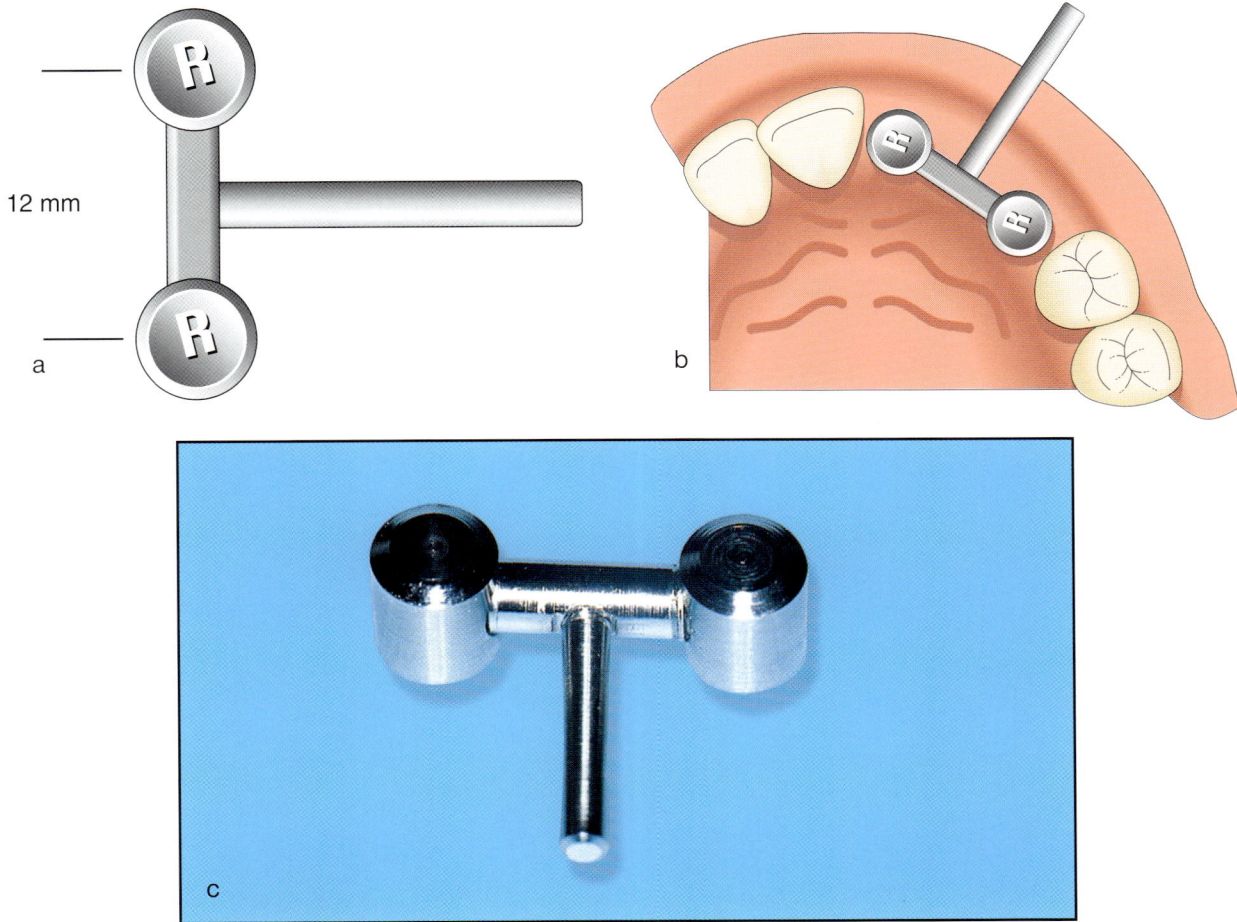

Fig 6-7 *(a to c)* Presurgical positioning guide used for a three-unit fixed partial denture supported by two implants. The distance from center to center is 12 mm. This guide can be used in combination with the three-unit guide to determine whether three or two implants will be placed to support the fixed partial denture.

The guides shown in Fig 6-8 are used to determine when it is possible to install a single-tooth restoration supported by one narrow-, regular-, or wide-platform implant. Figure 6-9 illustrates how to use the guides. It is obvious that in this patient, a narrow-platform implant must be used.

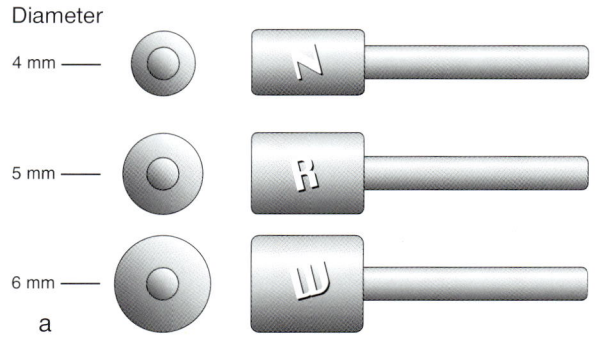

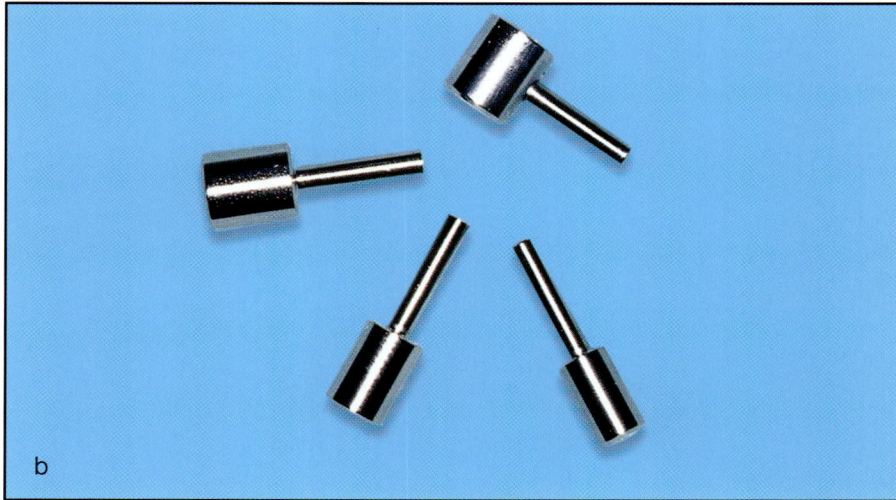

Fig 6-8 *(a and b)* Presurgical positioning guides used for single-tooth restorations. These guides correspond to narrow-, regular-, and wide-platform implants.

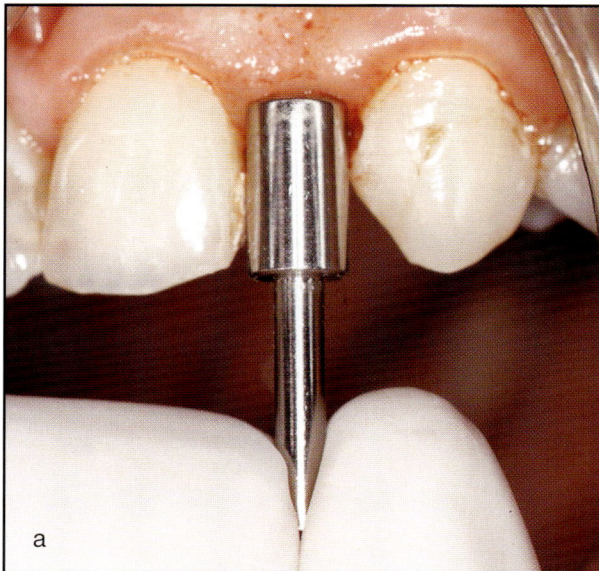

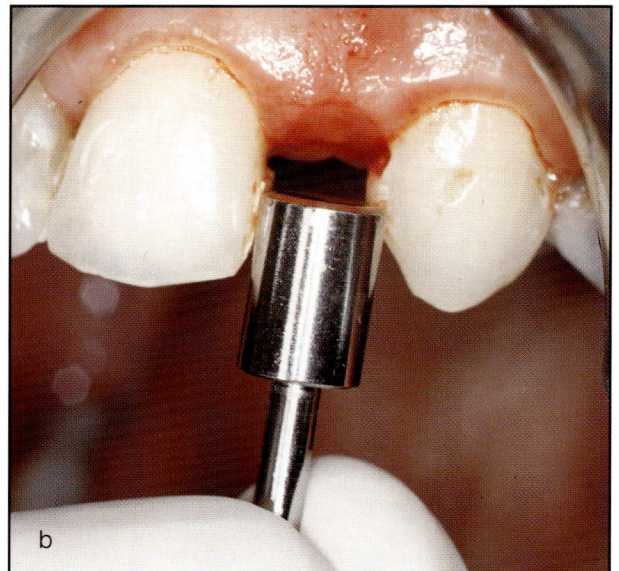

Fig 6-9 *(a and b)* When replacing a lateral maxillary incisor, the use of the presurgical positioning guide will allow the practitioner to select a regular or narrow platform. In this particular case, the selection of a narrow-platform implant is obvious.

The clinician can use presurgical positioning guides intraorally as early as the patient's first visit to get an overall idea of implant treatment (Fig 6-10). The guides can also be used on the cast to visualize treatment (Fig 6-11). This approach will facilitate the fabrication of a radiologic stent, a surgical guide stent, or both.

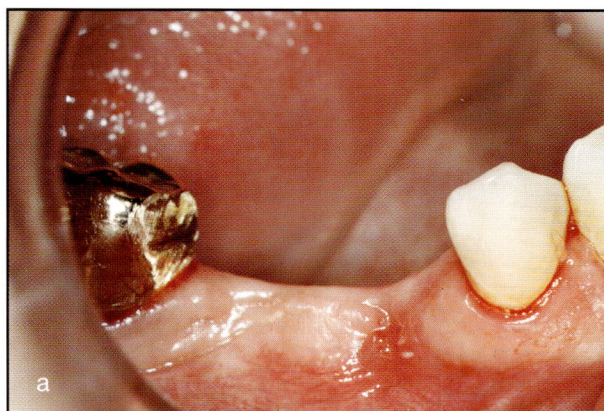

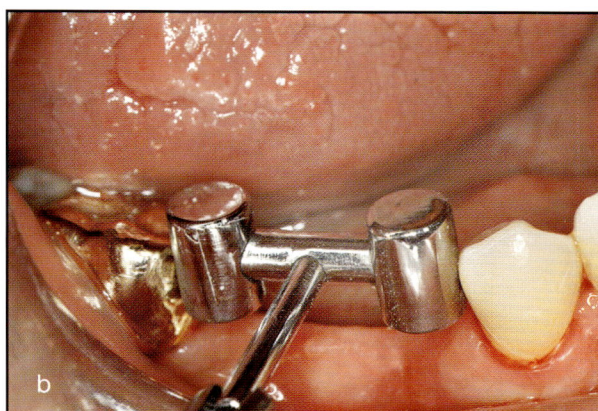

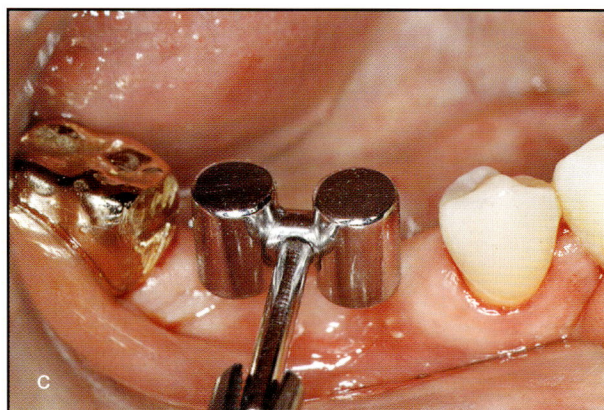

Fig 6-10 *(a to c)* At the first visit, the presurgical positioning guide is placed in an edentulous area to give an idea of different treatment options. In this case, two implants placed consecutively will be a better option than two implants separated by a pontic (the cylinders touch the adjacent teeth in such a situation).

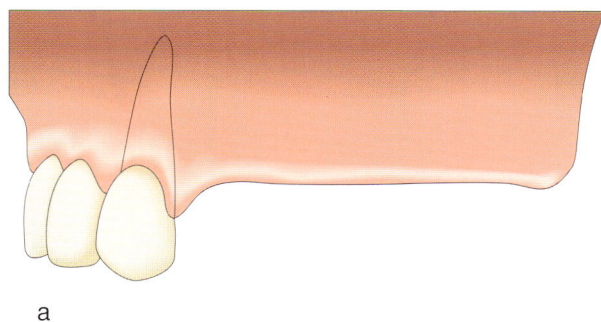

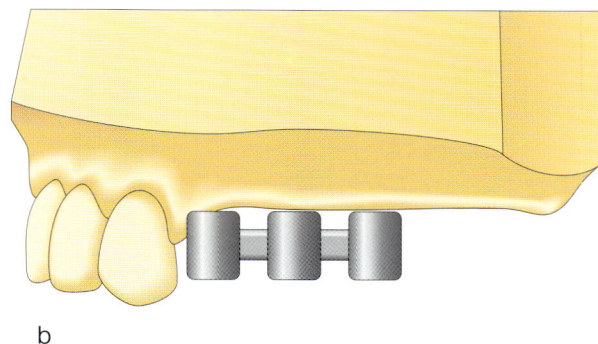

a

b

Fig 6-11 *(a and b)* In an edentulous region (for example, a maxilla missing premolars and molars), a presurgical positioning guide is placed intraorally, as well as on the cast, to illustrate the space to be occupied by the future prosthetic restoration.

Radiologic and surgical guide stents

The radiologic stent is designed with the use of presurgical positioning guides and according to the optimal position of the implants, which can be indicated by a radiopaque material in the stent (Fig 6-12). Intraoral placement of the radiologic stent during the radiographic examination (using, for example, the Scanora technique) yields objective information about the desired implant site and what is needed to place the implant in such a position (see Fig 6-12). When computer tomography is used, programs such as Dentascan will offer cuts with a scale of 1 to 1. Thus, the presurgical positioning guide can be placed directly on the radiographic film to identify the desired implant sites (Fig 6-13). In other words, the use of a radiologic stent can be avoided.

The surgical guide stent is designed and fabricated with the aid of the presurgical positioning guide. This means that the proper space between implants will be taken into consideration by the technician fabricating the guide stent. It must be stressed that presurgical positioning guides and implant-positioning guides are designed in such a way that they are complementary to each other (Fig 6-14).

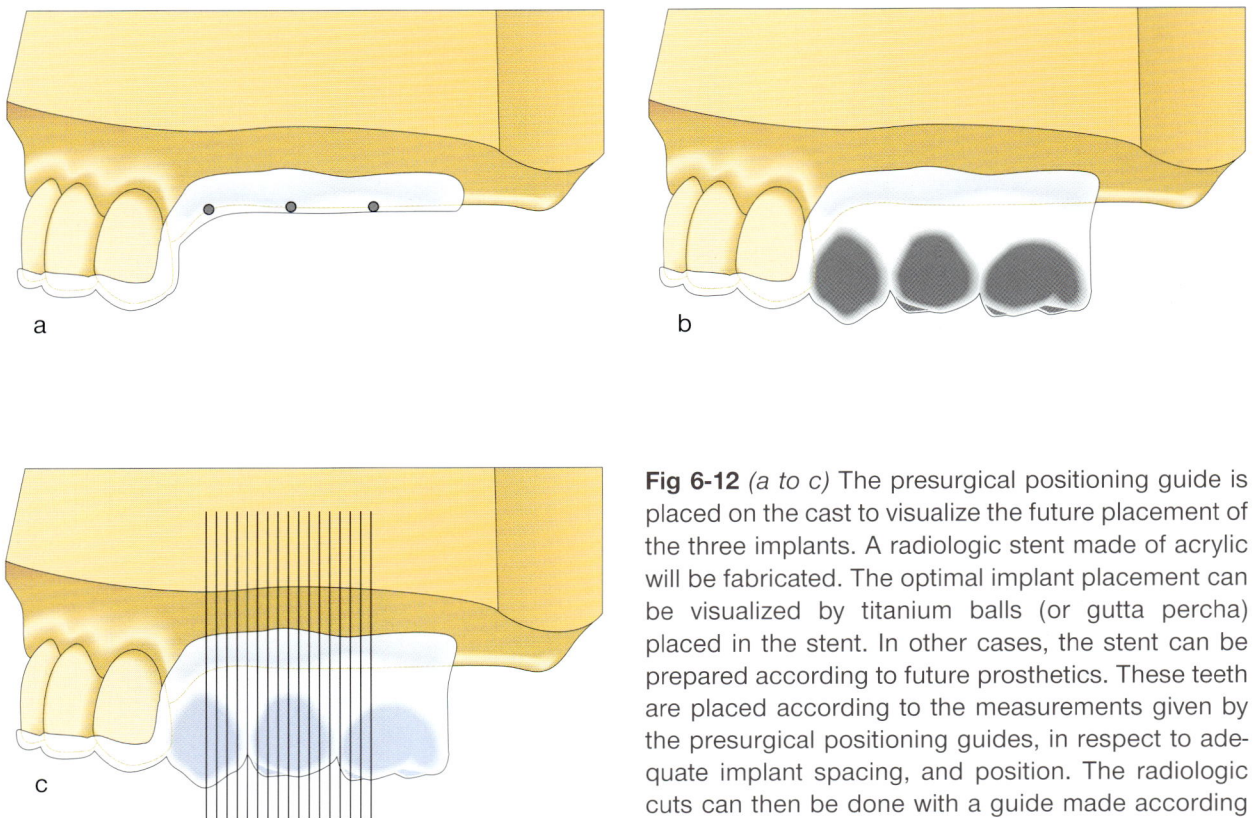

Fig 6-12 *(a to c)* The presurgical positioning guide is placed on the cast to visualize the future placement of the three implants. A radiologic stent made of acrylic will be fabricated. The optimal implant placement can be visualized by titanium balls (or gutta percha) placed in the stent. In other cases, the stent can be prepared according to future prosthetics. These teeth are placed according to the measurements given by the presurgical positioning guides, in respect to adequate implant spacing, and position. The radiologic cuts can then be done with a guide made according to the optimal placement.

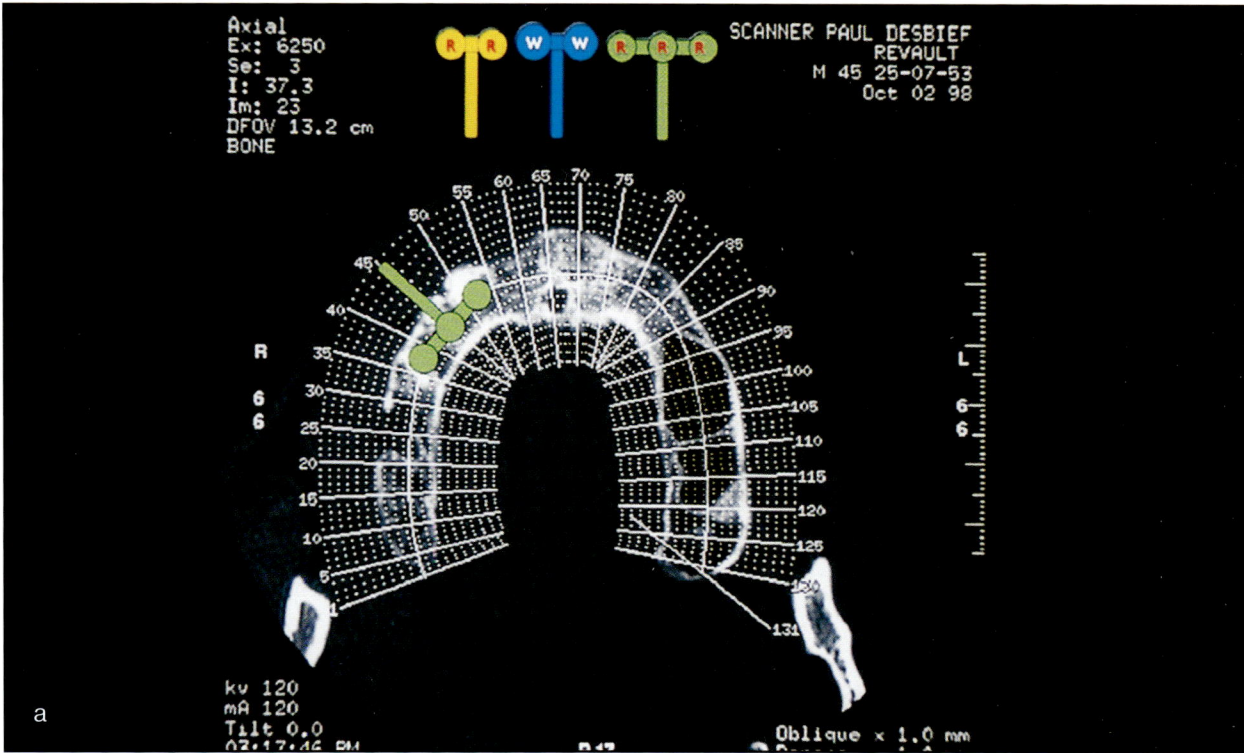

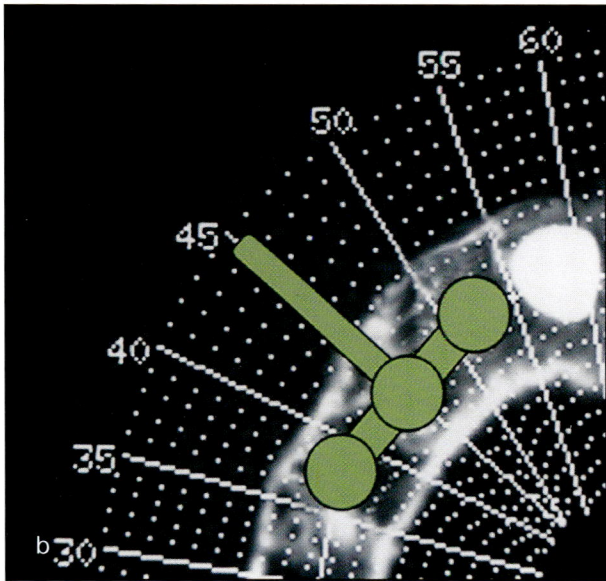

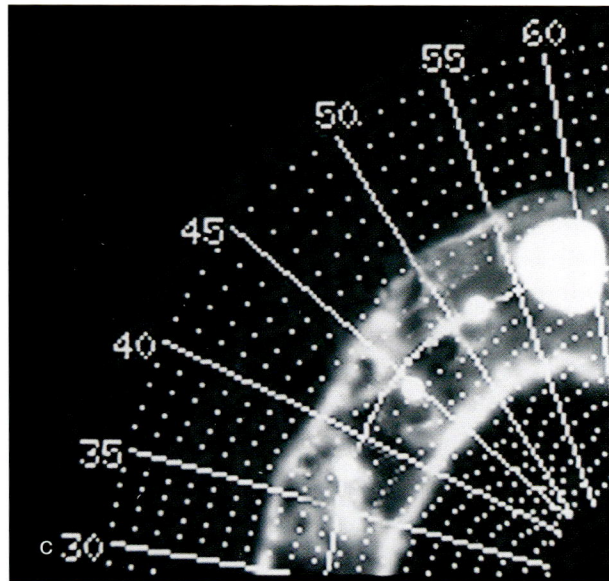

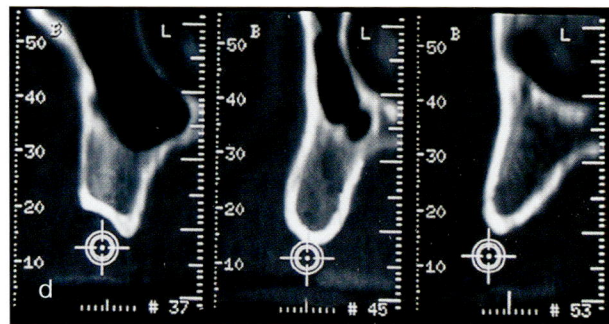

Fig 6-13 *(a to d)* In the case of three implants to be placed in the maxilla, the presurgical positioning guide is placed directly on the film. In such a case, the presurgical positioning guide placed over an occlusal view will help to locate the adequate cuts in relation to the future implant placement (cuts at teeth 37, 45, and 52).

Fig 6-14 *(a to c)* There is a close relationship between the situation on the cast and the clinical situation. The lab technician built the surgical guide according to adequate implant placement and not only according to teeth anatomy. The surgeon will be able to use implant positioning guides in conjunction with the surgical stents fabricated using the presurgical positioning guides. The communication between prosthodontist, lab technician, and surgeon is optimized by using this technique.

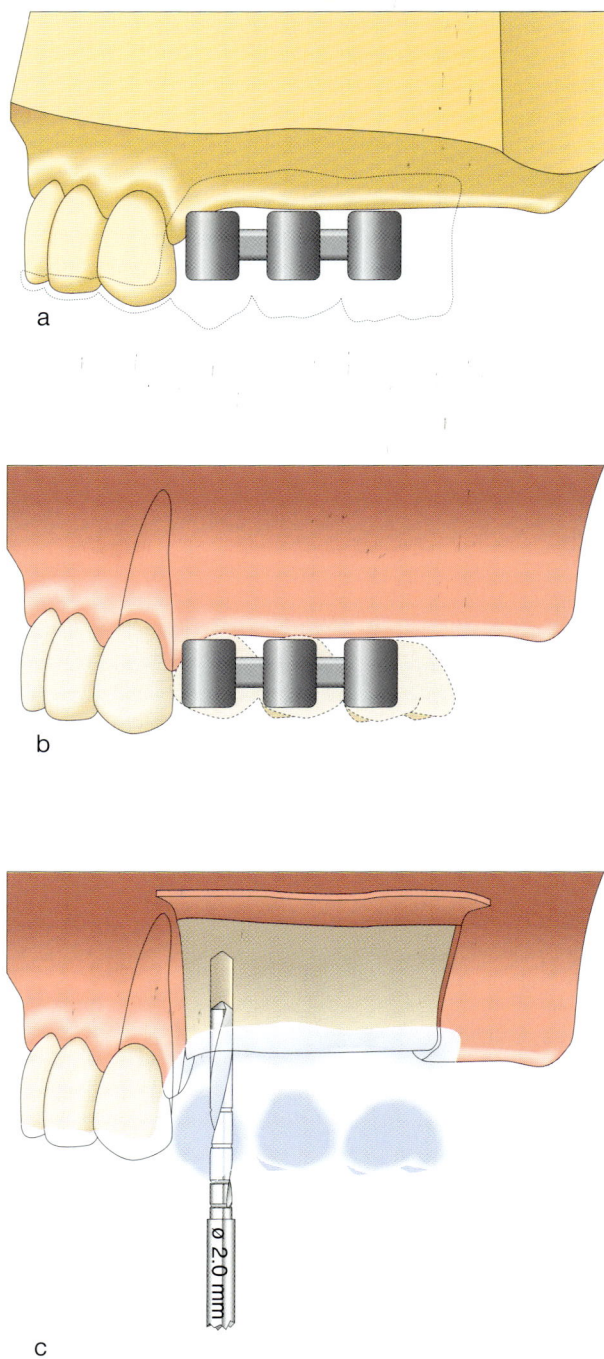

a

b

c

Implant-positioning Guides

The various components of the implant-positioning guides complement available direction indicators (Figs 6-15 and 6-16). Implant-positioning guides are available in three different shapes: "milestone," "short flag," and "long flag," with guidepin diameters of 2 or 3 mm to fit in a preparation (Fig 6-17).

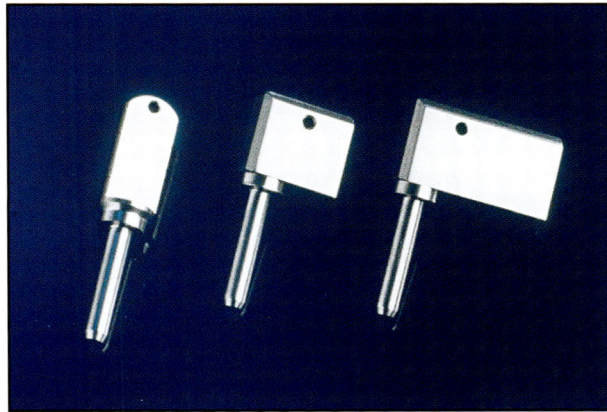

Fig 6-15 Implant-positioning guides: milestone, short flag, long flag.

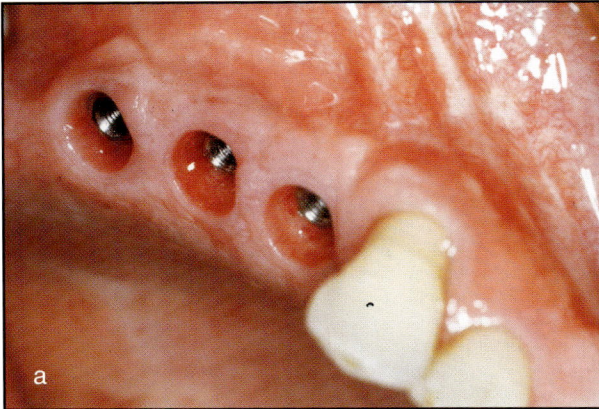

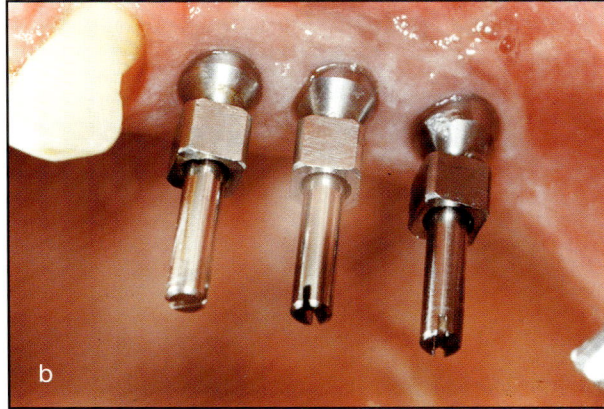

Fig 6-16 *(a and b)* Optimal placement of three maxillary implants. Adequate mesiodistal space as well as angulation is illustrated by the impression copings in place.

The milestone is primarily intended to give an image of the final prosthetic restoration (see Fig 6-17d), and the flags are intended to guide the surgeon in placing implants at a proper distance (at least 7 mm) from each other (see Fig 6-17e).

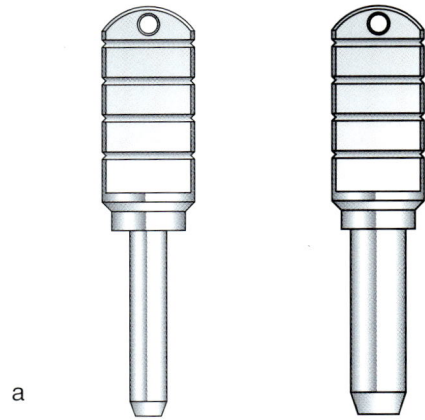

a

Fig 6-17 *(a)* The milestone is placed in position after drilling 2 and 3 mm. It gives a precise idea of the position, the angulation of the implant to be placed, and the position and angulation of the prosthetic restoration on top of the implant.

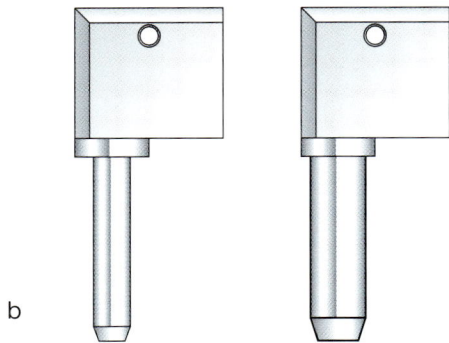

b

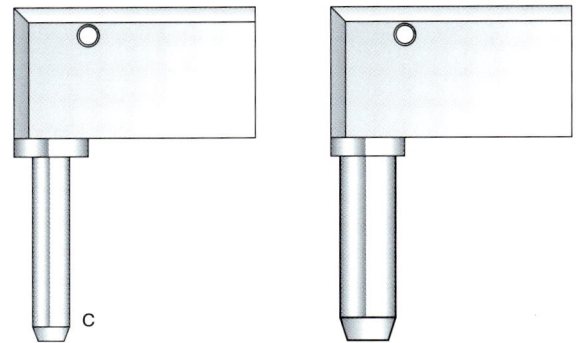

c

Fig 6-17 *(b and c)* Flags (short and long) help the surgeon to determine the adequate space between two implants. Short flags are used as a guide for the minimum space between two implants. Long flags correspond to the placement of two implants supporting a three-unit fixed partial denture with a pontic. These tools come in 2- and 3-mm diameters to be used at different stages of surgery.

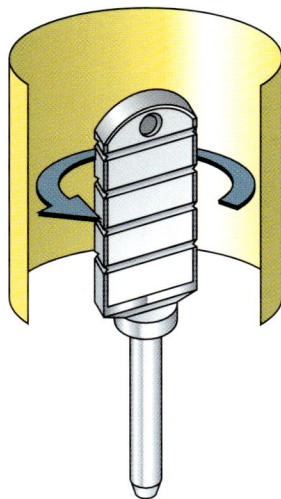

d

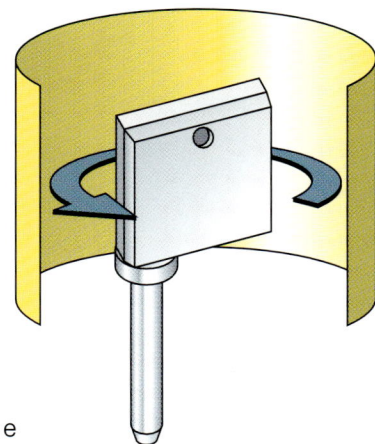

e

Fig 6-17 *(d and e)* Milestone and flag can be rotated for a specific use (emergence profile, tripod configuration, multiple-implant placement).

Optimal position and angulation are the keys to success in implant placement, especially in partially edentulous patients, where there is less room for error than in completely edentulous patients. For example, 1 mm in positioning, 10 degrees in angulation, or both can completely jeopardize a good final result (Figs 6-18 and 6-19). The green in the figures indicates optimal implant placement, whereas red indicates less-favorable placement. Figure 6-20 lists different implant positions and their influences on the final esthetic, biomechanical, and phonetic results, as well as the possibilities for good oral hygiene.

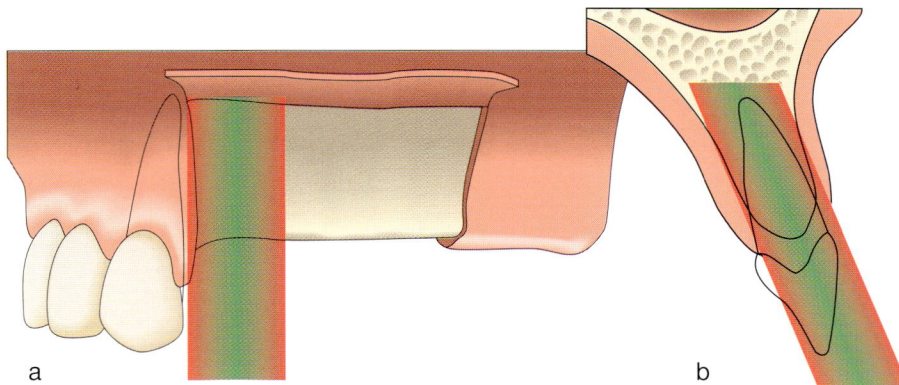

Fig 6-18 Potential implant-site positions. The green zone indicates the correct implant position, and the red zone indicates a more unfavorable position. Both mesiodistal *(a)* and buccolingual *(b)* aspects must be considered. When placing one implant, the first step is the use of a round bur. This will determine the future implant situation. For example, when placed too close to the adjacent tooth, this first hole will be the basis for a drilling sequence ending in poor esthetics, embrasures, and maintenance.

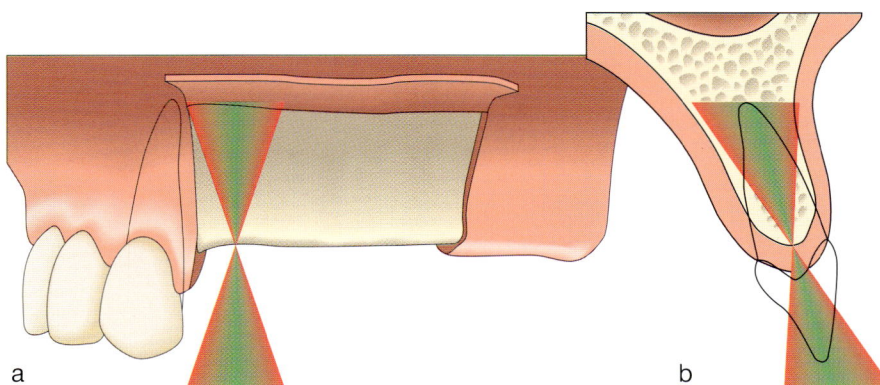

Fig 6-19 Potential implant angulations. The green zone represents correct implant angulation and the red zone unfavorable angulation (positioning). This has to be considered for mesiodistal, as well as buccolingual, aspects. The same concept is valuable when using the drills. Drilling angulation will directly influence the end result (insertion of the crowns or position of the access hole, for example).

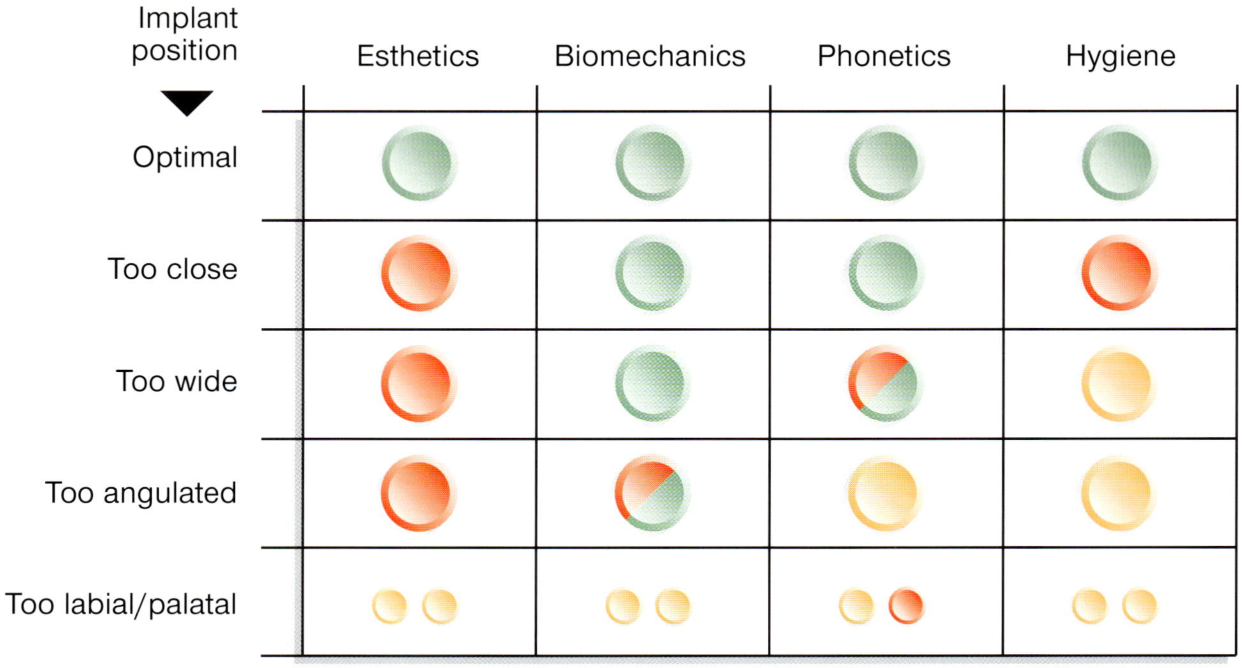

	Implant position ▼	Esthetics	Biomechanics	Phonetics	Hygiene
Optimal		🟢	🟢	🟢	🟢
Too close		🔴	🟢	🟢	🔴
Too wide		🔴	🟢	🔴🟢	🟡
Too angulated		🔴	🔴🟢	🟡	🟡
Too labial/palatal		🟡🟡	🟡🟡	🟡🔴	🟡🟡

Fig 6-20 Influence of implant position on final treatment results. Green circles indicate good prerequisites for acceptable treatment results, whereas yellow circles indicate difficulties in obtaining such results. Red circles indicate greater problems in obtaining acceptable treatment results. Sometimes an acceptable result cannot be achieved.

Figures 6-21 to 6-43 illustrate the various uses of the guides in optimal implant positioning. The sequence of treatment using the presurgical positioning guides will be presented in detail. The surgery starts using the surgical stent together with a round bur to locate the first implant placement. Then the 2-mm twist drill determines the angulation of this first implant. At this stage of the surgery, position and angulation can be modified freely; the milestone is of a great help in locating the future implant-supported restoration. The placement of the first implant will determine the placement of all the following implants. It is therefore important to double-check this position and angulation in order to avoid misplacement of all other implants. Figures 6-21 to 6-23 illustrate the drilling sequence using this method as well as different surgical options using presurgical positioning guides.

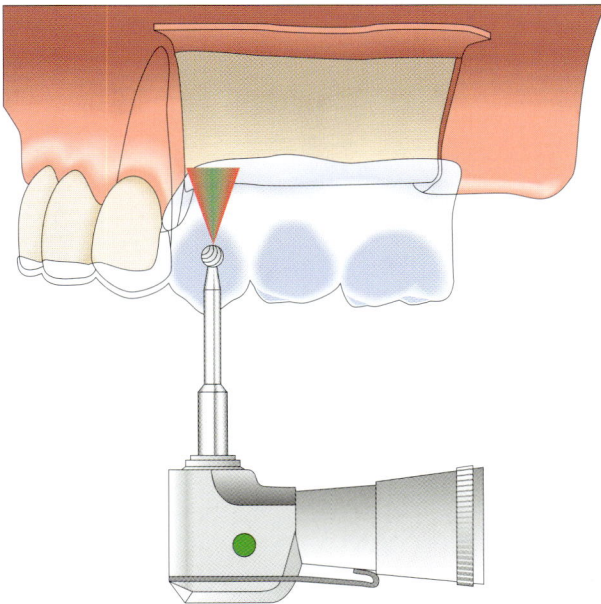

Fig 6-21 Individually designed guide stent placed in an edentulous area distal to the maxillary left canine. The stent will facilitate placement of the starting point for the implant-site preparation in the exposed cortical layer of the alveolar bone. A guide drill (round bur) is used for this preparation. The position of the starting point is more crucial with advanced bone resorption.

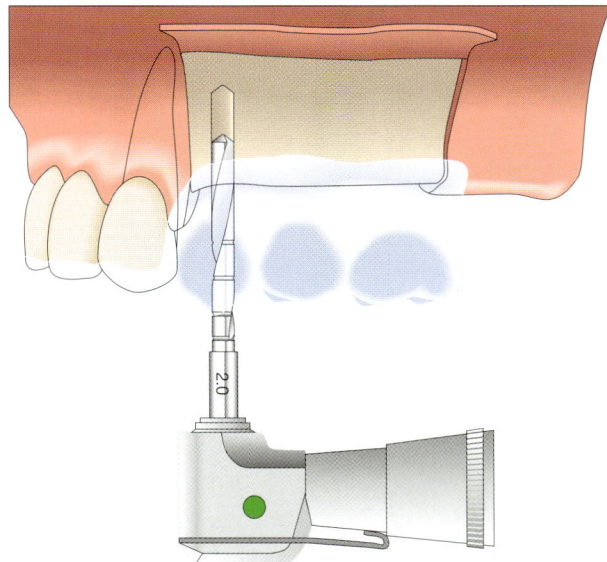

Fig 6-22 Use of a guide stent with the twist drill (diameter = 2 mm). The stent and the remaining left maxillary left canine guide the surgeon in reaching an acceptable position and angulation for implant-site preparation.

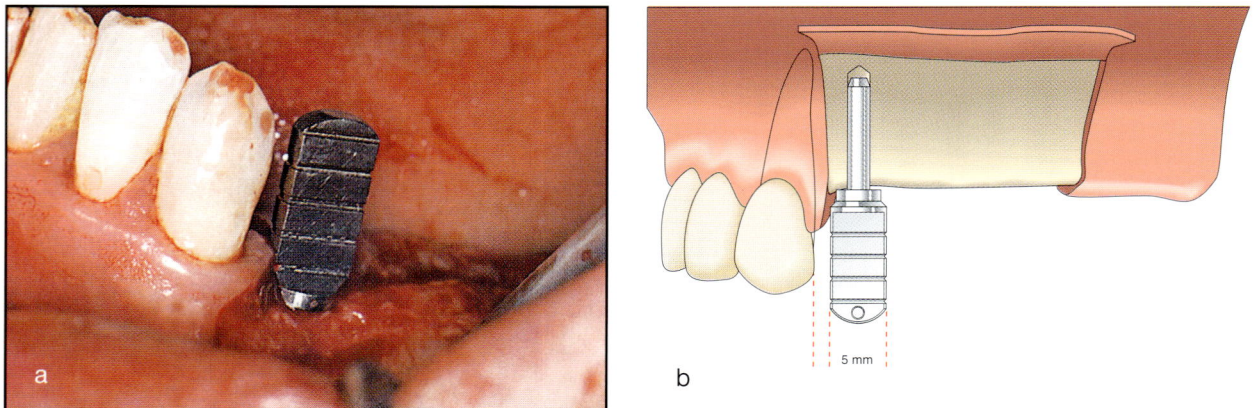

Fig 6-23 *(a and b)* Use of the milestone (diameter = 2 mm) facilitates confirmation of acceptable position and angulation of the initial implant-site preparation (at the 2-mm-diameter level). If corrections are necessary, it is preferable to use the guide drill and the twist drill (diameter = 2 mm) instead of the 3-mm twist drill. The base of the milestone is identical to the base of the abutment or the crown.

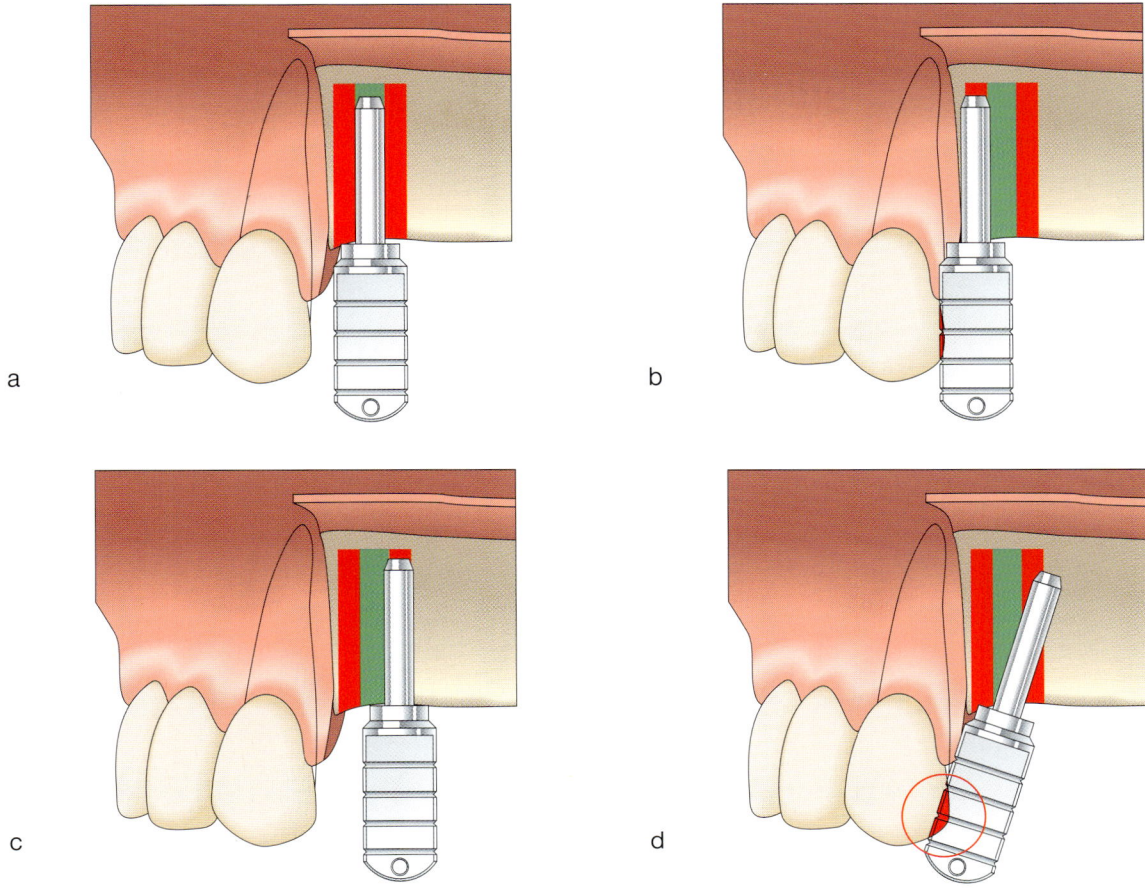

Fig 6-24 *(a)* Guide 1 can show the embrasure, as well as the image of the final crown restoration, when the position and angulation of the implant-site preparation is optimal. *(b)* When guide 1 is touching the neighboring tooth, the embrasure, as well as the shape of the final crown restoration, will be compromised. *(c)* When the space between the remaining tooth and guide 1 is too wide, difficulties in creating a good crown anatomy and embrasure may occur. *(d)* Use of guide 1 will reveal unfavorable angulation of the implant site. Such angulation may create difficulties in placement of the implant-supported prosthetic restoration.

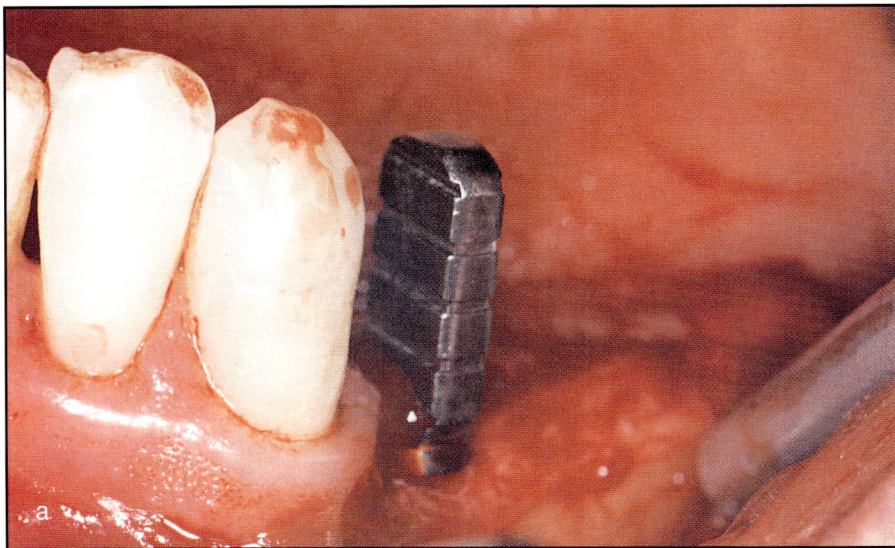

Fig 6-25a

Fig 6-25 *(a to c)* Milestone (guide 1) gives the clinician an image of the future outline of the crown restoration in the mesiodistal direction, as well as an image of the embrasure. Turning the guide 90 degrees will yield an image of the buccal crown outline. *(d and e)* When replacing a maxillary premolar, the placement of the milestone in the 2-mm-diameter hole will indicate the future overall volume of the prosthetic restoration in relation to the canine and the opposing arch, with the guide being placed in a labial-palatal direction. *(f and g)* The same concept is applicable in a mesiodistal direction even when the adjacent crown is prepared. This first preparation must be carefully planned, because it is the basis for the drilling sequence.

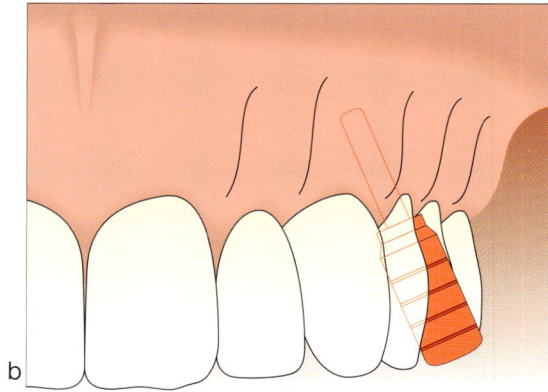

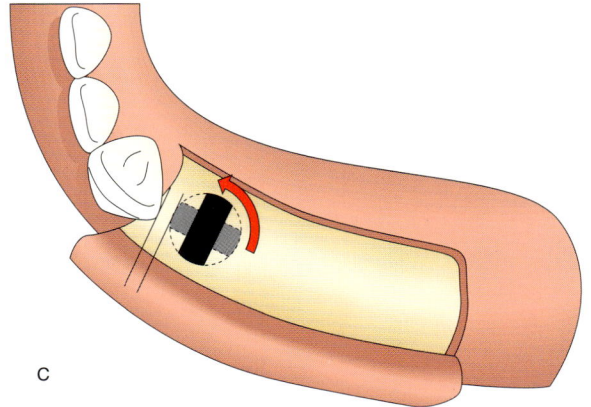

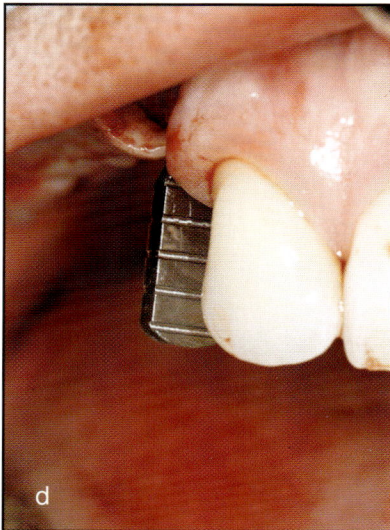

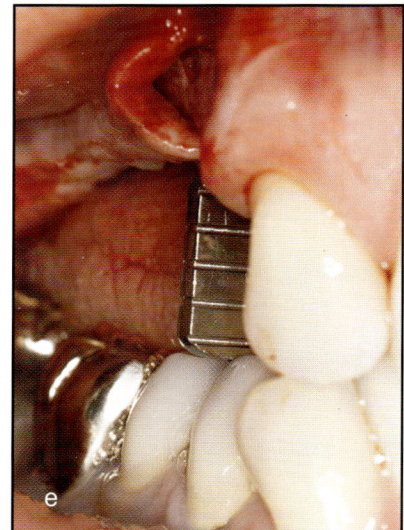

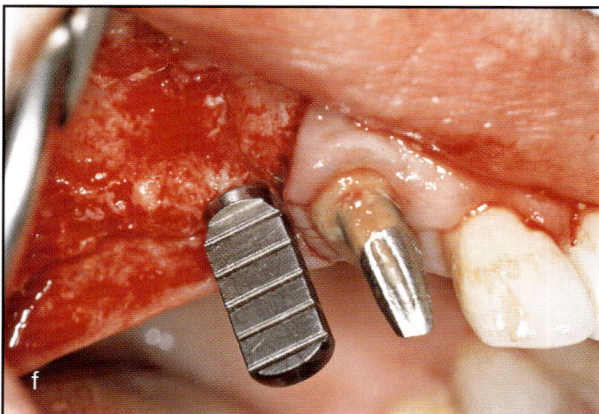

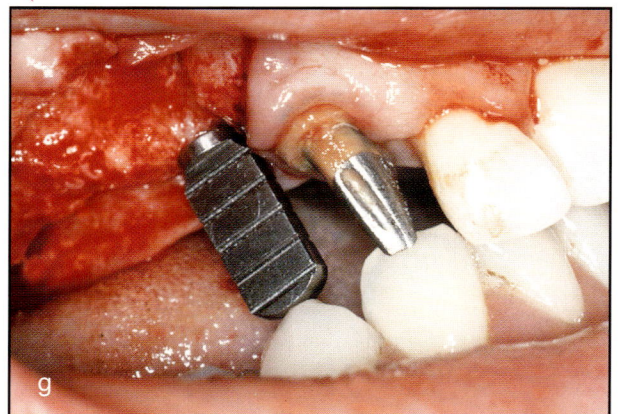

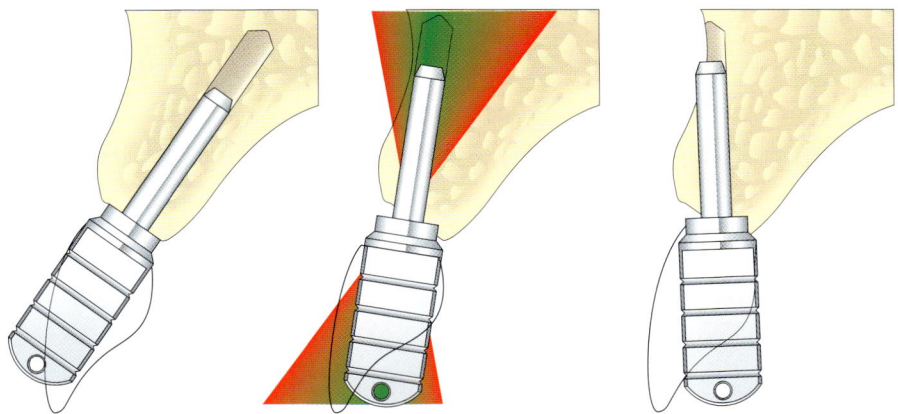

Fig 6-26 Guide 1 can be very useful in the anterior maxilla, where esthetic requirements are most important. If the implant-site preparation is too buccally angulated, the screw-access hole will appear on the buccal surface and create a potential esthetic complication. In addition, such an implant angulation is unfavorable from a biomechanical point of view. If the implant angulation is too palatal, then esthetic, biomechanical, and hygienic complications may occur. Correct inclination of the implant-site preparation is thus very important and reduces the need to use angulated abutments.

Maxilla   Mandible

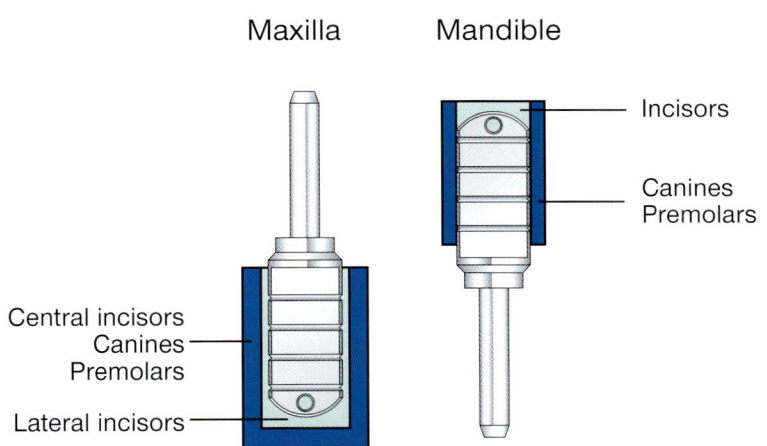

Incisors

Canines
Premolars

Central incisors
Canines
Premolars

Lateral incisors

Fig 6-27 Mesiodistal width of guide 1 in relation to the mean width of incisors, canines, and premolars.

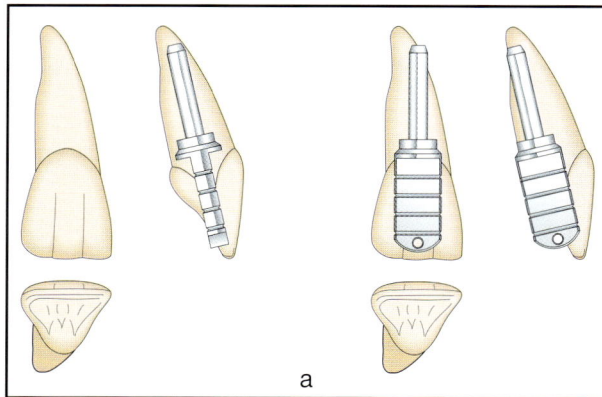

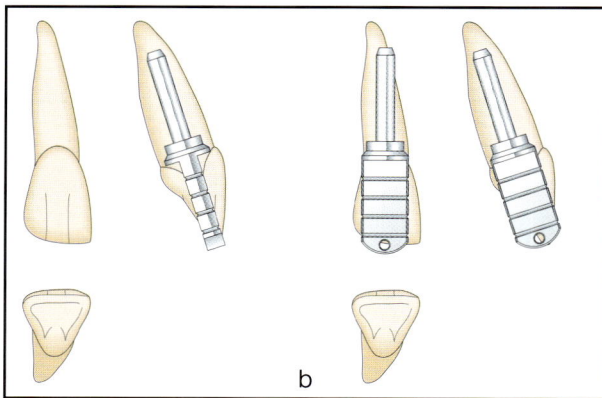

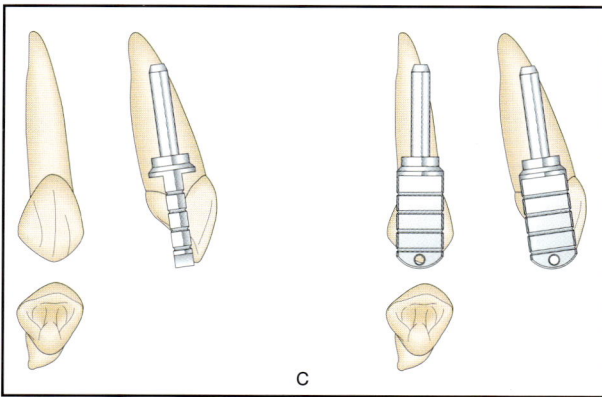

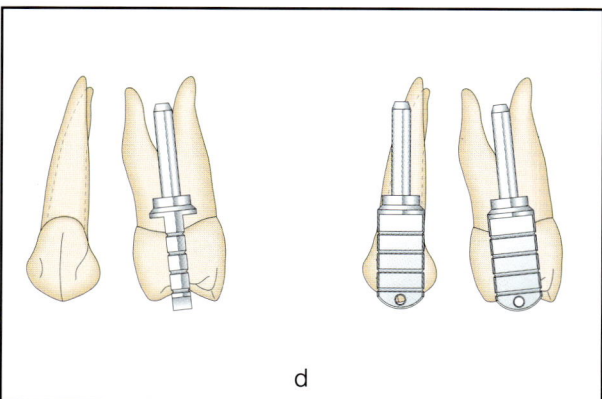

Fig 6-28 *(a and b)* Dimensional relationships between maxillary anterior teeth and the milestone in the mesiodistal and buccopalatal directions. The milestone can be used for several teeth and the flat surfaces give a good image of the crown volume, placement, and angulation. For detailed information regarding mean crown dimensions, see Table 4-1 in Chapter 4.

Fig 6-29 *(a and b)* Use of the short flag (guide 2) to start implant-site preparation in an adequate position. This use results in a center-to-center distance of 7 mm between implant-site preparations, which allows for a good design of the final fixed prosthesis. Furthermore, this 7-mm distance between centers makes adequate soft tissue manipulation possible at abutment connections. The amount of tissue allows the surgeon to create inter-implant papillae with favorable anatomy and proper blood supply, if necessary. This tissue manipulation is described in detail in Chapter 8.

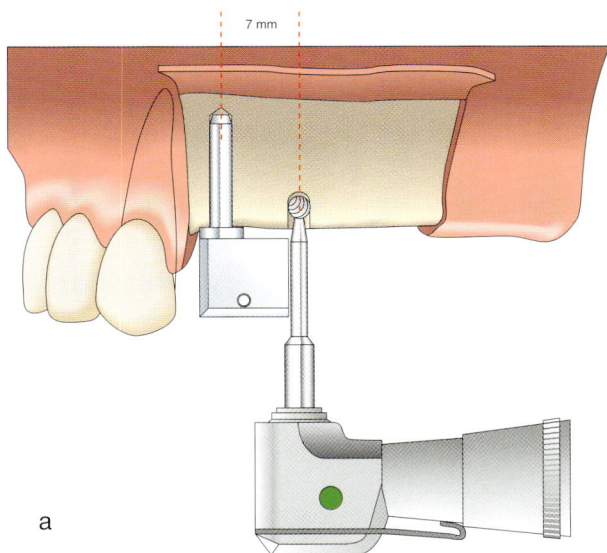

a

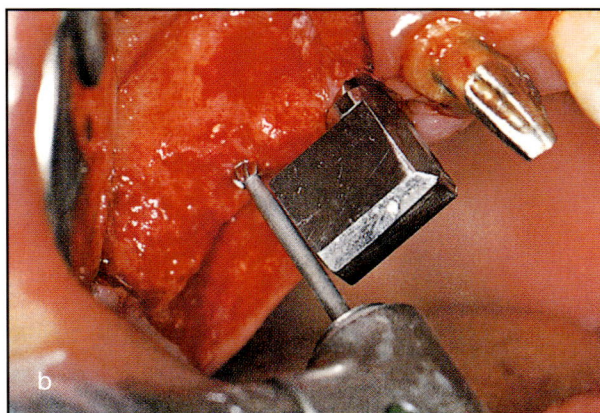

b

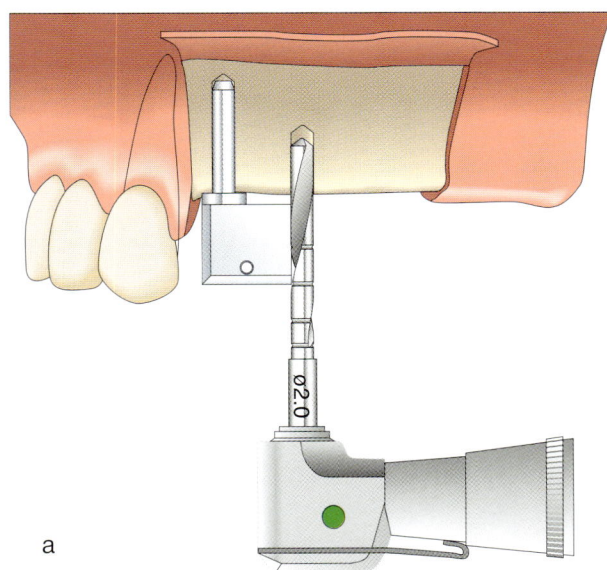

a

Fig 6-30 *(a and b)* Use of flags (either short or long) not only helps the surgeon find an acceptable position for an implant but also facilitates a parallel implant-site preparation.

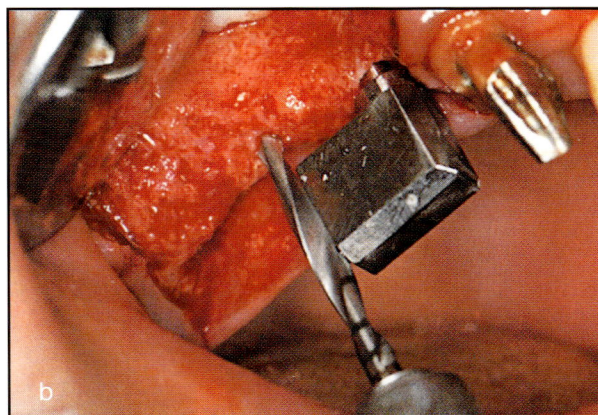

b

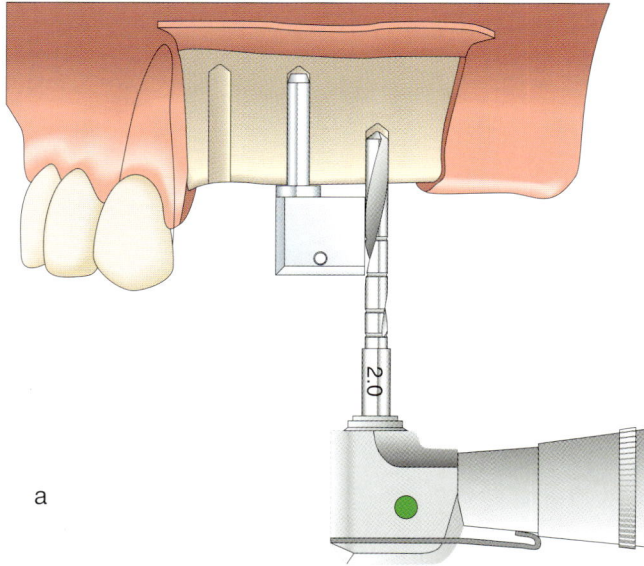

Fig 6-31(a to c) The procedure can be repeated for placement of all subsequent implants.

a

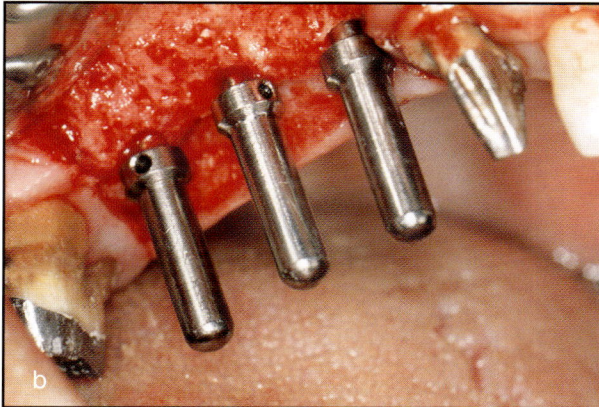

b

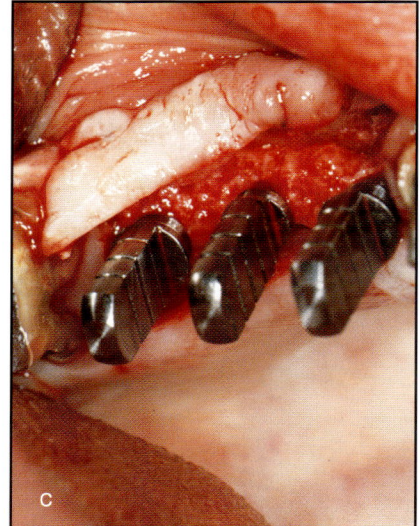

c

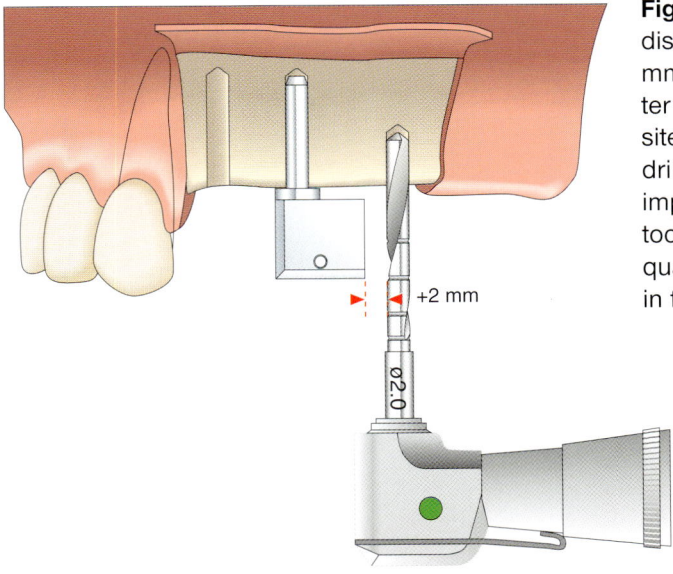

Fig 6-32 When a molar must be placed on the most distal implant, site preparation should start about 2 mm distal to the short flag, resulting in a center-to-center distance of 9 mm. After preparation of all implant sites using the twist drill (diameter = 2 mm), the pilot drill (diameter = 3 mm), and the 3-mm twist drill, implants can be placed according to the standard protocol (Adell et al 1985). A double-check of the adequate position can be done by placing the milestones in future implant sites.

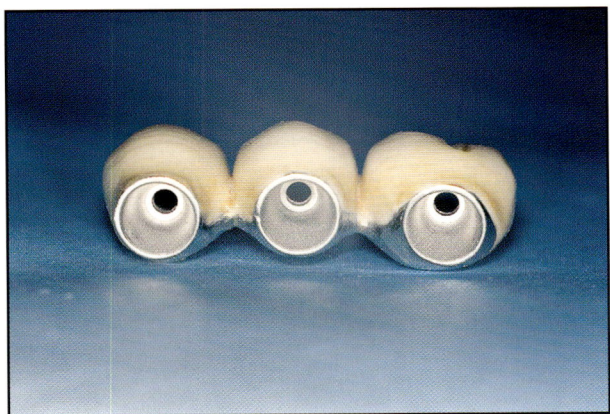

Fig 6-33 Clinical view illustrating the concept described in Figs 6-30 to 6-32 resulting in adequate shape of the crowns as well as embrasures.

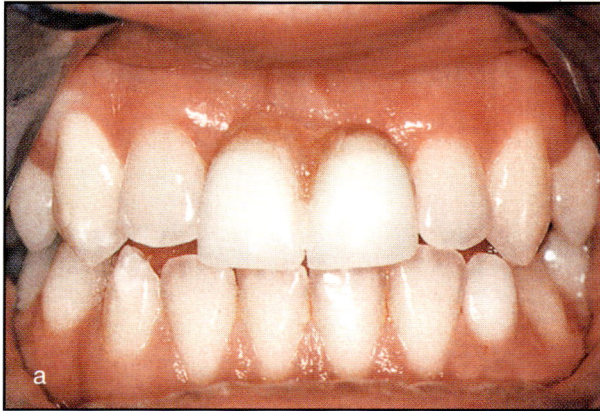

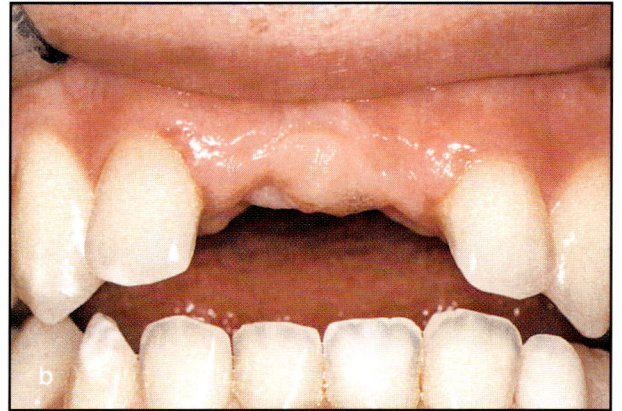

Fig 6-34 *(a and b)* Missing maxillary central incisors to be replaced by two implant-supported restorations. *(c to i)* Clinical use of implant-positioning guides in combination with conventional direction indicators.

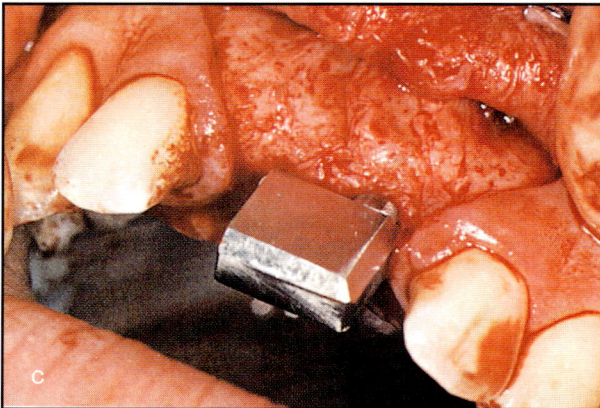

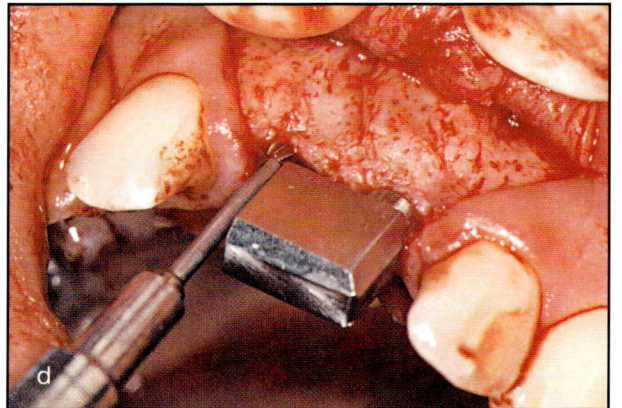

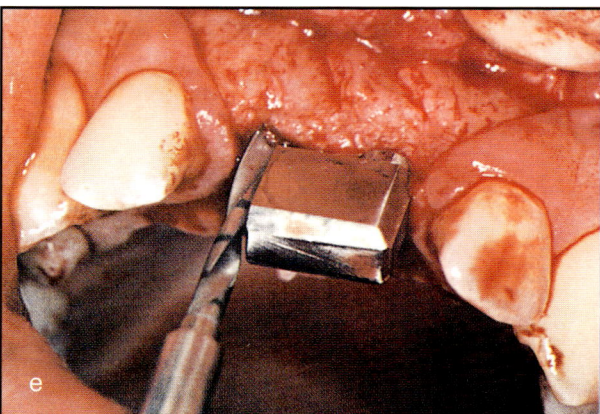

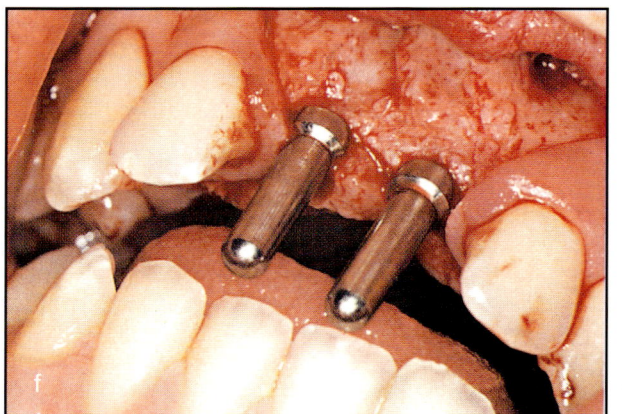

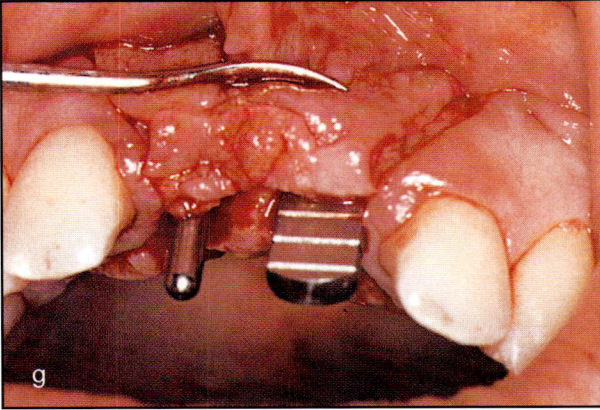

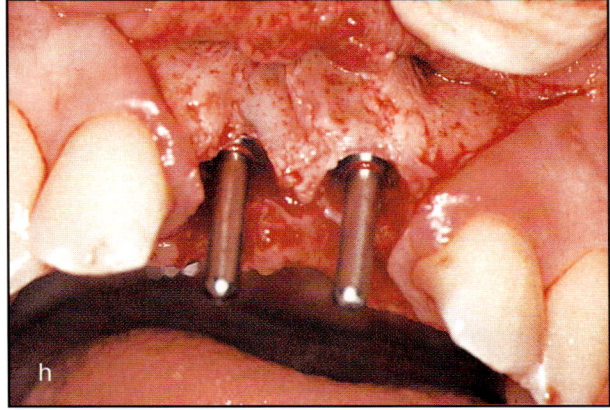

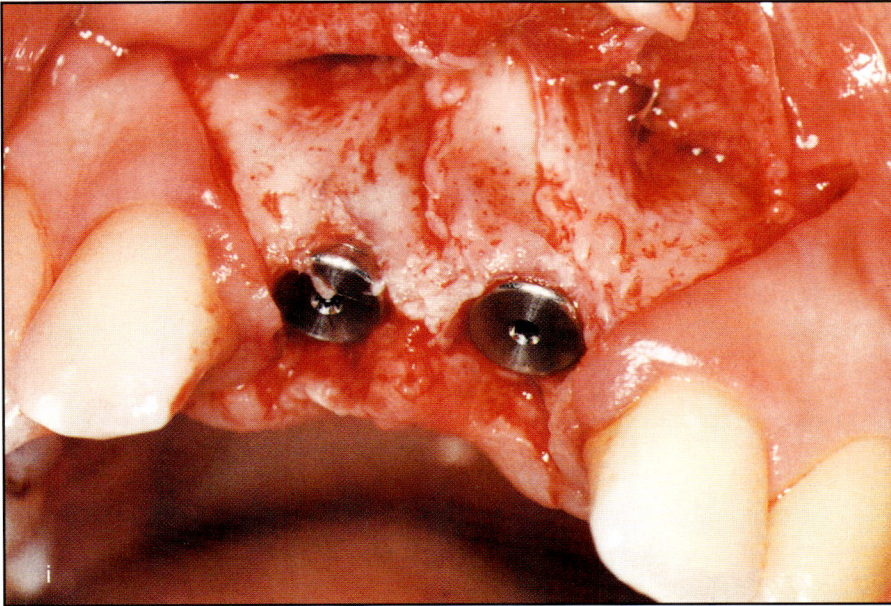

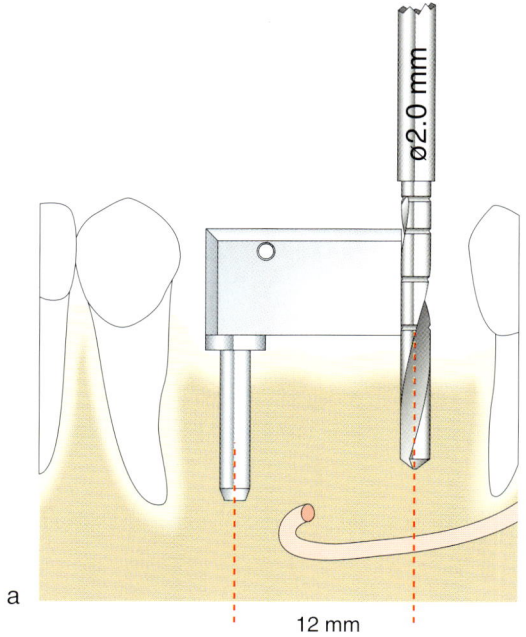

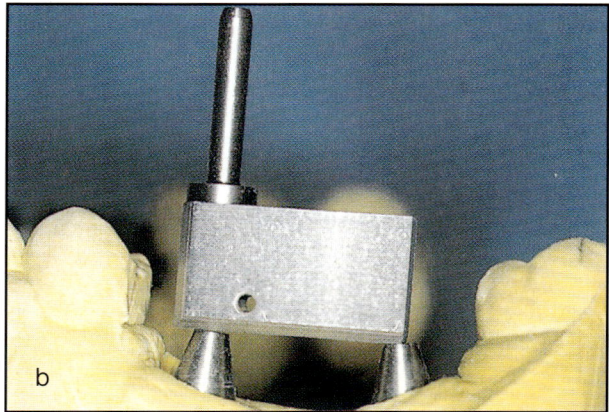

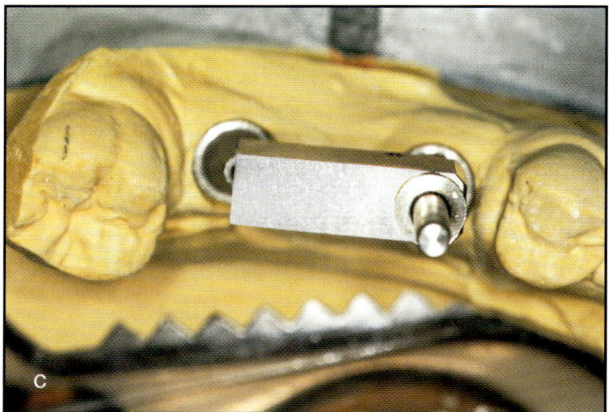

Fig 6-35 *(a to c)* Where treatment planning with presurgical positioning guides has indicated problems in placing three implants because of limited space, a pontic is placed between the implants. The use of the long flag (in accordance with the description of short flag use) will result in a minimum center-to-center distance of 12 mm between implant-site preparations. This is a minimum distance for placing a pontic between two implants to obtain a good esthetic result and conditions for proper oral hygiene. Where more than 14 mm between the centers of the sites is available, it is preferable, from both biomechanical and esthetic points of view, to place another implant rather than extending another pontic.

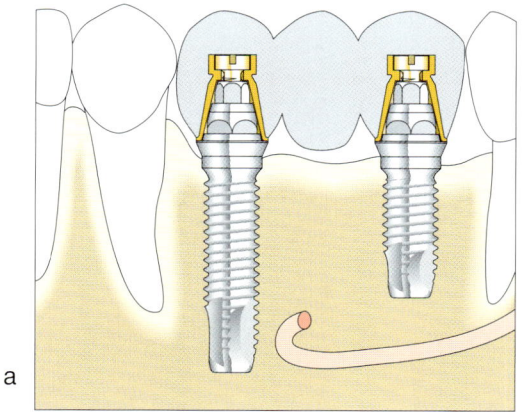

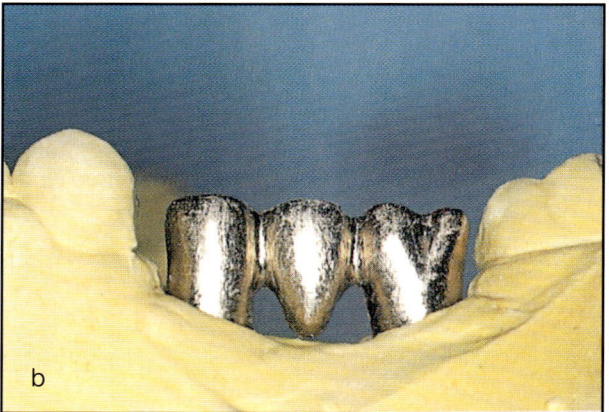

Fig 6-36 *(a and b)* Three-unit prosthesis supported by two implants.

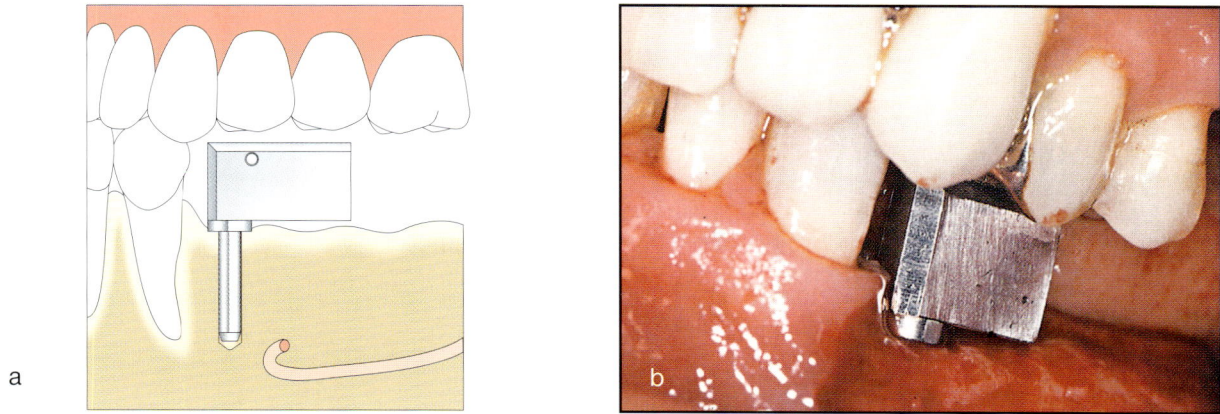

Fig 6-37 *(a and b)* Use of long and short flags to visualize the occlusal plane.

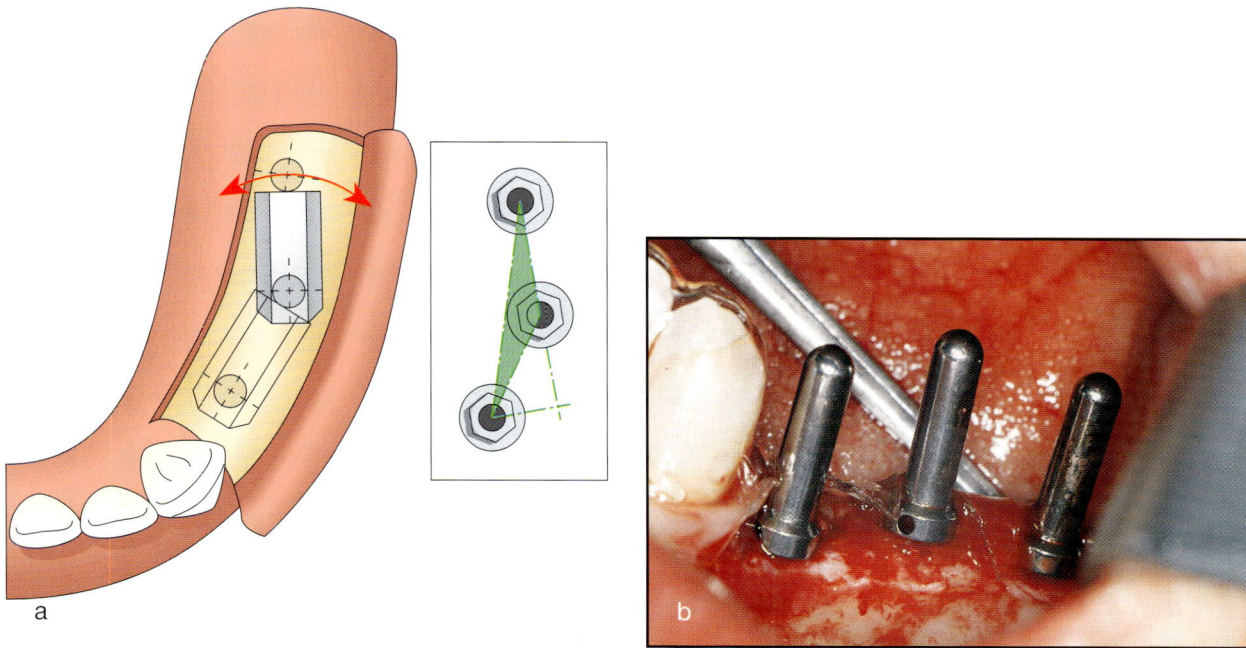

Fig 6-38 *(a)* Technique for visualizing a tripod (see Chapter 3) using flags. *(b)* Clinical example of a tripod configuration in a posterior mandible region.

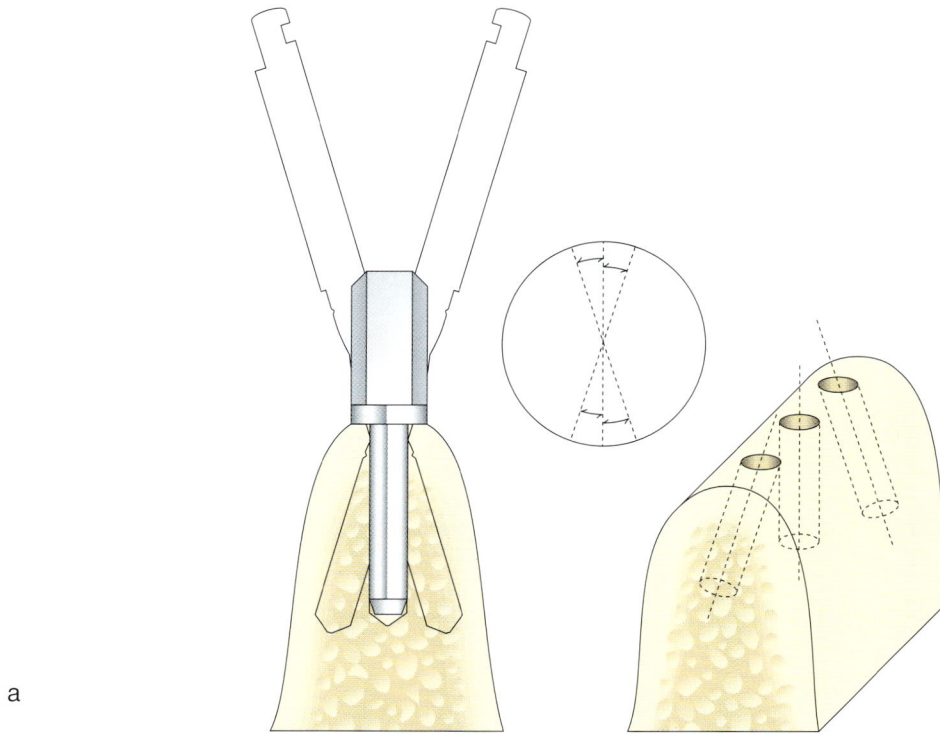

a

Fig 6-39 *(a)* Technique for using flags to visualize a controlled interimplant inclination in mesiodistal and buccolingual directions. *(b)* The flag can be used to control the degree of disangulation between implants, as well as to secure proper space between implants. The biomechanical importance of inclination and tripod configuration is discussed in Chapter 3. *(c)* When placing three implants in the maxilla, the most distal implant can be placed, using the cortical layer of the anterior wall of the sinus as an anchor. In this case a bony flap has been elevated, and sinus membrane has been reflected allowing a good visualization of the anterior wall of the sinus. The flag will help the clinician to control space and angulation between implants.

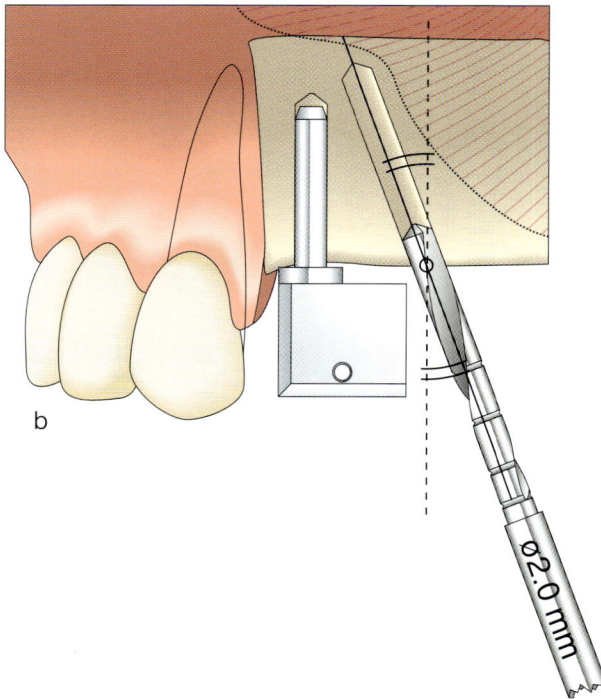

b

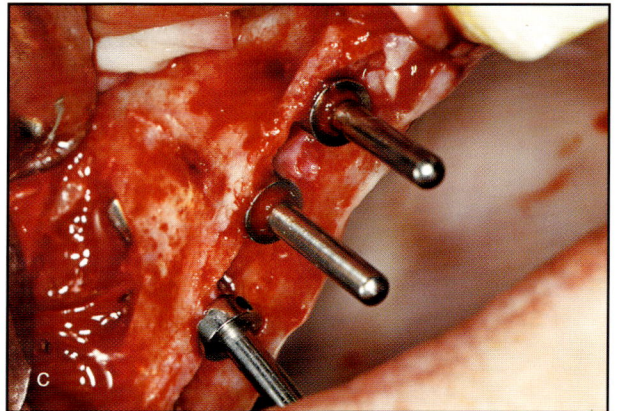

c

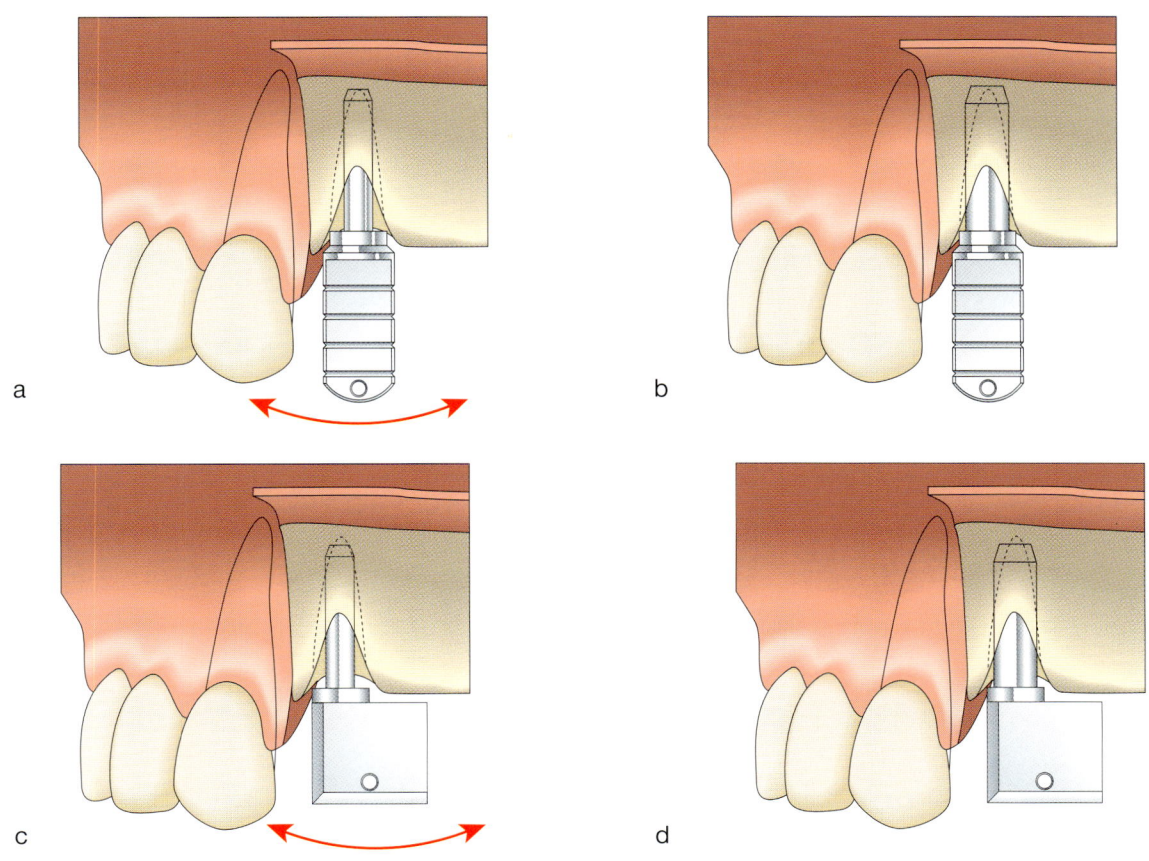

Fig 6-40 *(a to d)* Implant site with a bony defect (for example, an extraction socket, dehiscence). In such a situation, the potential implant site must be widened to 3 mm before proper stability of the implant-positioning guide (diameter = 3 mm) can be achieved.

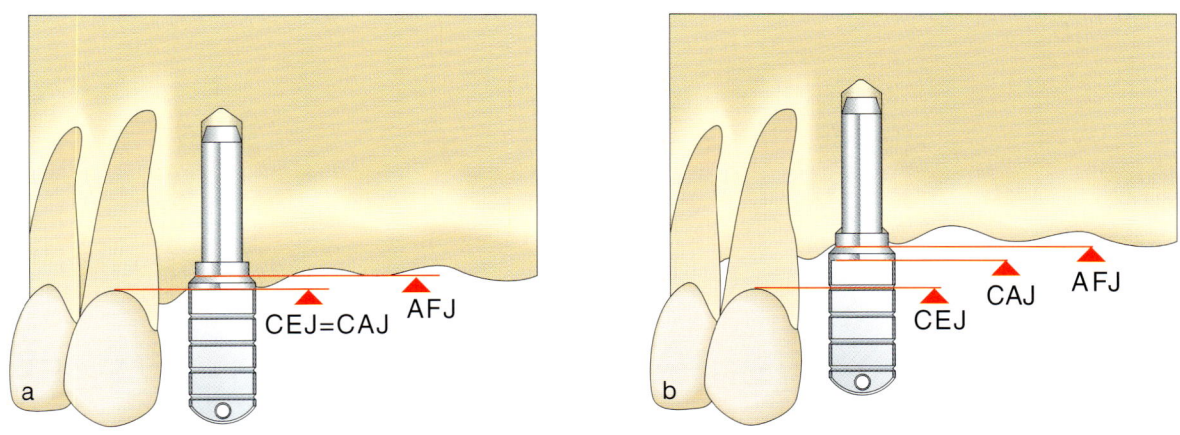

Fig 6-41 *(a and b)* Use of guide 1 (diameter = 3 mm) following countersinking to enhance vertical implant positioning related to the cementoenamel junction of adjacent teeth demonstrating intact and reduced periodontal tissue support, respectively. CEJ indicates cementoenamel junction; CAJ, crown-abutment junction; and AFJ, abutment-fixture junction. This topic is discussed in Chapter 4.

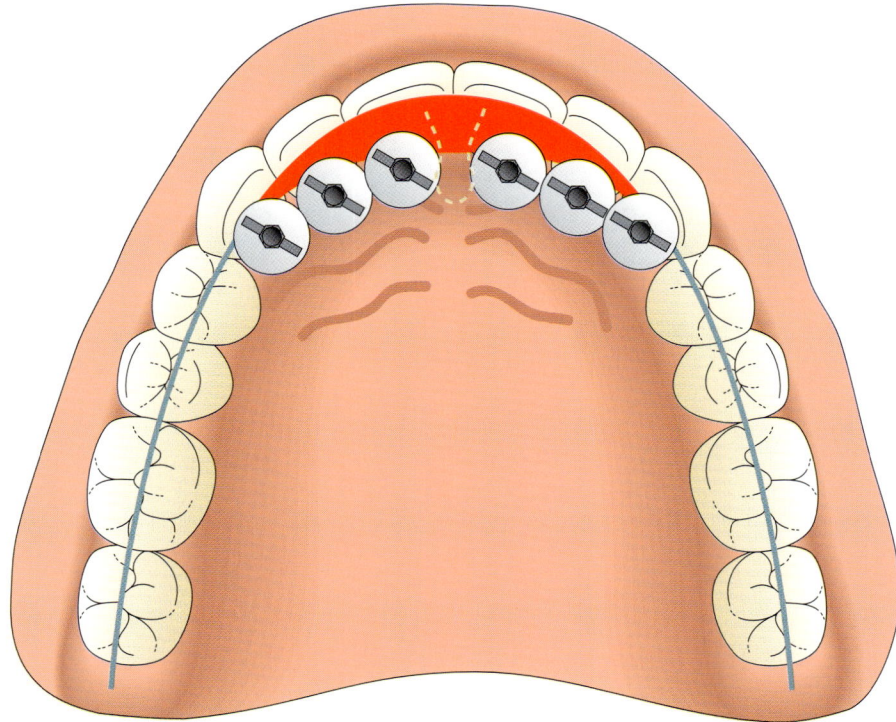

a

Fig 6-42 *(a and b)* Optimal implant positioning in the anterior maxilla when sufficient bone quantity is available. For example, when replacing six anterior teeth, the use of six implants is inadequate, because implants have to be placed in a palatal position and will be too proximal because of ridge resorption. A solution can be to place four implants in a lateral position, avoiding problems related to placement in the central position. In this manner the anterior ridge will be easier to manage and adequate lip support will be created.

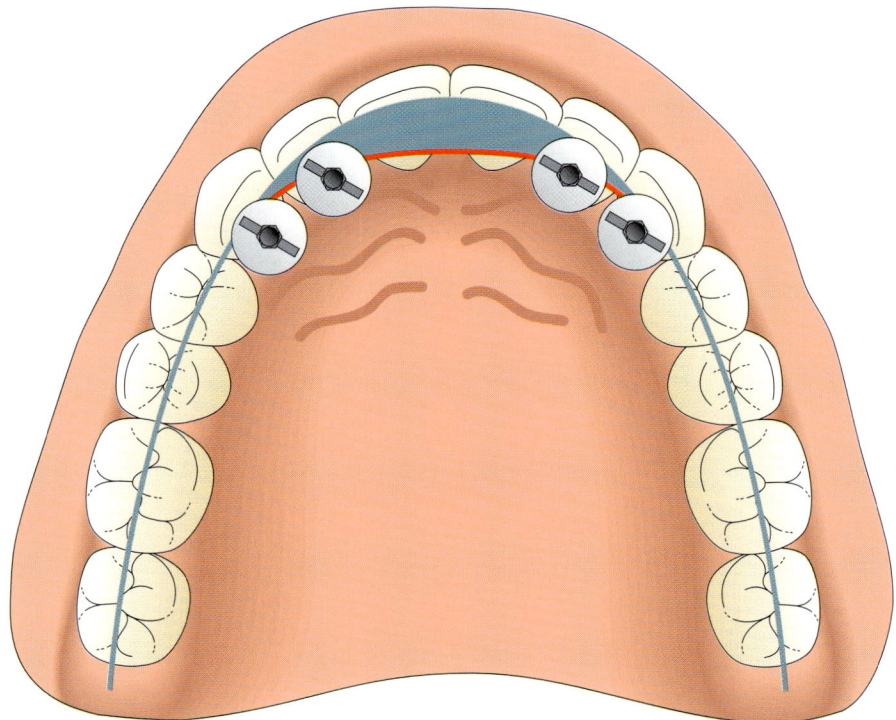

b

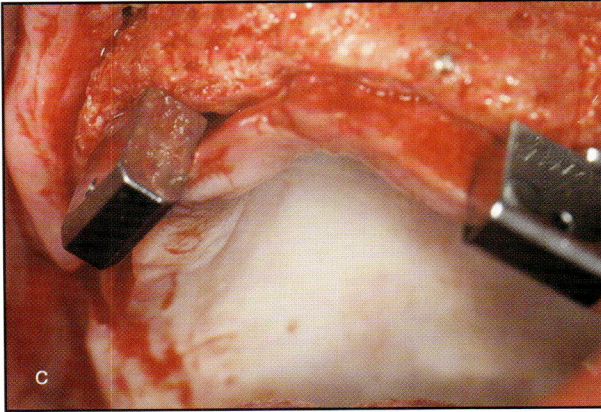

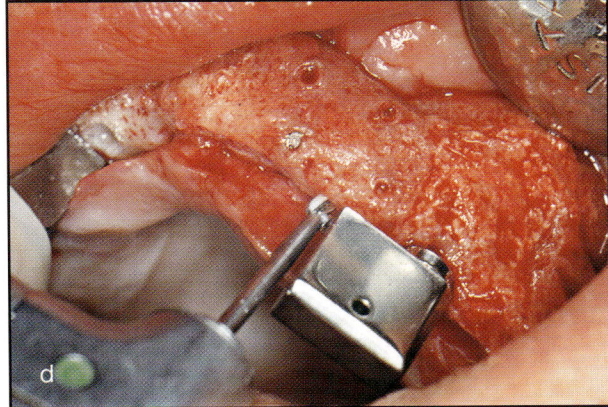

Fig 6-42 *(c and d)* When dealing with a maxilla, the drilling sequence can start in the canine area. Angulation can be checked using the milestone, then flags are used to locate the lateral incisor positions.

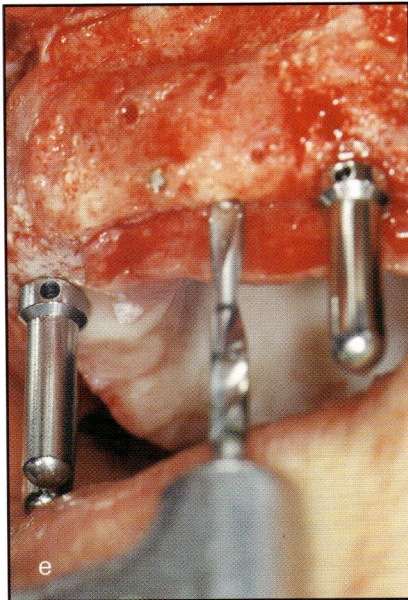

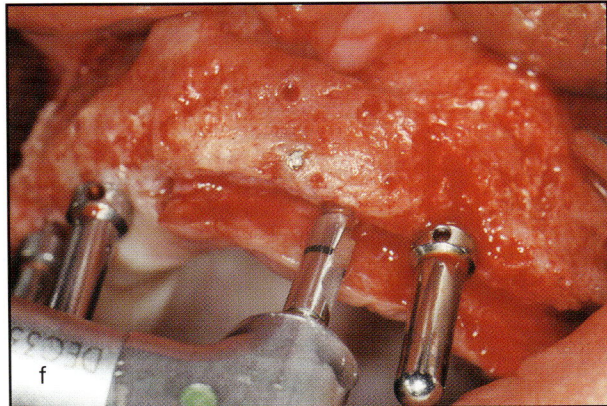

Fig 6-42 *(e and f)* The drilling sequence continues in the usual manner.

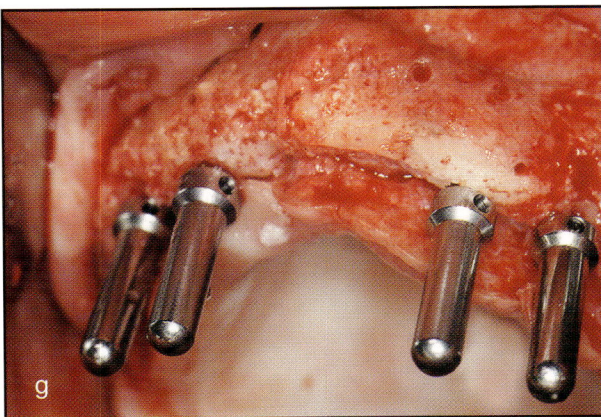

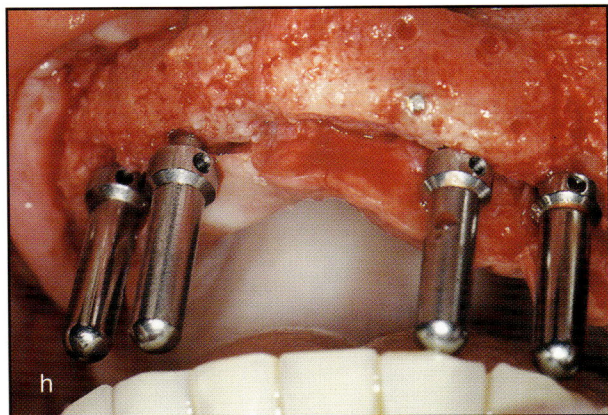

Fig 6-42 *(g and h)* By using implant-positioning guides, the surgeon can be sure there is adequate space between the implants as well as correct angulation. The distal implants will be placed using the same protocol.

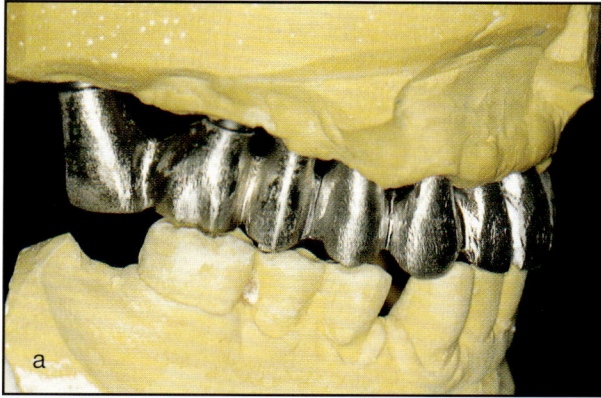

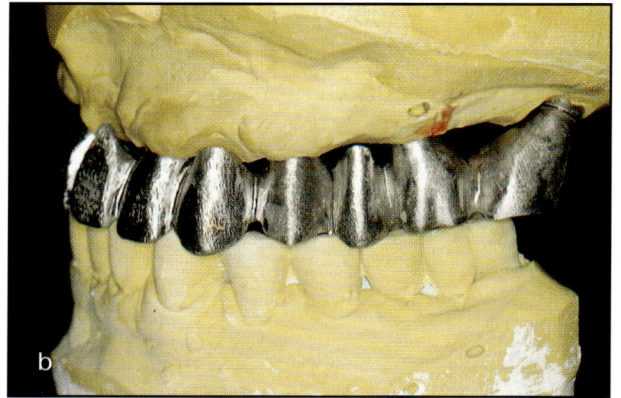

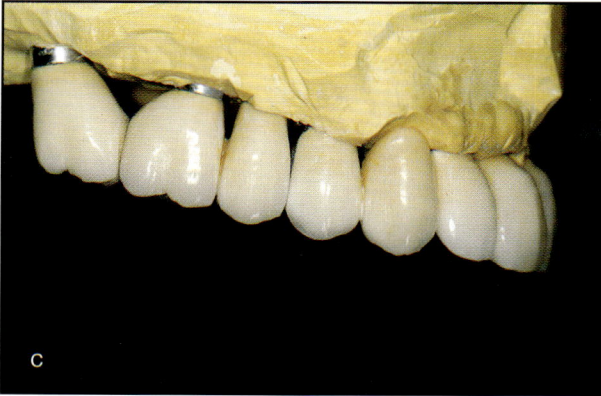

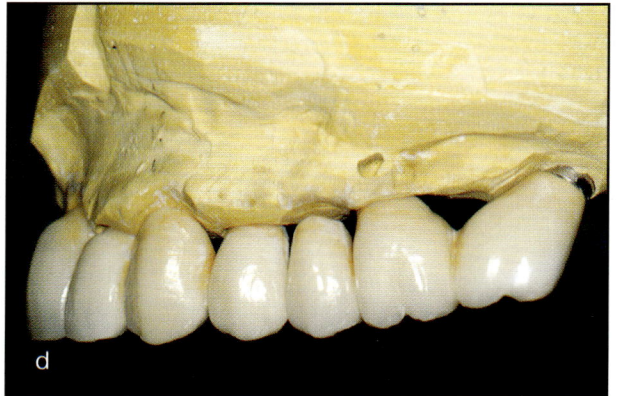

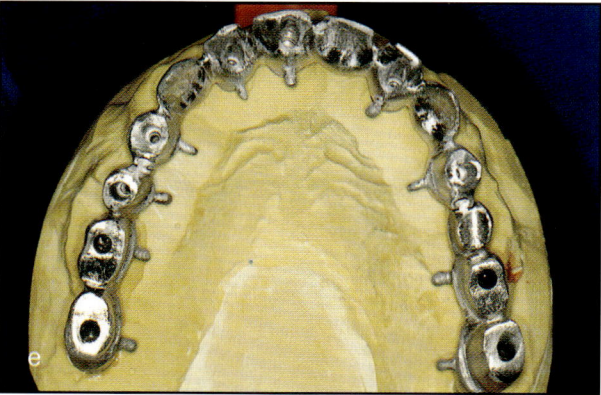

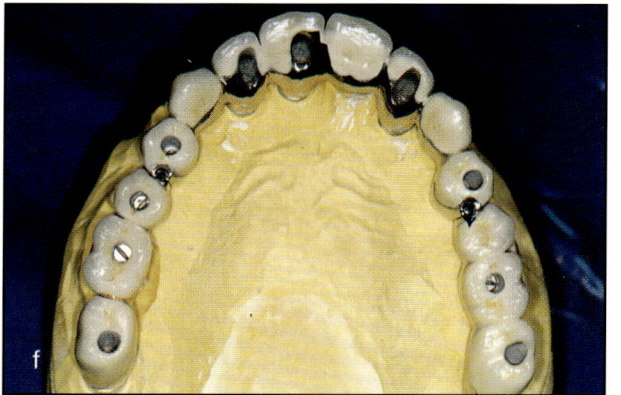

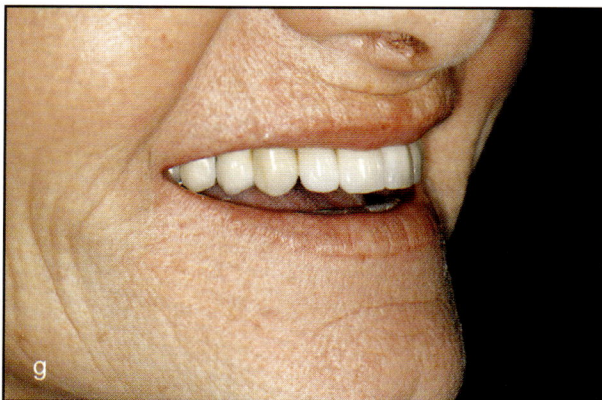

Fig 6-43 *(a and b)* Optimal implant positioning concept is illustrated on this cast of a maxillary implant restoration. *(c to f)* The lab technician can then build physiologic embrasures of teeth with a harmonious shape. Note the mesial angulation of the more distally placed implant and access holes located in the center of the future crowns. *(g)* Finished prosthesis in place. Note the adequate lip support.

Conclusion

Presurgical positioning guides and fixture positioning guides have been developed not only to simplify implant surgery but also to increase precision in implant placement. These tools are highly related to the implant placement philosophy:

– Respect of space between implants, allowing papilla formation and preservation, adequate embrasures, and good esthetics
– Optimal angulation of the implants being in relation with biomechanics as well as esthetics and function

A systematic use of these tools will provide the surgeon and the prosthodontist a reliable and reproducible treatment plan, avoiding problems and misunderstanding between the practitioners. Optimal implant positioning is becoming a reality for most of the treatment cases.

Reference

Adell R, Lekholm U, Brånemark P-I. Surgical procedures. In: Brånemark P-I, Zarb GA, Albrektsson T (eds). Tissue-Integrated Prostheses: Osseointegration in Clinical Dentistry. Chicago: Quintessence, 1985:211–232.

Chapter 7

Minor Bone Augmentation Procedures

Peter Moy, DMD, and Patrick Palacci, DDS

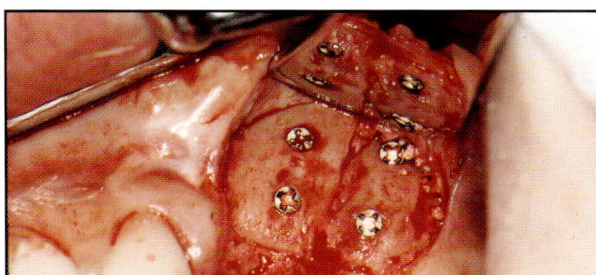

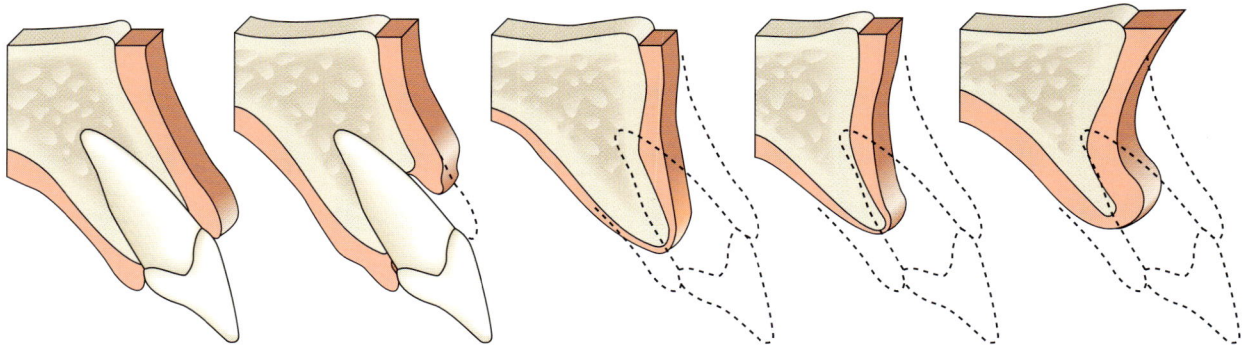

Fig 7-1 Resorption pattern often found in the anterior maxilla because of periodontal disease or trauma.

The progression of periodontal disease and traumatic injuries frequently result in tooth loss, as well as recession of hard and soft tissue. The resultant defective alveolar ridge presents a difficult problem for implant placement in the anterior maxilla. When the volume or contour of bone is inadequate, bone augmentation procedures are necessary to reconstruct the deficient alveolar ridge, thus allowing adequate osseous anchorage and permitting the placement of dental implants in the proper position and alignment.

Diagnosis of Deficient Osseous Ridges

Lekholm and Zarb (1985) classified the edentulous arch based on the amount of bone loss and the ratio of cortical to cancellous bone. In the partially edentulous arch, careful examination of the horizontal dimension of the edentulous ridge is critical to optimize the esthetic result of the implant-retained restoration (Figs 7-1 and 7-2). The anterior maxilla classification of Palacci and Ericsson (see Chapter 5) addresses horizontal and vertical tissues defects and should be considered in the surgical management of the anterior "esthetic zone." The loss of teeth, as well as change in osseous ridge contour, results in inadequate lip support (Fig 7-3).

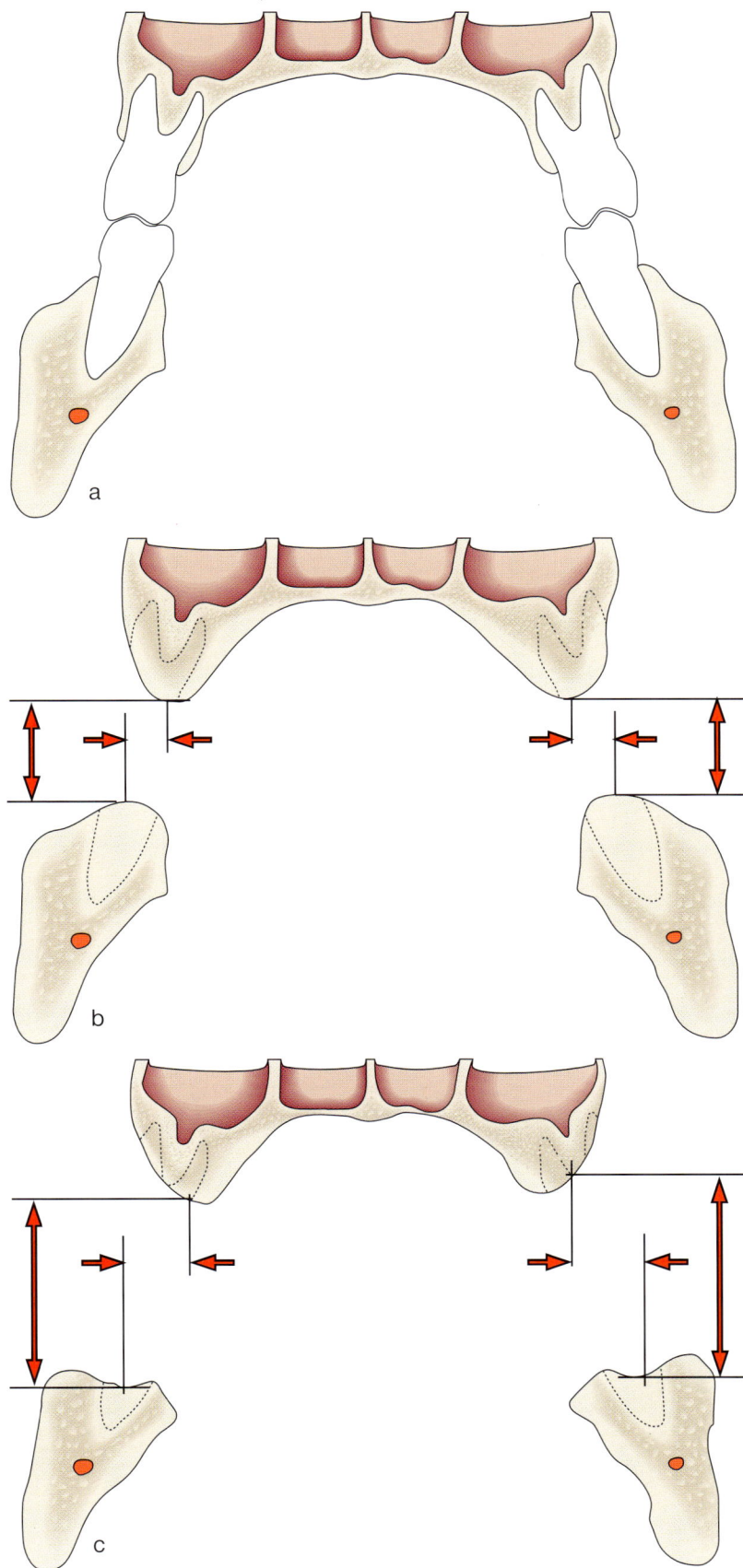

Fig 7-2 *(a)* Normal relationship of alveolar ridges when dentition is present. *(b)* Moderate resorption of alveolar ridges and the effects on the horizontal and vertical relationships of the ridges. *(c)* Severe resorption of alveolar ridges demonstrating an exponential increase in the vertical compared with the horizontal relationship.

To properly evaluate the volume of the residual ridge, a complete clinical examination that includes ridge mapping must be performed and the appropriate radiographs obtained. If a computed tomography (CT) scan is obtained, the use of a radiographic template will increase the amount of information obtained (Fig 7-4). The radiographic template may be converted into a surgical template and used during implant surgery (Fig 7-5). The positions of the pontic teeth are identified by radiopaque material (barium sulfate powder mixed with self-curing acrylic powder in a ratio of 1:3). The radiopaque tooth form is visualized on the axial views of the CT scans, giving the clinician additional information on the extent of horizontal bone loss in relationship to the shape of the crown, as well as on the appropriate implant position and angulation (Fig 7-6). Based on this information, the surgeon will be able to inform the patient about the specific osseous tissue-grafting procedure planned and discuss the various grafting materials that can be used.

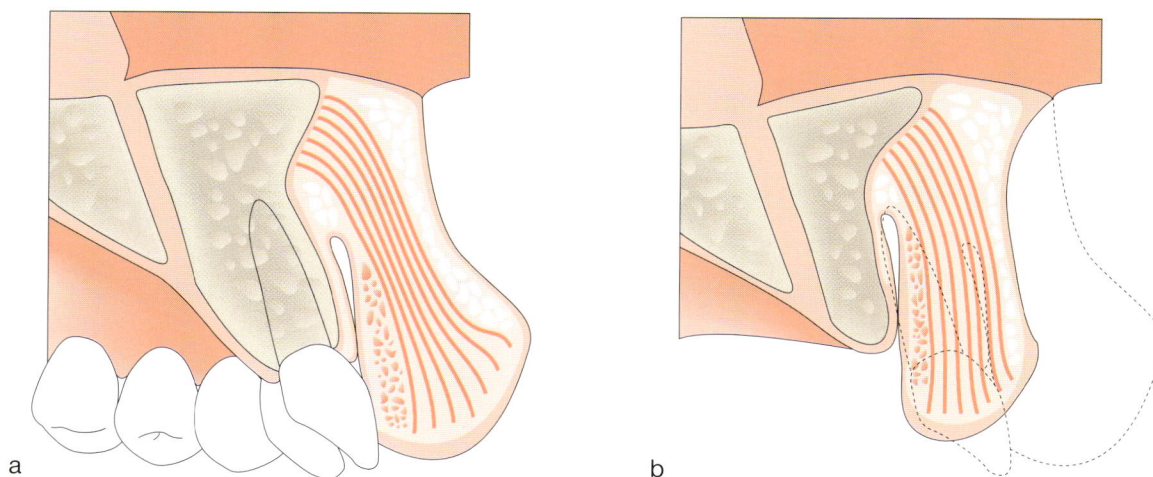

Fig 7-3 *(a)* Natural anatomical structures providing support for the upper lip. *(b)* Loss of lip support when teeth and/or alveolar ridge anatomy is lost.

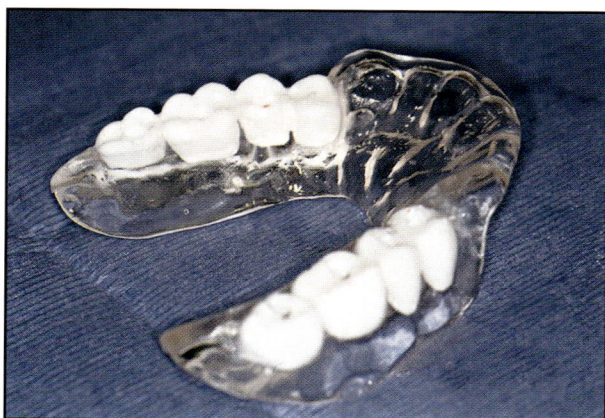

Fig 7-4 Radiographic template using barium sulfate powder.

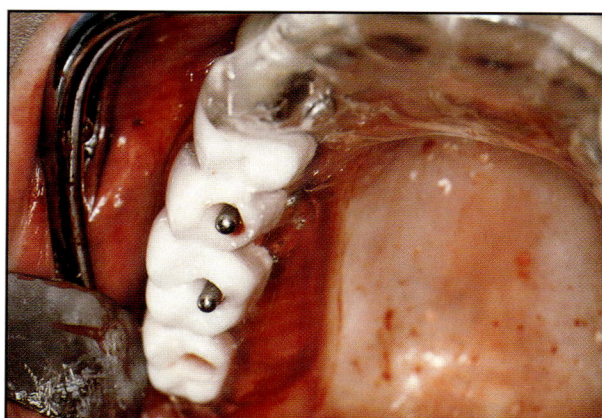

Fig 7-5 Converting a radiographic template into a surgical guide.

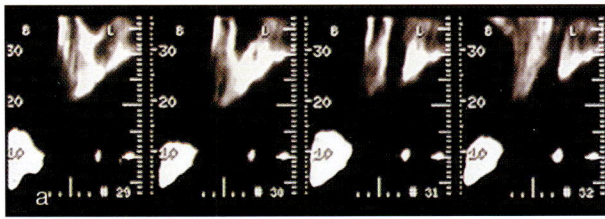

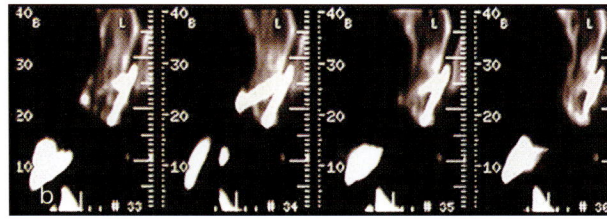

Fig 7-6 *(a)* Computed tomography scan revealing ridge volume that is inadequate for proper implant placement. *(b)* Computed tomography scan after an augmentation procedure increasing the ridge to permit ideal implant placement.

Bone-grafting Materials

A variety of donor sources have been used to provide osteoinduction or osteoconduction for bone-grafting procedures (Tolman 1995). The "gold standard" today for maxillary sinus augmentation and site development is autogenous bone, which may be harvested from either extraoral or intraoral sites. Other sources include allogenic and alloplastic materials.

Autogenous material

The advantages of using autogenous bone are its high osteogenic or osteoinductive potential; the rapid healing time of the grafted bone and of conversion to vital bone; and the ability of autogenous bone to yield various shapes (block form, saddle, or particulated), as well as particles large enough for use. The use of autogenous bone also has disadvantages. A secondary surgical site is required for harvesting donor bone. The pain and morbidity associated with the donor site, the increased surgical time, and the potential for a prolonged recuperation period are further disadvantages.

Extraoral donor sites

Typical extraoral donor sites of autogenous bone include the iliac crest (Keller et al 1987), tibia (Beirne and Brånemark 1980), or calvaria (Zins and Whitaker 1983). These donor sites are selected when the reconstruction involves large defects or alveolar ridges with severe bone loss. The disadvantages of using extraoral donor sites include the potential for increased morbidity (longer recuperation period, reduced ambulatory capacity, or external scarring), the need for two surgical sites, and the need for general anesthesia in the majority of cases. Advantages include the large quantity of available bone for harvesting, the increased osteogenic activity with this form of donor bone, and the ability to customize the donor bone to a variety of forms or shapes.

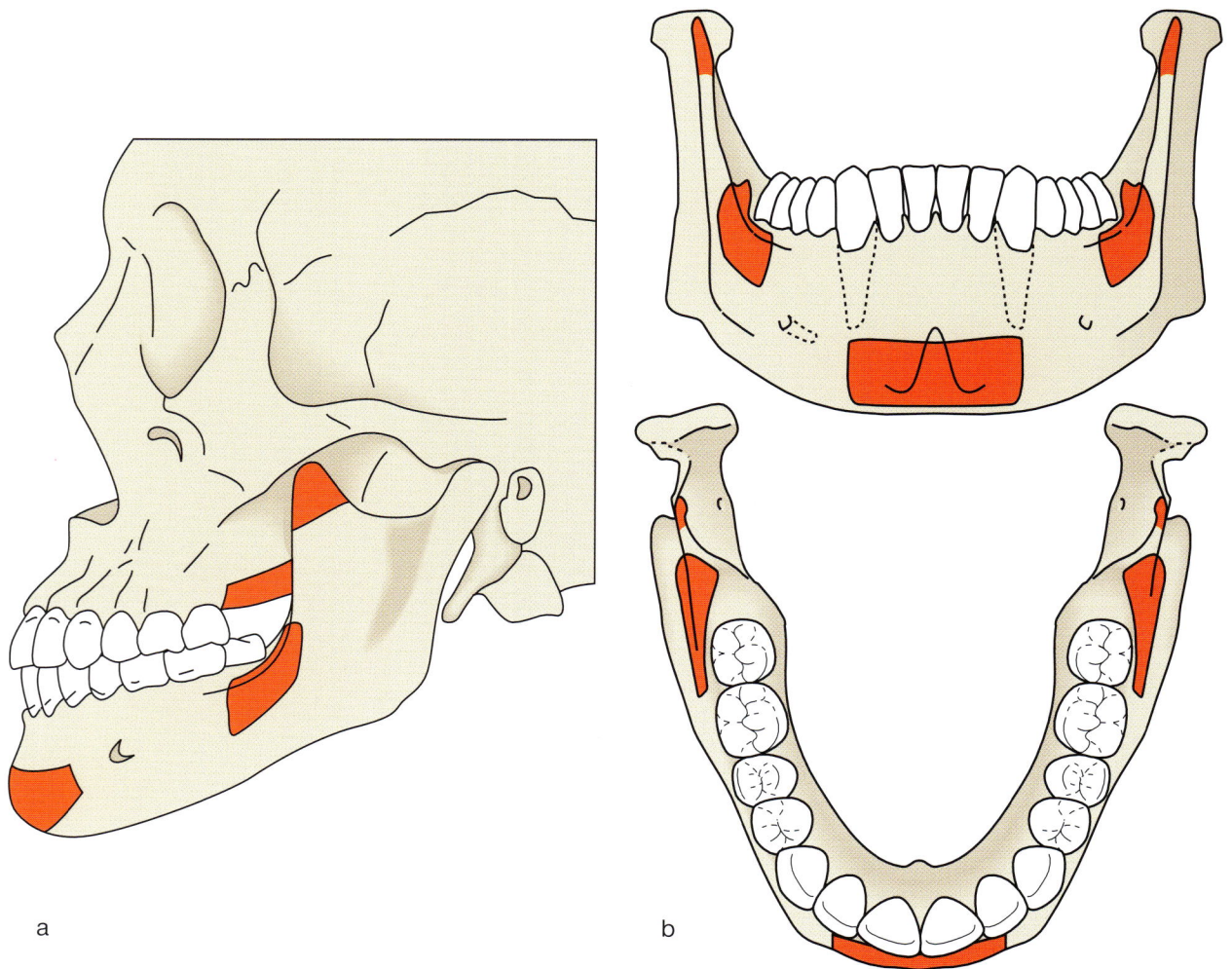

Fig 7-7 *(a)* Intraoral donor sites. *(b)* Intraoral donor sites in the mandible.

a

b

Intraoral donor sites

Intraoral bone donor sites include the tuberosity area or, more frequently, the chin (Wood and Moore 1988) or lateral ramus regions (Fig 7-7). Several techniques for harvesting bone in the chin area can be selected according to the size and type of defect to be treated. For narrow defects (for example, single-tooth loss), a vertical rectangular block is harvested from the midline of the chin (Fig 7-8a). For larger defects, one or two blocks can be harvested bilateral to the midline (Fig 7-8b). Several cores of bone can be harvested using a trephine and then particulated in a bone mill (Fig 7-8c).

A similar approach can be applied when harvesting bone from the ramus area, although a trephine technique is not recommended there. Because the ramus region has a thin buccolingual dimension, the use of a trephine would increase the risk of nerve injury. To minimize the risk of trauma to the neurovascular bundle, a thin fissure bur (for example, a No. 701 fissure bur) is recommended in performing the ostectomy. Thin cuts are made through the lateral cortical layer only. The rectangular cortical block of donor bone is removed using straight elevators.

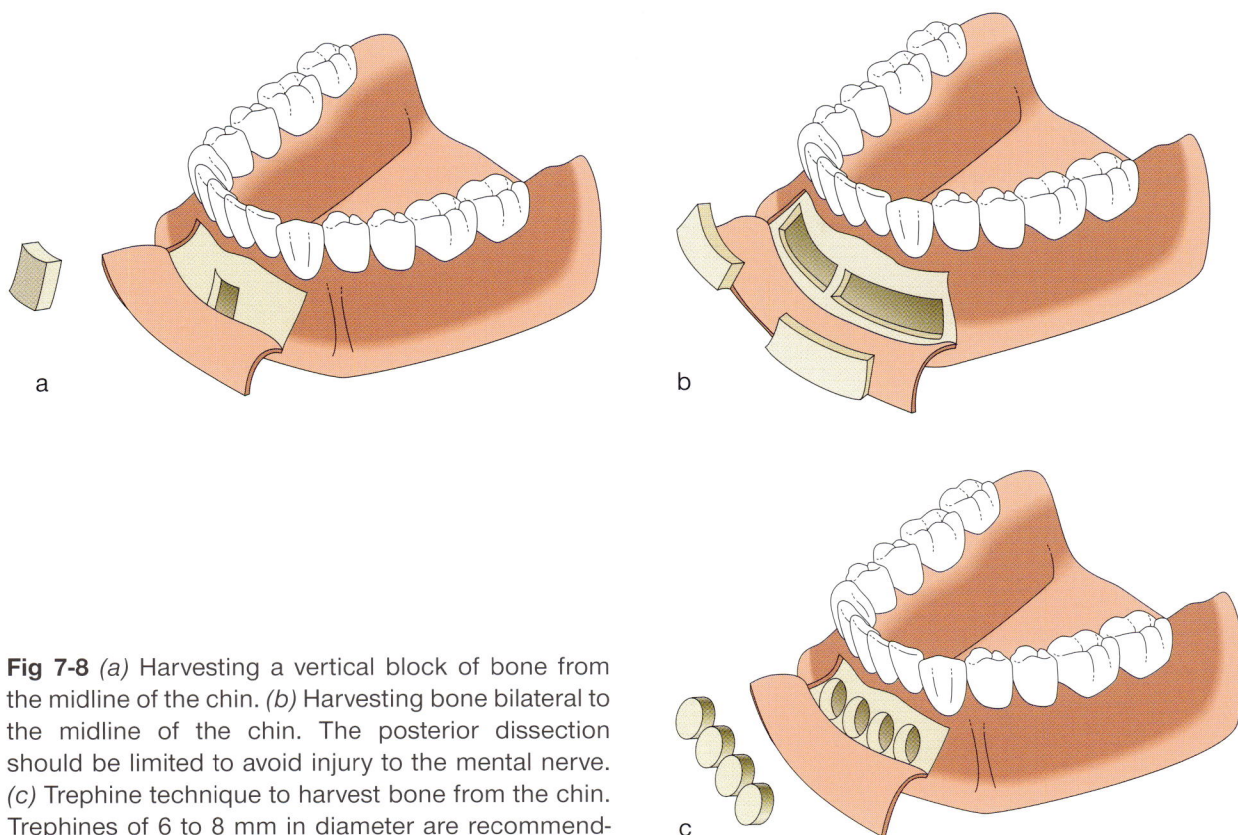

Fig 7-8 *(a)* Harvesting a vertical block of bone from the midline of the chin. *(b)* Harvesting bone bilateral to the midline of the chin. The posterior dissection should be limited to avoid injury to the mental nerve. *(c)* Trephine technique to harvest bone from the chin. Trephines of 6 to 8 mm in diameter are recommended.

The disadvantages of using intraoral donor sites are the limited volume of available bone and the anatomical limitations (risk of injury to neurovascular structures or dentition). However, there are several advantages of using intraoral donor sites. Both the donor and recipient sites are located intraorally. Lower morbidity is associated with an intraoral procedure (faster recovery period, less blood loss, and no visible scarring). Finally, general anesthesia is typically not required.

Intraoral donor sites are the primary choice in cases of limited defects (for example, unilateral sinus-grafting procedures) or moderate resorption of the alveolar ridges. In the reconstruction of larger defects or in bilateral situations, harvesting from a combination of intraoral donor sites may be necessary (ramus plus chin or bilateral ramus regions).

Allogenic material

Allogenic bone (freeze-dried or lyophilized) has been used extensively for intraoral augmentation procedures, especially in conjunction with grafting procedures around dental implants (Landsberg et al 1994). Early work by Urist (1965) showed that osteoinduction with formation of viable bone was possible using freeze-dried bone allograft (FDBA). Further studies by Urist and coworkers (1968) revealed that FDBAs induce new bone formation by an inductive substratum, later termed *bone morphogenetic protein* (BMP). Freeze-dried bone allografts have been used for both maxillary sinus augmentation and augmentation of deficient alveolar ridges.

The use of FDBA has several advantages. It eliminates the need to create a second surgical site, thus shortening the surgical time and recovery period. It is readily available in a variety of particle sizes and in unlimited volume. Finally, it is cost-effective. One of the disadvantages of using FDBA is the time required for the osteoinduction phase (generally twice as long as for autogenous bone). Also, only the particulate form of FDBA is used intraorally to correct defects, thus limiting the ability to correct certain contour deficits. Freeze-dried bone allografts also carry a potential, although a very low probability, for an antigenic response.

Alloplastic material

A third source of donor material is alloplastic material. This category includes the hydroxyapatites (Holmes and Hagler 1988), tri-calcium phosphates (Jarcho 1986), and xenograft materials (Bio-oss and Osteograft) (Haas et al 1998). Alloplastic material has the same advantages as FDBA; in addition, the use of alloplastic material eliminates the risk of a possible antigenic response. The major disadvantage of the use of alloplastic material is that it is only osteoconductive. Because the material lacks viable cells and is unable to release BMP, alloplastic particles can act only as a scaffold or matrix to assist in the bone formation process. Alloplastic material is most often used as an additive material with autogenous bone to increase the volume of donor bone.

Management of Maxillary Ridge Deficiencies

The correction of alveolar ridge deficiencies in the maxilla can be separated into two categories because of differences in anatomy, masticatory forces, and resorption patterns.

These variations have resulted in different osseous defects in the posterior versus the anterior maxilla. Thus, surgical procedures to correct osseous deficiencies must be customized for the particular region of the maxilla.

Posterior maxilla

The posterior maxilla is unique in that the masticatory forces are predominantly vertical, leading to loss of osseous ridge height from the occlusal perspective and less so from the horizontal perspective. The presence of the maxillary sinus cavity and the descending floor of the cavity because of pneumatization as the patient ages further reduce the ridge height (Fig 7-9). Onlay or inlay techniques are the treatment of choice in the posterior maxilla.

Onlay technique

The onlay technique (Fig 7-10) is indicated when resorption has occurred at the crest of the ridge with no supraeruption of the opposing dentition. This technique is contraindicated in the presence of supraerupted molars in the opposing arch, because interocclusal space is limited. The onlay technique requires a cortical-cancellous block of bone, autogenous bone being the donor material of choice. Particulated donor material is not indicated, because the particulate graft is unable to withstand the compressive forces generated during mastication.

The intraoral cavity is the donor site of choice for harvesting a cortical-cancellous block for use as an onlay graft. The ascending ramus, which usually provides a graft 3 to 4 mm thick, is an appropriate donor site. Careful radiologic examination to precisely locate the mandibular nerve will avoid any nerve injury during harvesting (Fig 7-11). This type of graft will provide the additional ridge height necessary to correct the vertical defect in the deficient posterior maxilla, as well as to resist

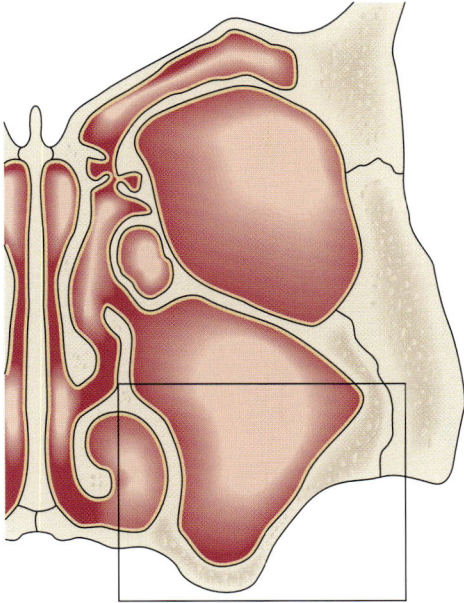

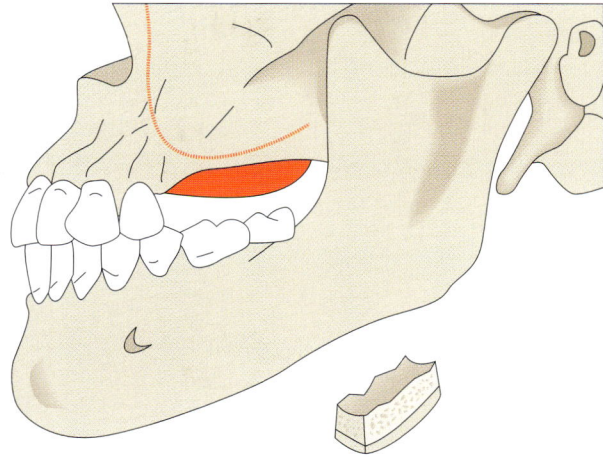

Fig 7-9 Pneumatization process of the maxillary sinus. The floor of the sinus has dropped below the nasal floor into the superior aspect of the residual alveolar ridge.

Fig 7-10 A posterior onlay graft is indicated when resorption has occurred within the alveolar ridge and the opposing molars have not supraerupted.

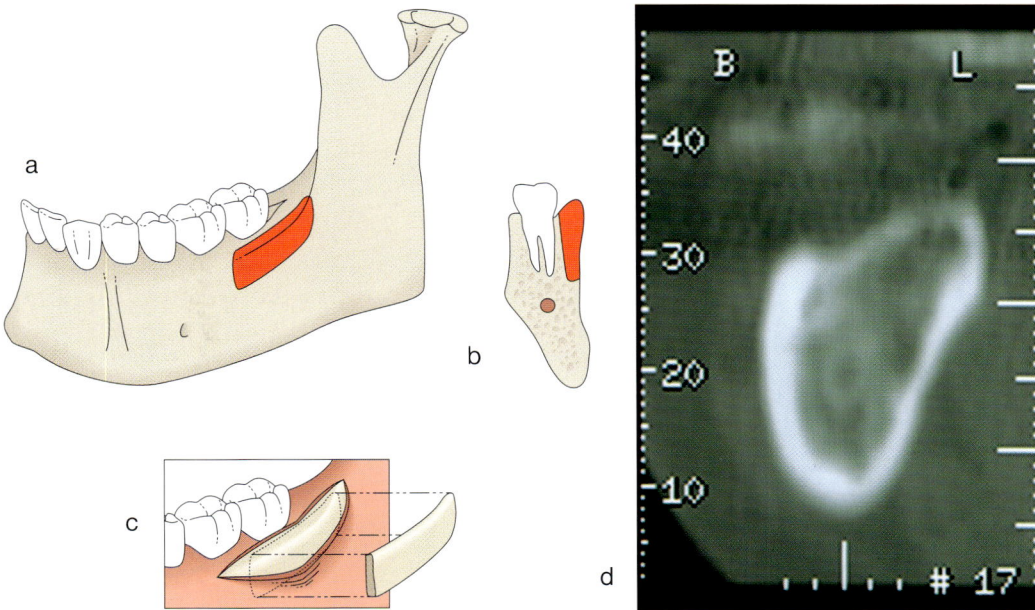

Fig 7-11 *(a to c)* Donor site in the ramus region. The graft is harvested laterally from the second molar area in a distal direction. *(d)* Location of the inferior alveolar nerve in relationship to the lateral ramus.

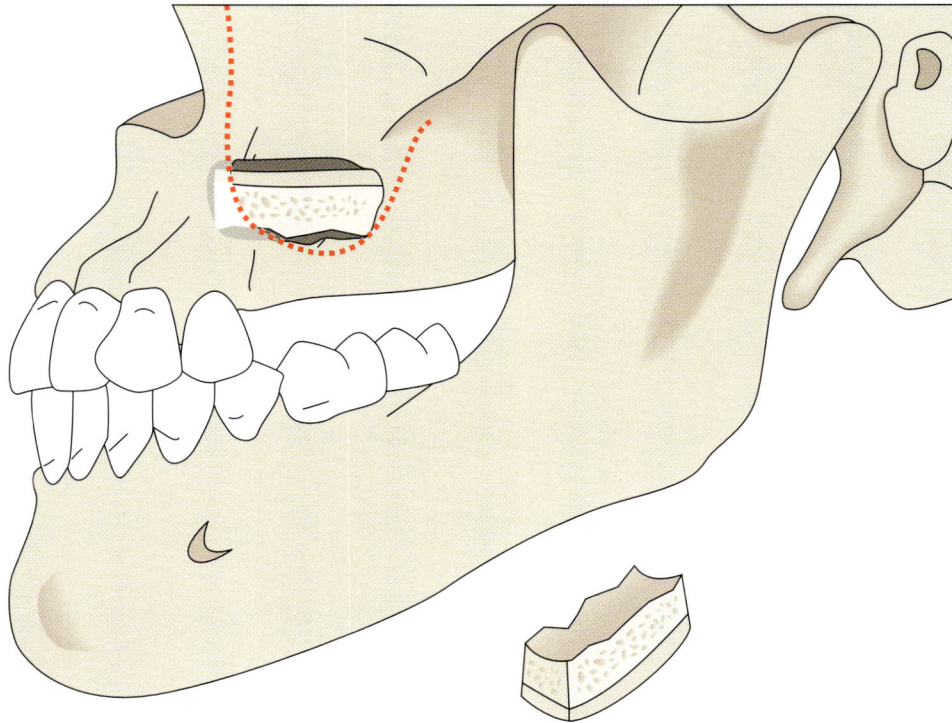

Fig 7-12 A sinus inlay graft is indicated when resorption is mainly caused by pneumatization and the opposing molars have supraerupted.

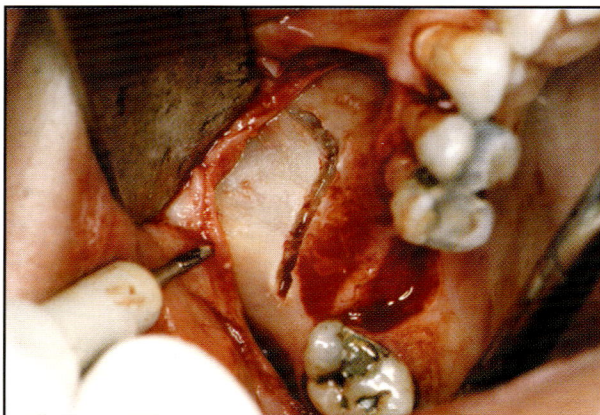

Fig 7-13 Osteotomy of the lateral wall of the maxillary sinus using a fissure bur.

resorption that is due to vertical masticatory forces.

Inlay technique

When resorption of ridge height is minimal but bone volume is lacking (Fig 7-12), a sinus inlay graft is indicated. Placing the bone graft into the sinus cavity adds height but does not reduce the interocclusal space. The use of a variety of donor materials, as well as combinations of materials, has been reported for the augmentation of the sinus cavity. Although studies have shown new bone formation with many of these materials, the material of choice remains autogenous bone (Jensen and Sennerby 1998).

Sinus augmentation technique

An osteotomy using a round or fissure bur with copious irrigation will create a rectangular window in the lateral wall of the maxillary sinus (Fig 7-13). Optimum care must be used to avoid cutting through the medial side and damaging the sinus membrane of the maxillary sinus. An infractured technique, in which

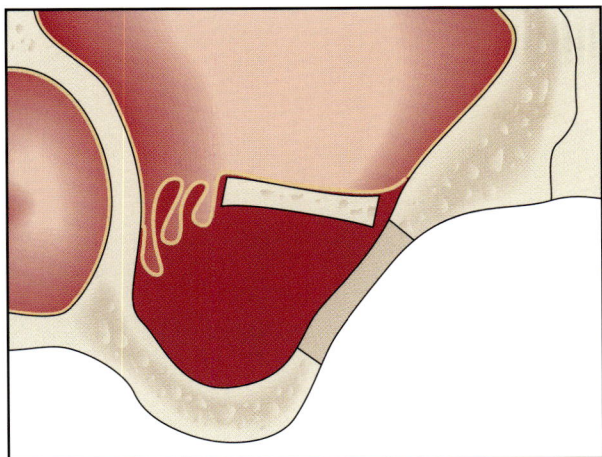

Fig 7-14 Approach to the maxillary sinus using infractured technique.

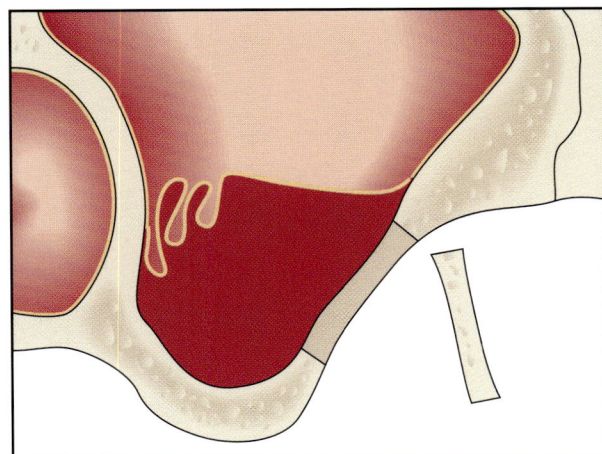

Fig 7-15 Classic approach to the maxillary sinus by removing the lateral osseous window.

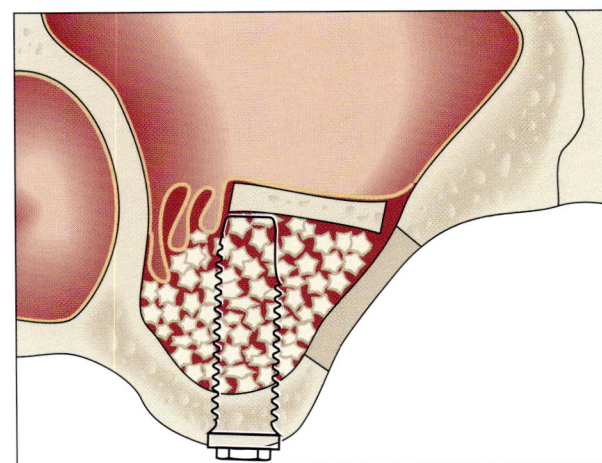

Fig 7-16 The elevation of the sinus membrane permits placement of graft material to maximize the height gain.

the osseous window is pushed inward, may be used. This bony window remains attached to the membrane and is deflected medially, the membrane being elevated from the medial side of the sinus cavity (Fig 7-14). For greater visibility, this bony window can also be removed before elevation of the sinus membrane (Fig 7-15). After the osteotomy has been completed, a smooth curette is used to gently lift the osseous window off the membrane. The dissection of the membrane from the medial wall continues with a Freer-type dissector. The main advantage of this technique (Boyne and James 1980) is the unobstructed access to the elevation of the sinus membrane, which will reduce the incidence of membrane tearing. The donor bone can be particulated or left as a cortical-cancellous block when placed in the sinus cavity (Fig 7-16).

Advantages of the block graft are resistance to resorption and ease of handling (Keller et al 1999). However, the difficulty in obtaining a perfect fit of the block of bone to the contour variations within the sinus cavity may result in undesirable spaces at the bony interface. The advantages of particulated autogenous bone are faster resorption, which leads to an earlier osteoinduction phase of bone formation, and the ability to compress the particulate graft into the sinus cavity to fill in the contour variations, thus reducing the number of spaces between the recipient bed and the donor material. Another benefit of particulating the donor material is the ability to mix the autogenous bone with other synthetic alloplastic materials. This technique increases the total volume of donor material available to fill in the larger sinus cavities. Particulated donor bone is most often used in sinus augmentation procedures because of the ability of the cavity to contain the particulated material.

Sinus augmentation, as well as posterior ridge augmentation, permits placement of

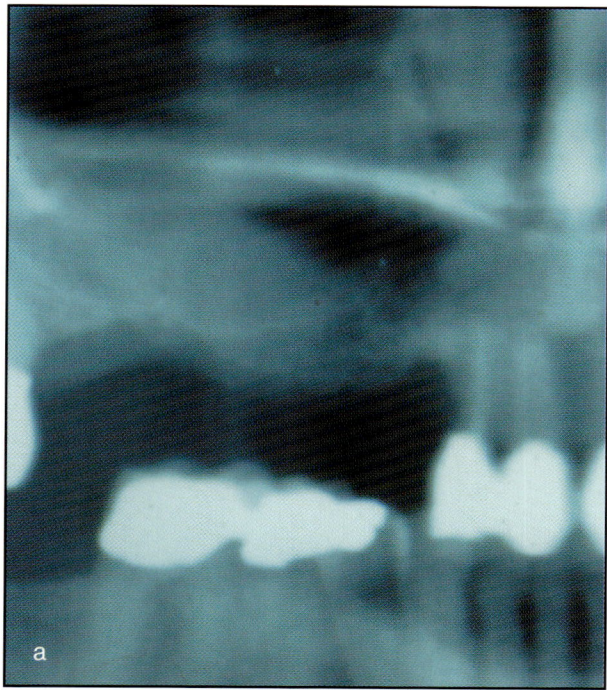
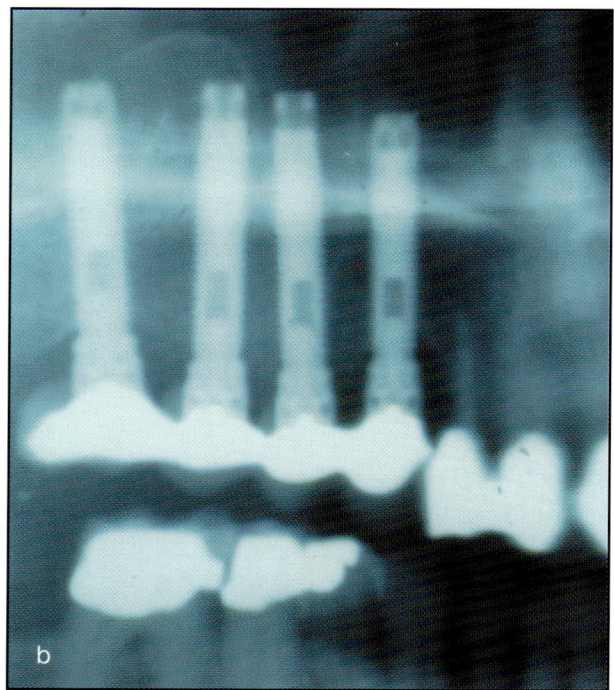

Fig 7-17 (a) Panoramic radiograph revealing a pneumatized sinus with less than 2 mm of residual alveolar ridge. (b) Post-treatment radiograph showing maximum vertical augmentation permitting the placement of 20-mm implants.

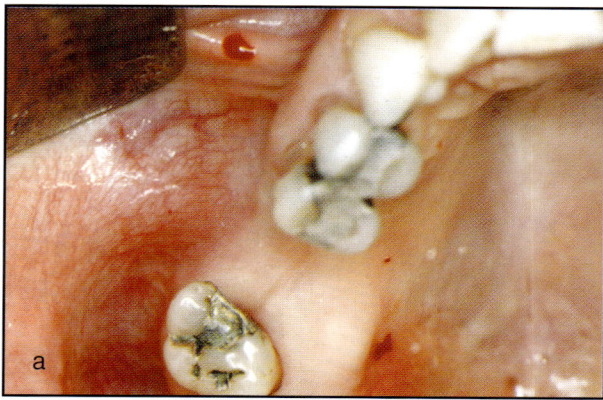
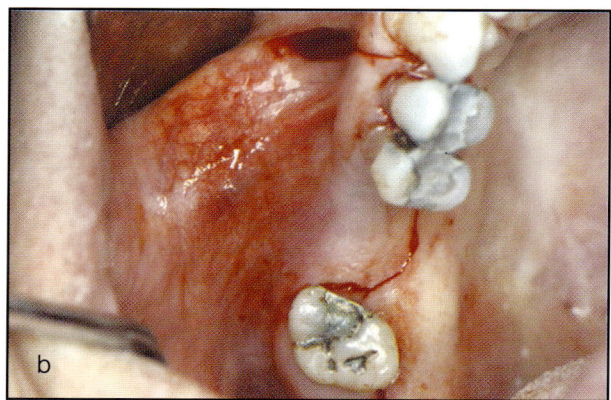
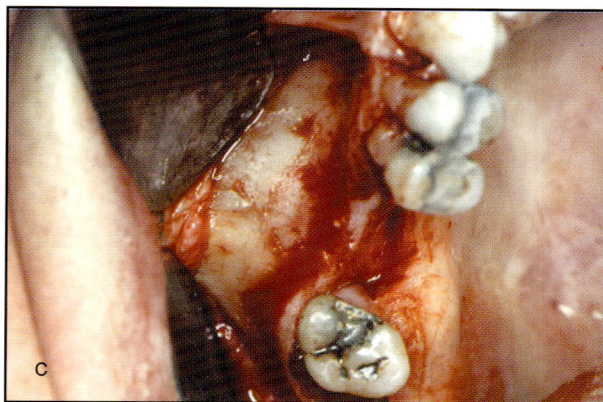

Fig 7-18 (a) Edentulous zone to be treated by implant placement. Bone resorption and sinus pneumatization are such that bone augmentation is necessary to place an implant. (b) Palatal incision. The releasing incisions are located distal to the second molar and anterior to the first premolar. (c) A full-thickness flap is reflected to expose the labial plate of the ridge.

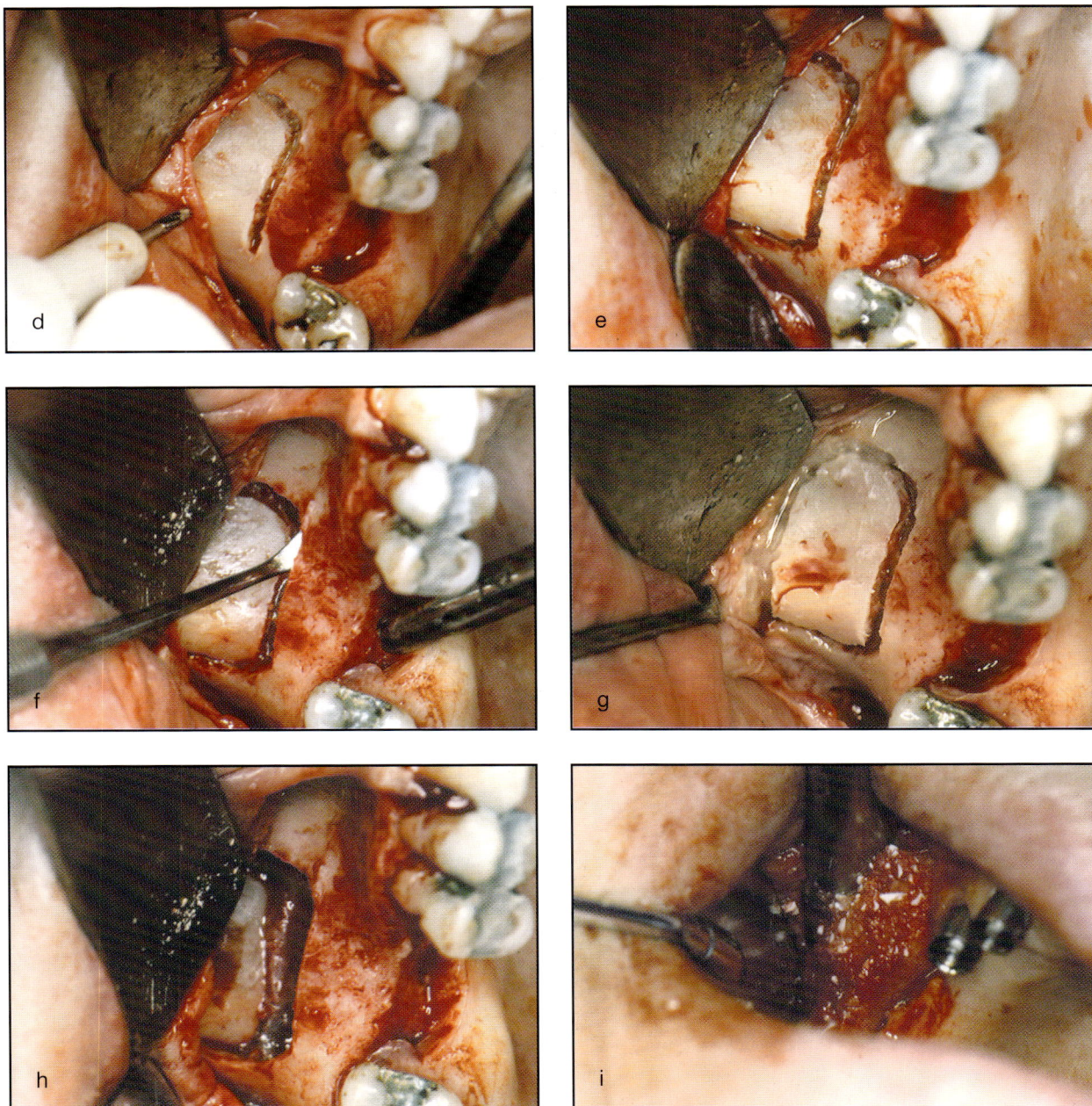

Fig 7-18 *(d and e)* Using a fissure bur, an osteotomy will create a window in the lateral wall of the sinus. *(f to h)* The sinus membrane is carefully lifted using a smooth curette. *(i)* Clinical view of the grafted site with autogenous bone graft.

implants in sites where implant placement was previously not possible (Fig 7-17a). It also permits the placement of longer implants and creates a more favorable biomechanical situation by reducing the implant-to-crown ratio (Fig 7-17b). When properly planned and executed, these surgical techniques allow the treatment of the severely atrophic posterior maxillary ridge using a predictable, fixed prosthetic restoration (Fig 7-18).

Anterior maxilla

Grafting in the anterior maxilla requires a different approach and techniques. Restoration in the esthetic zone often requires augmentation in both a horizontal and vertical dimension. However, the alveolar crest does not provide a natural cavity to contain the particulated graft materials, as the sinus cavity does. Therefore, donor bone must have strength and rigidity, as well as permit fixation of the graft with a secure fit in the recipient bed (Fig 7-19). Therefore, a cortical-cancellous block is most often used for grafting in the anterior maxilla. The three techniques most frequently used are: the veneer graft (Fig 7-20), onlay graft (Fig 7-21), and saddle graft (Fig 7-22). Each type of graft is used to augment the ridge in different directions, depending on the type of defect. For example, veneer grafts are used to restore isolated horizontal defects, and onlay grafts correct vertical deficiencies. In short, inlay grafts correct volume deficiencies; veneer grafts, width deficiencies; and onlay grafts, height deficiencies. Saddle grafts correct deficiencies in both height and width. To correct problems in height, width, and contour, combination grafts are used.

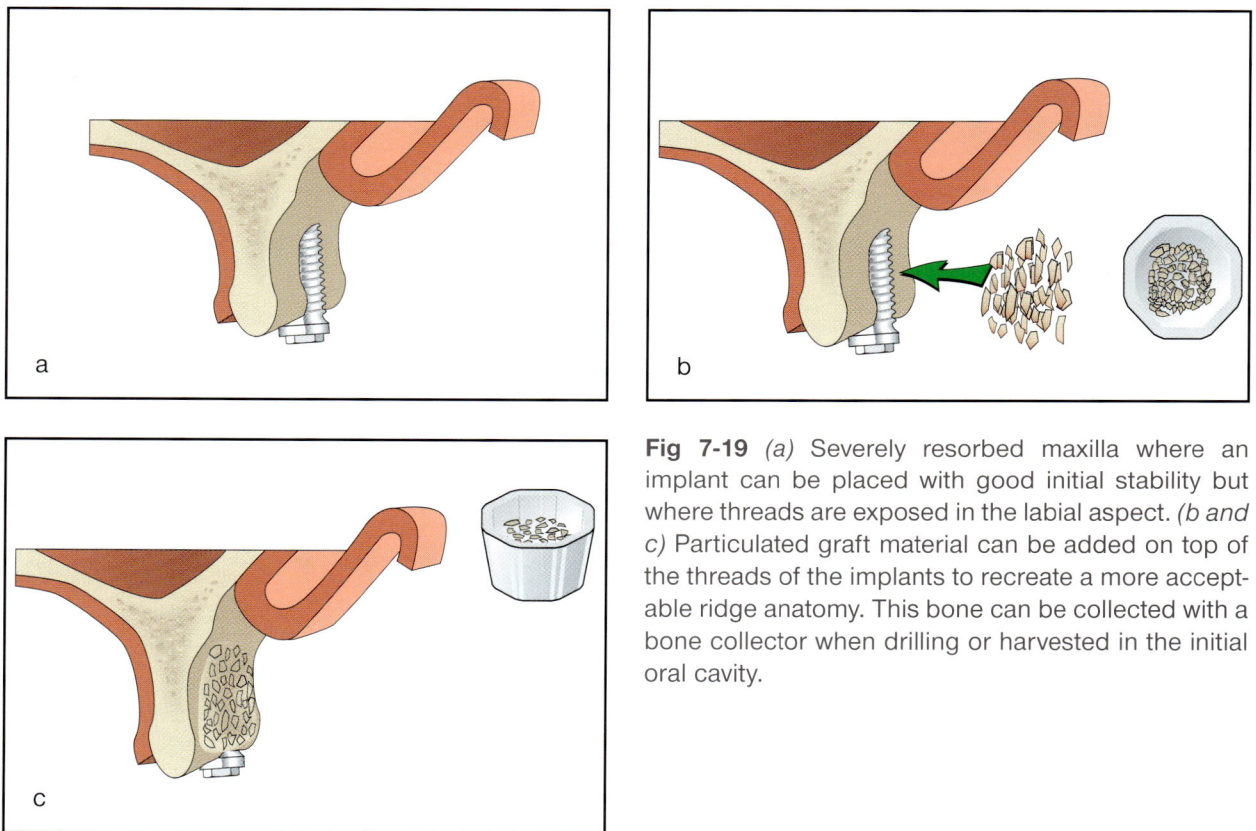

Fig 7-19 *(a)* Severely resorbed maxilla where an implant can be placed with good initial stability but where threads are exposed in the labial aspect. *(b and c)* Particulated graft material can be added on top of the threads of the implants to recreate a more acceptable ridge anatomy. This bone can be collected with a bone collector when drilling or harvested in the initial oral cavity.

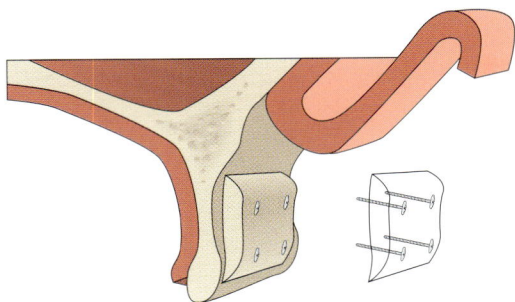

a

Fig 7-20 *(a)* A schematic drawing illustrating a veneer graft.

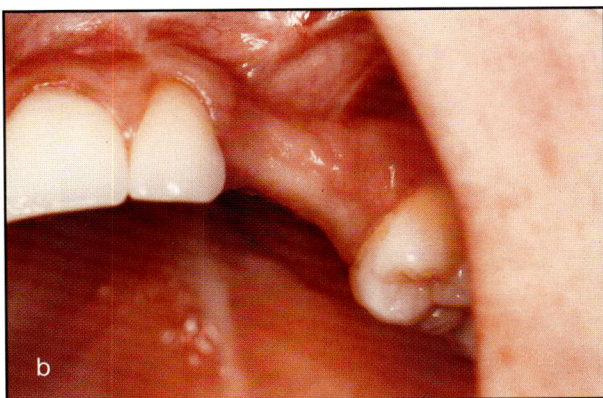

b

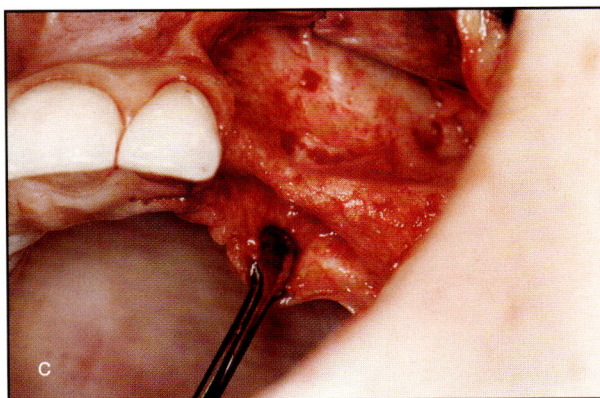

c

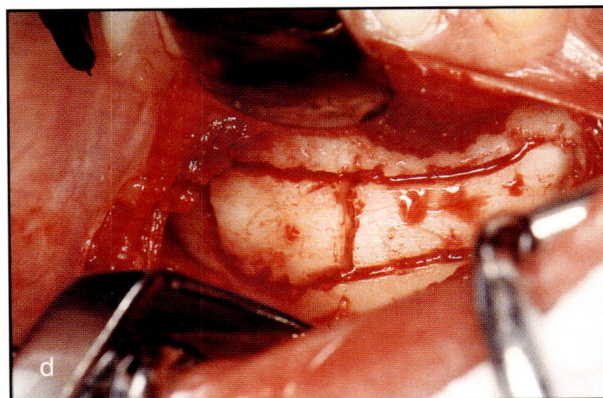

d

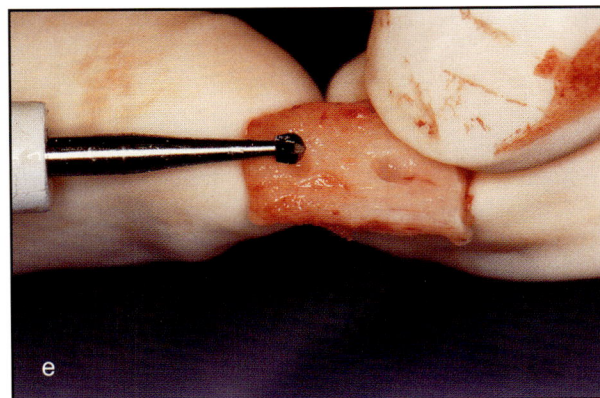

e

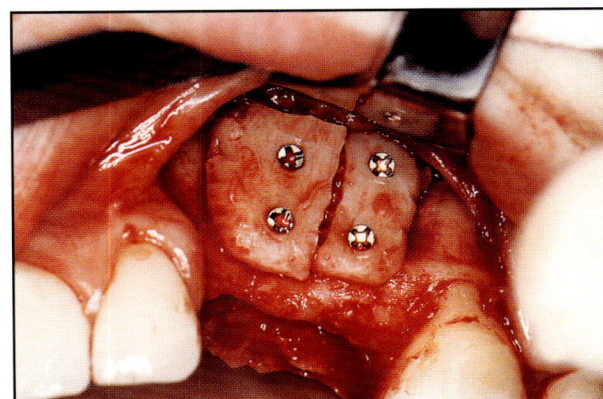

Fig 7-20 *(b and c)* Severely resorbed, horizontally deficient maxillary ridge. Full-thickness flap is reflected to expose the atrophic, partially edentulous ridge. *(d)* Harvesting of block graft from the chin area. *(e and f)* Shaping the donor bone to fit properly in the recipient bed. A small round bur is used to countersink the cortical layer so the heads of the fixation screws will be flush with the cortical bone surface. Veneer grafts are fixed securely to the recipient bed using 1.5-mm-diameter fixation screws.

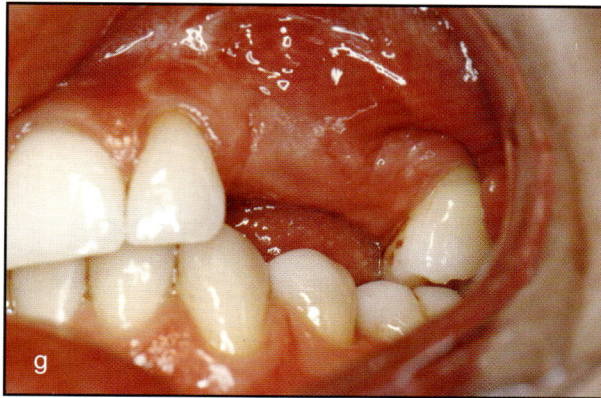

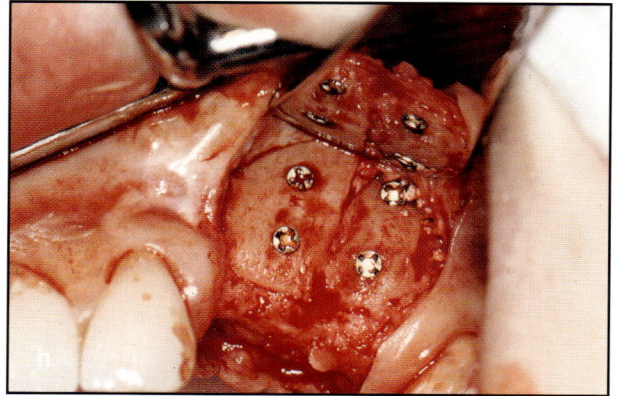

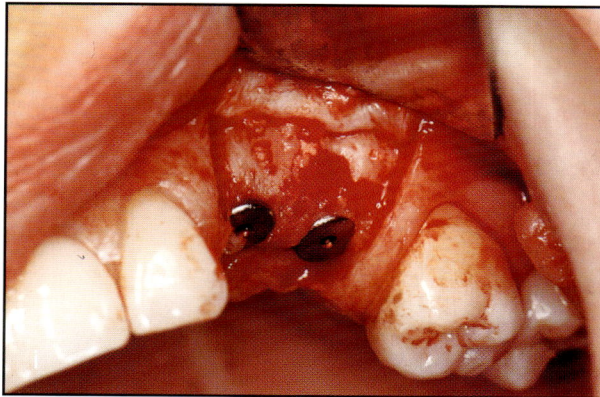

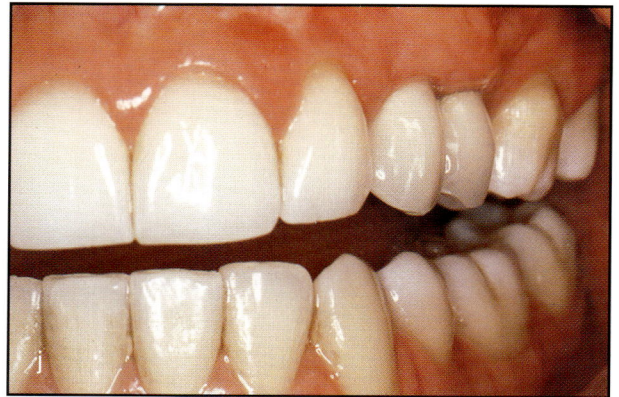

Fig 7-20 (g) Six months after augmentation of the deficient maxillary ridge. (h) Elevation of the soft tissue flap to reposition the consolidated bone graft during the implant placement procedure. (i) The fixation screws have been removed and the implants secured in position. (j) Frontal view of final restorations. (k) Lateral view of final restorations. Note the re-establishment of the natural contours of osseous and gingival tissue.

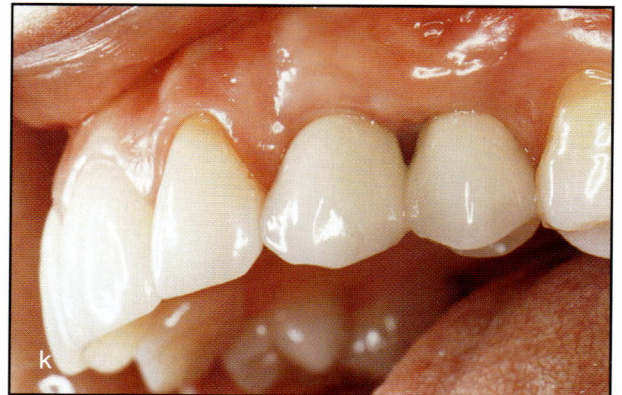

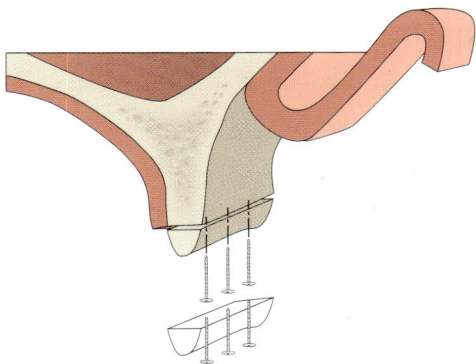

a

Fig 7-21 (a) Schematic drawing illustrating an onlay graft.

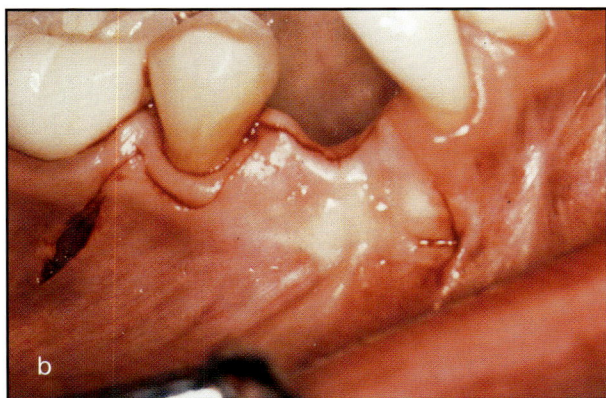

b

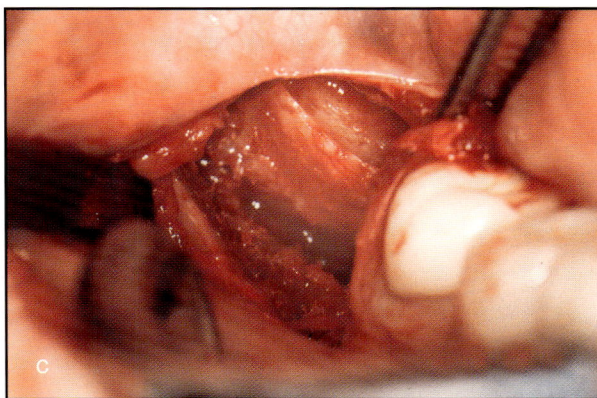

c

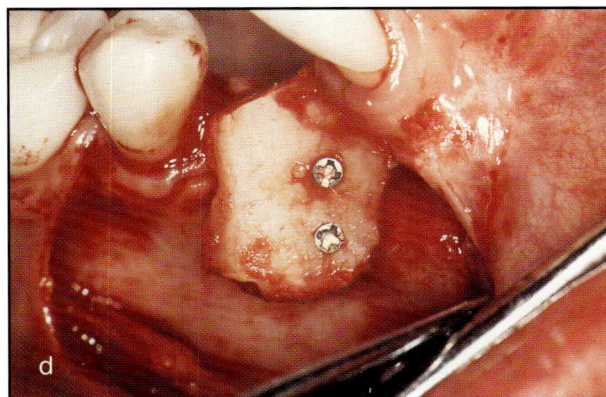

d

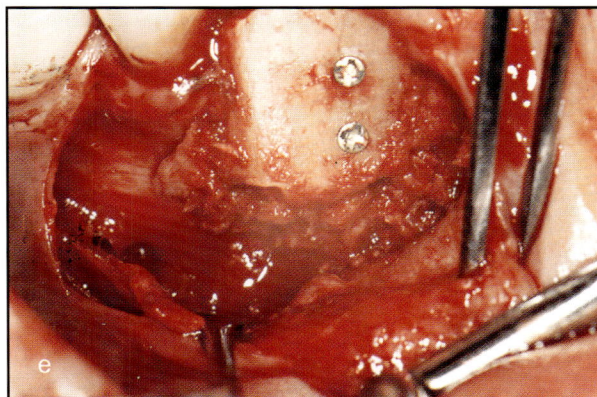

e

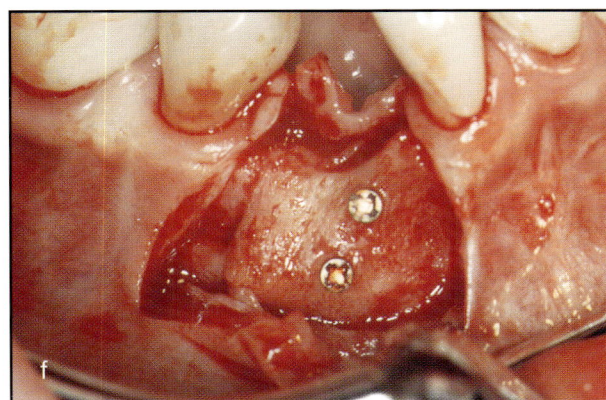

f

Fig 7-21 (b) Severely resorbed mandibular ridge after the traumatic loss of a canine. (c) Flap designed to avoid deflection of periodontal tissue from adjacent natural dentition. (d) Harvesting autogenous bone from the lateral ramus region limits the anterior portion of bone cut distal to the second molar. (e) Donor bone adapted to the recipient bed and secured in position with 1.5-mm-diameter rigid fixation screws. (f) Residual areas of the alveolar defect corrected with the remaining cancellous bone and cortical chips.

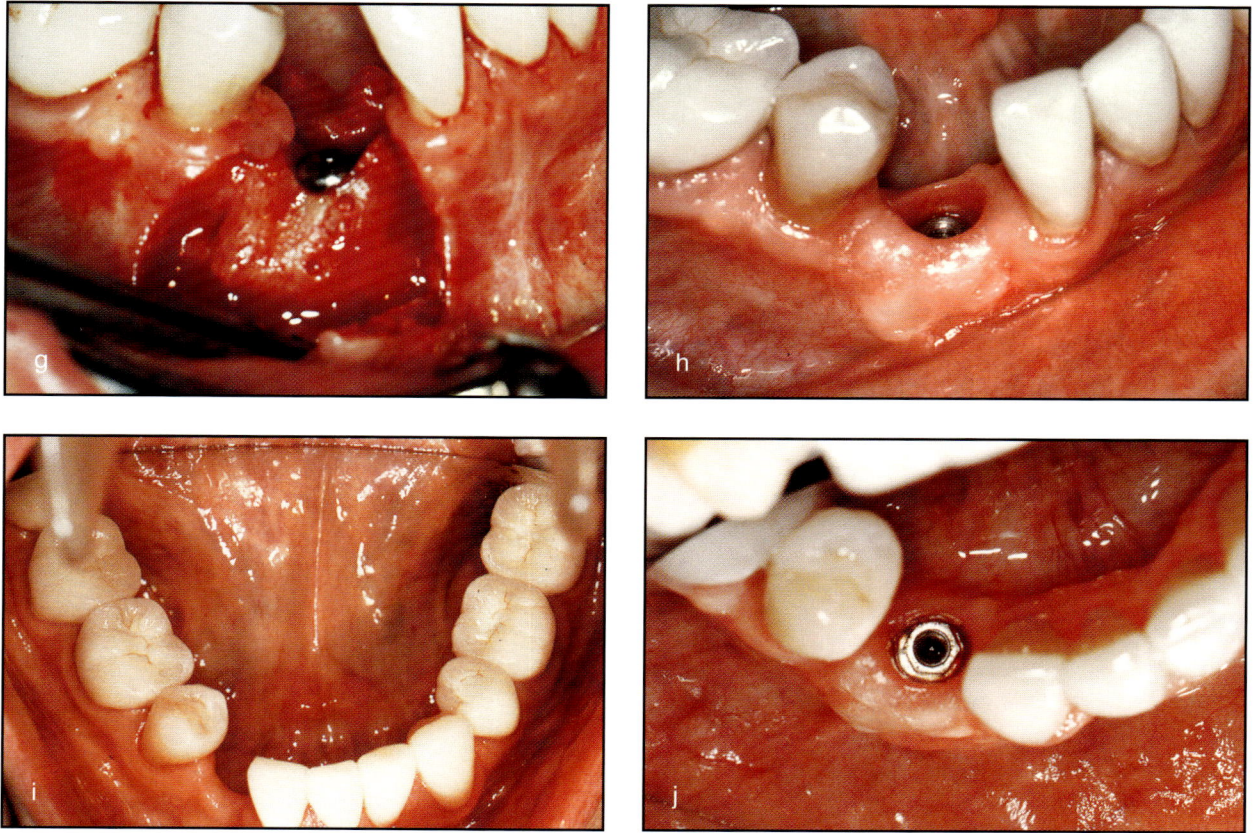

Fig 7-21 *(g)* A small saddle graft fixed with 1.5-mm-diameter fixation screws. *(h)* Occlusal view of the saddle with the implant seated in the proper position. *(i and j)* Labial view revealing the gain in height and width with the saddle graft. *(k)* Three months after delivery of the final restoration. Note the correction of the labial deficiency. *(l)* Close-up view. Note the re-establishment of interproximal tissue.

To rigidly stabilize the cortical-cancellous block of donor bone, both the graft and the recipient bed must be prepared properly to minimize the gap or dead space between donor bone and recipient site. The recipient bed should be relatively flat and decorticated (Fig 7-23). Fixation screws must be placed in sufficient numbers and be inserted in the proper positions (triangulated when possible) to ensure rigid stabilization of the graft (Fig 7-24). Drilling through both cortices with a 1-mm fissure bur will create vascular channels. These bleeding sites from the recipient bed will hasten neovascularization of the graft and enhance adherence of the overlying soft tissue. Increasing vascularity will enhance platelet adhesion, thus improving the stability of the grafted bone and reattachment of the periosteal layer of the soft tissue flap. Bone chips may be added to the edges of the grafted bone to fill in spaces or open areas between the bone graft and recipient bed (Fig 7-25). A clinical case is shown in Fig 26.

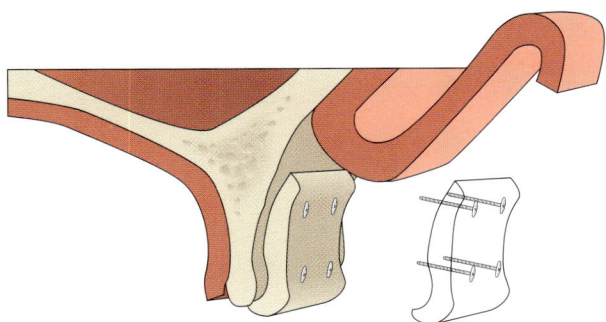

Fig 7-22 Schematic drawing illustrating a saddle graft.

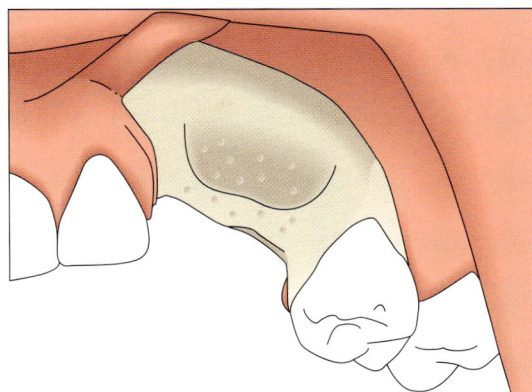

Fig 7-23 Preparation of the recipient bed: decorticating the buccal surface and creating vascular channels.

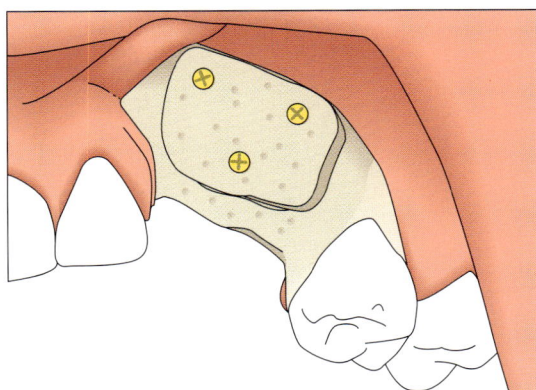

Fig 7-24 Fixation of donor bone. Placement of fixation screws in a triangulated position maximizes the rigidity of the graft.

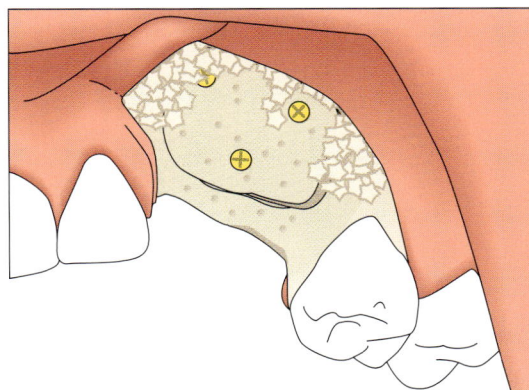

Fig 7-25 Wedging the mixture of particulated donor material to fill in spaces and exposed corners of donor bone.

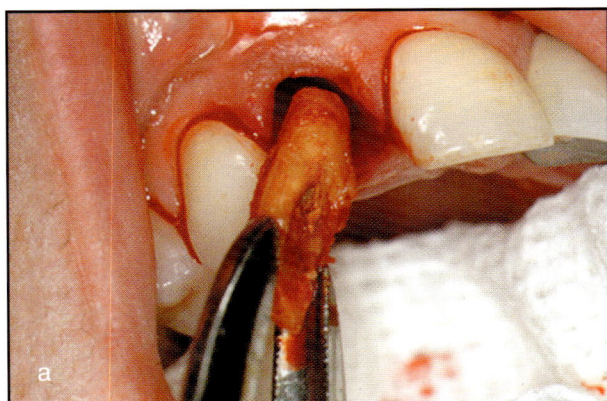

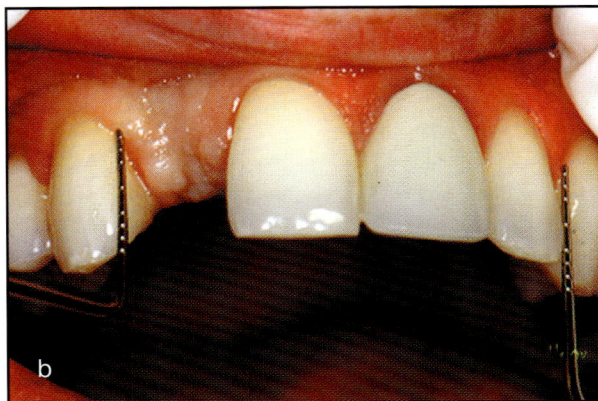

Fig 7-26 *(a)* Removal of a fractured, lateral incisor. *(b)* Presurgical measurements of soft tissue height and contours. This charting will assist the surgeon in determining the need for hard and/or soft tissue grafting and recommending the appropriate grafting technique.

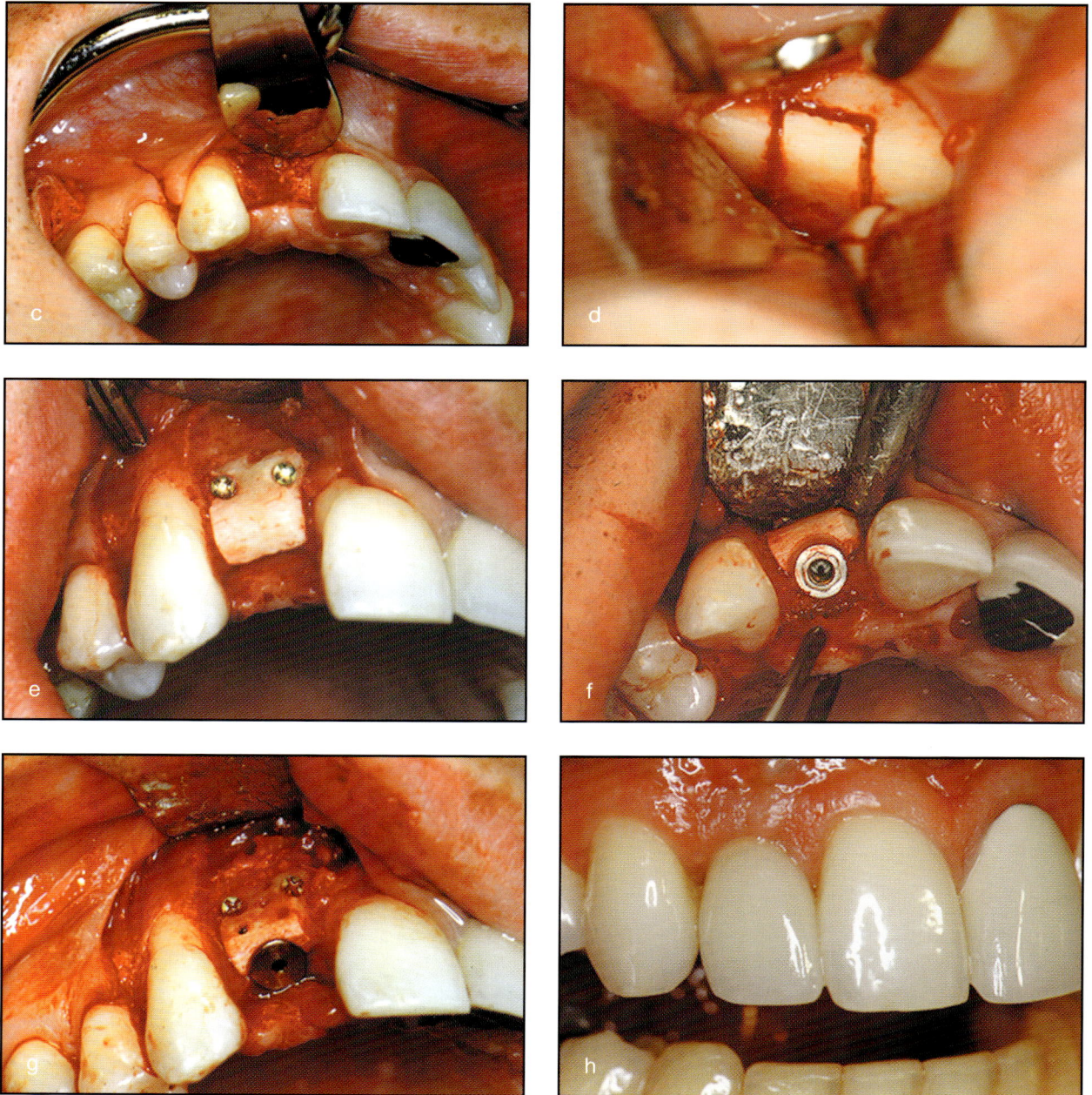

Fig 7-26 *(c)* The horizontal incision is placed on the palatal aspect to avoid scarring on the labial aspect and visualization of the scar, especially in patients with high smile lines. *(d)* Harvesting of donor bone from the lateral ramus. A No. 701 fissure bur was used to create the osteotomy through the buccal cortical plate. *(e)* A small saddle graft is fixed with 1.5-mm-diameter fixation screws. *(f)* Occlusal view of the saddle with the implant seated in the proper position. *(g)* Labial view revealing the gain in height and width with the saddle graft. *(h)* Three months after delivery of the final restoration. Close-up view. Note the correction of the labial deficiency and the re-establishment of interproximal tissue.

Other Considerations

Healing

The average healing time for a bone graft varies from 3 to 6 months, depending on the need for the grafted material to support the implant. When basal bone is available to provide initial stability for the implant, healing time for the graft is shorter.

Complications are related to two major factors: inadequate fixation of the graft and inadequate soft tissue closure and poor vascularization. Any undesired micromovements of the graft material during healing may result in the formation of connective tissue between graft and recipient bed, leading to graft failure.

Soft tissue closure

The soft tissue flap must be reapproximated over the graft without tension. Releasing incisions of the flap should be extended apically and diagonally to maximize the blood supply by creating a broader base. Tension in the flap may be released further by horizontal scores in the periosteal layer. Suturing should start using 2-0 silk in a vertical mattress fashion to resist any tension or muscle pull on the flap. A continuous running 4-0 chromic suture is then used to achieve watertight closure of the soft tissue edges.

Predictability

Among the various surgical techniques mentioned, the most predictable is the inlay graft. The other techniques are less predictable and may have resorption rates up to 20% of the total volume. With combinations of onlay, veneer, and saddle grafts, the final outcomes are difficult to predict. Several additional surgeries may be required to obtain an acceptable end result with these grafting procedures.

Conclusions

To properly reconstruct lost contours and anatomy in the deficient osseous ridge, the surgeon must have a full understanding of the requirements for correct work-up, making an accurate diagnosis, and applying the proper surgical technique to achieve harmony and success in the management of osseous defects. Different surgical techniques are indicated depending on the shape and size of the hard and/or soft tissue defect, as well as the location of the defect (maxilla vs mandible—anterior vs posterior). The variety of surgical techniques (inlay, onlay, veneer, and saddle grafts) provides the surgeon with specific approaches for treating specific anatomic defects. The goal of osseous tissue augmentation is to optimize the esthetic and functional results of the final dental restoration. With this in mind, the surgeon must select the most appropriate osseous grafting procedure to maximize the enhancement of the soft tissue contours and gingival architecture. By maintaining this goal throughout treatment, the surgeon will be able to achieve ideal esthetics and restore proper function for the dental invalid.

References

Beirne U, Brånemark P-I. Reconstruction of alveolar jaw bone: an experimental and clinical study of immediate and preformed autologous bone grafts in combination with osseointegrated implants. Scand J Plast Reconstr Surg 1980;14:23–48.

Boyne P, James RA. Grafting of the maxillary sinus with autogenous marrow and bone. J Oral Surg 1980; 38:613–616.

Haas R, Donath K, Fodinger M, Watzek G. Bovine hydroxyapatite for maxillary sinus grafting: comparative histomorphometric findings in sheep. Clin Oral Implants Res 1998;9:107–116.

Holmes R, Hagler H. Porous hydroxyapatite as a bone graft substitute in maxillary augmentation: a histometric study. J Craniomaxillofac Surg 1988;16: 199–205.

Jensen OT, Sennerby L. Histologic analysis of clinically retrieved titanium microimplants placed in conjunction with maxillary sinus floor augmentation. Int J Oral Maxillofac Implants 1998;13:513–521.

Jarcho M. Biomaterial aspects of calcium phosphates. Dent Clin North Am 1986;30:25–47.

Keller EE, Tolman DE, Eckert S. Surgical-prosthodontic reconstruction of advanced maxillary bone compromise with autogenous onlay block bone grafts and osseointegrated endosseous implants: a 12-year study of 32 consecutive patients. Int J Oral Maxillofac Implants 1999;14:197–209.

Keller EE, Van Rockel NB, Desjardins JP, Tolman DE. Prosthetic-surgical reconstruction of severely resorbed maxilla with iliac bone grafting and tissue-integrated prostheses. Int J Oral Maxillofac Implants 1987;2:155–165.

Landsberg CJ, Grosskopf A, Weinreb M. Clinical and biologic observations of demineralized freeze-dried bone allografts in augmentation procedures around dental implants. Int J Oral Maxillofac Implants 1994;9:586–592.

Lekholm U, Zarb GA. Patient selection and preparation. In: Brånemark P-I, Zarb GA, Albrektsson T (eds). Tissue-Integrated Prostheses: Osseointegration in Clinical Dentistry. Chicago: Quintessence, 1985:199–209.

Tolman DE. Reconstructive procedures with endosseous implants in grafted bone: a review of the literature. Int J Oral Maxillofac Implants 1995;10: 275–294.

Urist MR. Bone: formation by autoinduction. Science 1965;150:893–899.

Urist MR, Dowell TA, Hay PH, Strates BS. Inductive substrates for bone formation. Clin Orthop 1968; 59:59–96.

Wood RM, Moore DL. Grafting of the maxillary sinus with intraorally harvested autogenous bone prior to implant placement. Int J Oral Maxillofac Implants 1988;3:209–214.

Zins JE, Whitaker LA. Membranous vs endochondral bone autografts: implications for craniofacial reconstruction. Plast Reconstr Surg 1983;72:778–785.

Chapter 8

Peri-implant Soft Tissue Augmentation Procedures

Patrick Palacci, DDS

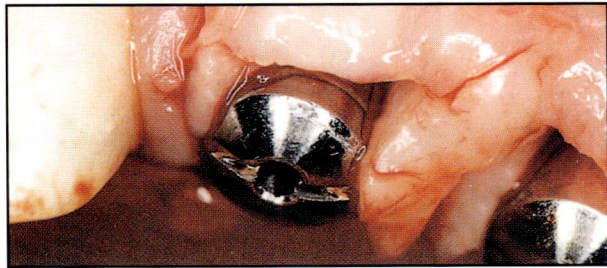

According to the literature, soft tissue augmentation of the alveolar ridge can be performed predictably (for a review see Seibert and Lindhe 1997). The roll and pouch procedure, as well as interpositional and onlay graft procedures, can be used to add ridge width and height for optimal esthetic outcome following treatment of the natural dentition. Similar ridge augmentation concepts can be applied in implant treatment. These procedures can be used in conjunction with the papilla regeneration technique described later. A more favorable clinical situation can be expected at second-stage surgery when creating papillaes. Optimal results can then be expected.

Ridge Augmentation

Soft tissue augmentation can be performed (1) prior to implant placement, (2) at the time of implant placement, (3) at the time of abutment connection (in conjunction with the papilla regeneration technique), or (4) after prosthetic insertion. The first three procedures can be performed with predictable outcomes, whereas the fourth is more of a rescue surgery and has lower predictability. Where the amount of bone is sufficient for proper implant placement but ridge volume is insufficient, soft tissue augmentation can be performed during implant placement to avoid additional surgical procedures.

The keys for success in soft tissue augmentation are careful preparation of the recipient site, selection of an adequate donor site, meticulous preparation of the graft, precision in placement of the graft, and an adequate suturing technique.

Preparation of the recipient site

Following elevation of the mucoperiosteal flap, the apical portion of the flap is split by cutting through the periosteum (Fig 8-1). This technique minimizes tension and does not jeopardize the survival of the graft. The dissection can be extended laterally to allow optimal adaptation of the lateral portions of the flap to the adjacent sites.

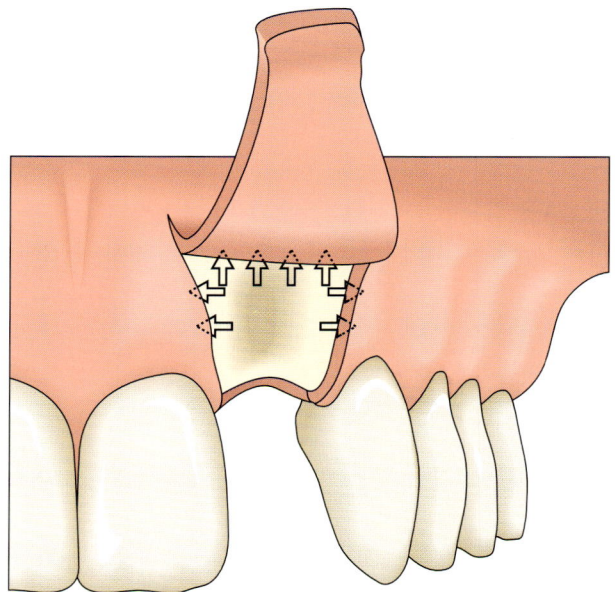

a

Fig 8-1 (a) When performing soft tissue augmentation, a full-thickness flap is elevated. Careful releasing incisions are made laterally and apically in order to gain flexibility in the tissues.

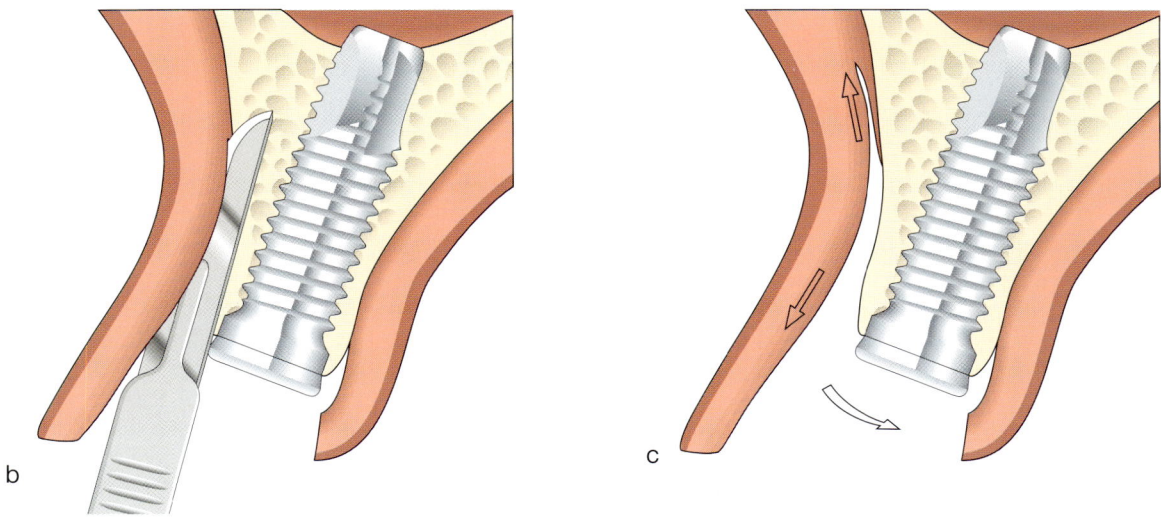

Fig 8-1 *(b and c)* In the apical direction, a split-thickness flap is elevated, releasing the tissues in a coronal direction. One should avoid any tension when suturing back the flap.

Selection of donor site

The most frequently used donor sites are *(1)* the palatal area mesial to the first molar, *(2)* the posterior ridge areas, and *(3)* the maxillary tuber areas (Fig 8-2). In the palatal area mesial to the first molar, a split-thickness flap is elevated, and the underlying connective tissue covering the bone is harvested (Fig 8-3). Insufficient thickness of the tissue in this region can be a contraindication for the use of this site as a donor site. In the posterior ridge areas, a wedge technique is applied (Fig 8-4). Several edentulous areas can be selected in the same patient.

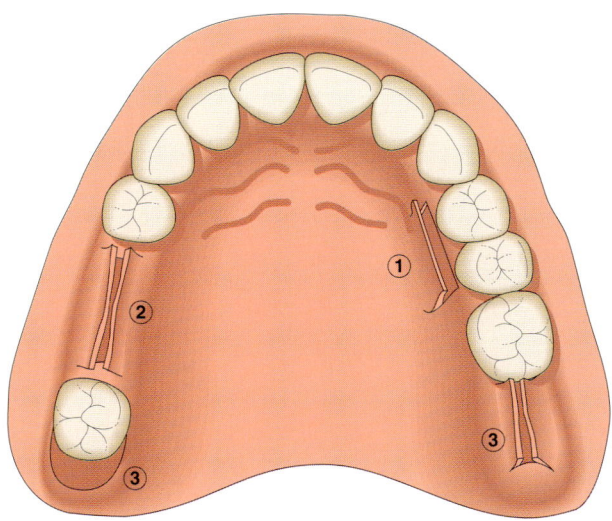

Fig 8-2 Location of the different intraoral donor sites: 1, Palatal; 2, ridge (edentulous area); 3, tuberosity.

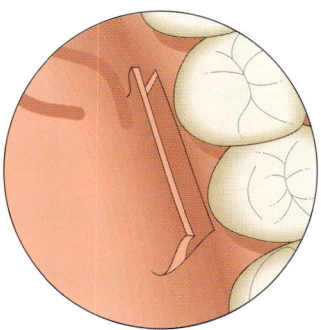

Fig 8-3 In the palatal area a bevel incision is done, the flap is elevated, and the connective tissue remaining between the internal side of flap and the bone is reflected.

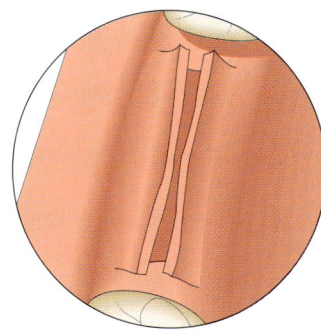

Fig 8-4 In a ridge area, two bevel incisions in labial and palatal direction are made, the tissue located at the top of the ridge and laterally will be used as graft material.

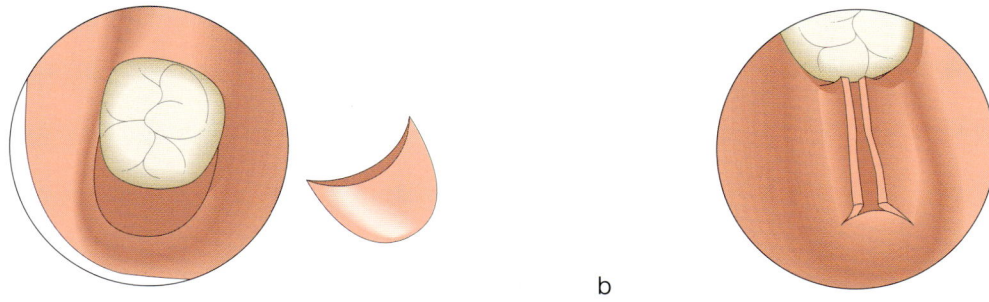

Fig 8-5 In the tuber area, according to the quantity of connective tissue available, one can choose between a gingivectomy *(a)* or a distal wedge *(b)* to harvest the graft.

According to the thickness of the tissue in the maxillary tuber areas, a wedge or gingivectomy technique can be used (Fig 8-5). When the gingivectomy technique is used, the epithelial layer of the grafting tissue portion must be removed before its placement at the recipient site. Usually a graft harvested from one tuber area can be used to recreate an adequate ridge corresponding to one tooth (Fig 8-6). When an extensive area is to be augmented, several donor sites can be used in combination.

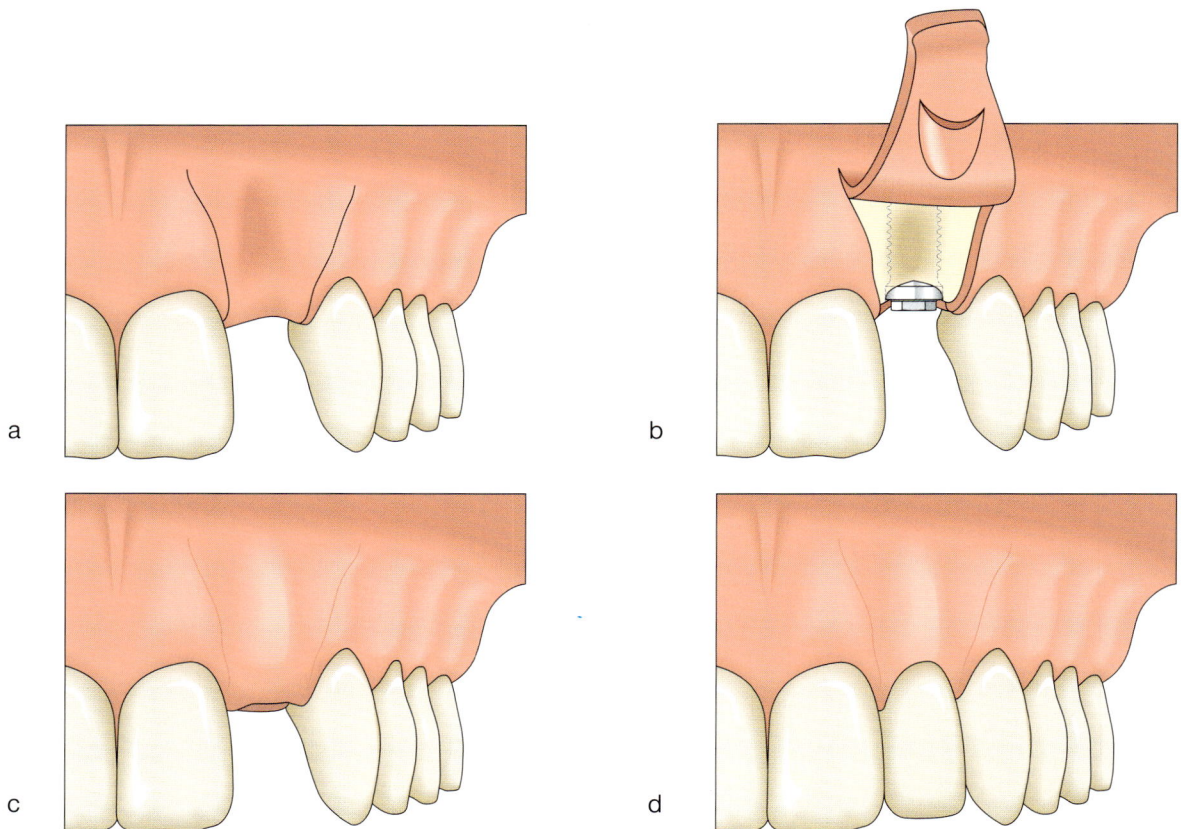

Fig 8-6 In a case of a single-tooth replacement, the ridge may present some resorption *(a)*. At the time of or before implant placement, the ridge can be corrected by adding connective tissue in the inner part of the flap. The shape and quantity of donor material harvested from the tuber area corresponds to one missing tooth *(b to d)*.

Preparation of the graft

The harvested graft must be placed in the recipient site to enable visualization of its proper size and position. If needed, the graft is trimmed before permanent placement and subsequent adaptation and suturing of the flap (Fig 8-7).

Placement of the graft

According to the need for augmentation (in the horizontal or vertical direction), the graft can be placed and sutured in a more or less apical portion of the inner surface of the flap (Fig 8-8).

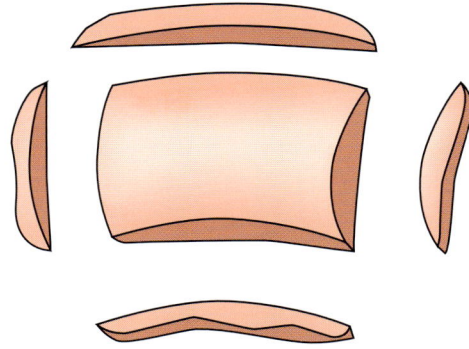

Fig 8-7 Trimming of the graft to precisely fit the recipient site.

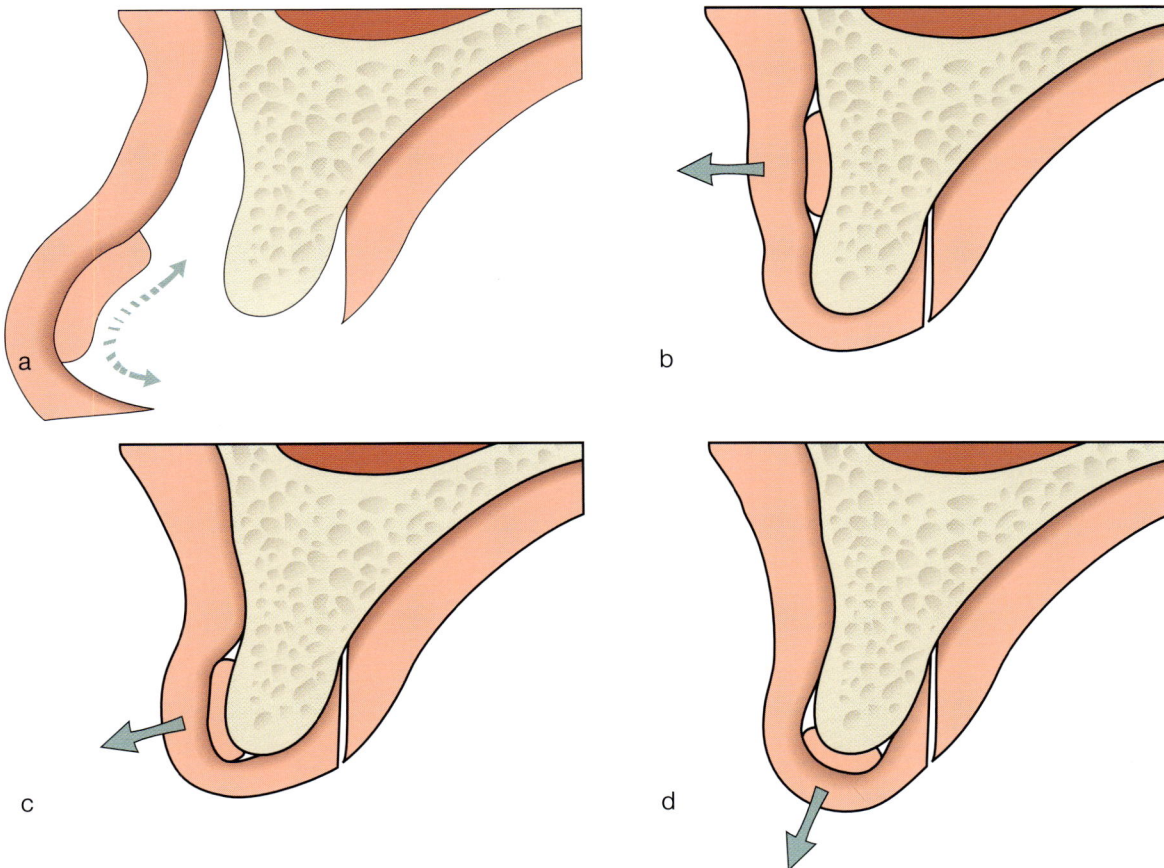

Fig 8-8 The soft tissue graft can be placed according to the desired ridge augmentation *(a)*. If the ridge has to be augmented in a horizontal direction, the graft should be sutured apically. It should be sutured in a more coronal position if the need is to augment the ridge in a more vertical direction *(b to d)*.

Suturing of the graft

Optimal stabilization of the graft is essential to obtain an adequate end result. After adequate positioning, the graft will be sutured to the flap according to Fig 8-9. When the area of augmentation is wider, several pieces of connective tissue can be sutured together before being stabilized to the flap.

Figures 8-10 and 8-11 present, respectively, cases where a first maxillary premolar and a maxillary right lateral incisor have to be replaced.

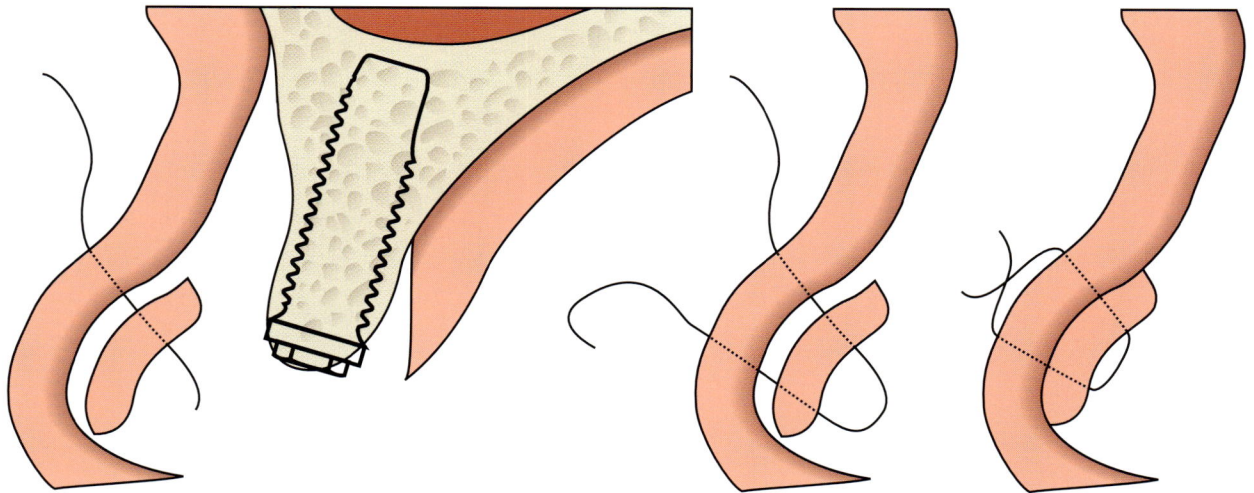

Fig 8-9 Suturing the connective tissue can be simplified by stabilizing the graft against the inner part of the flap as shown.

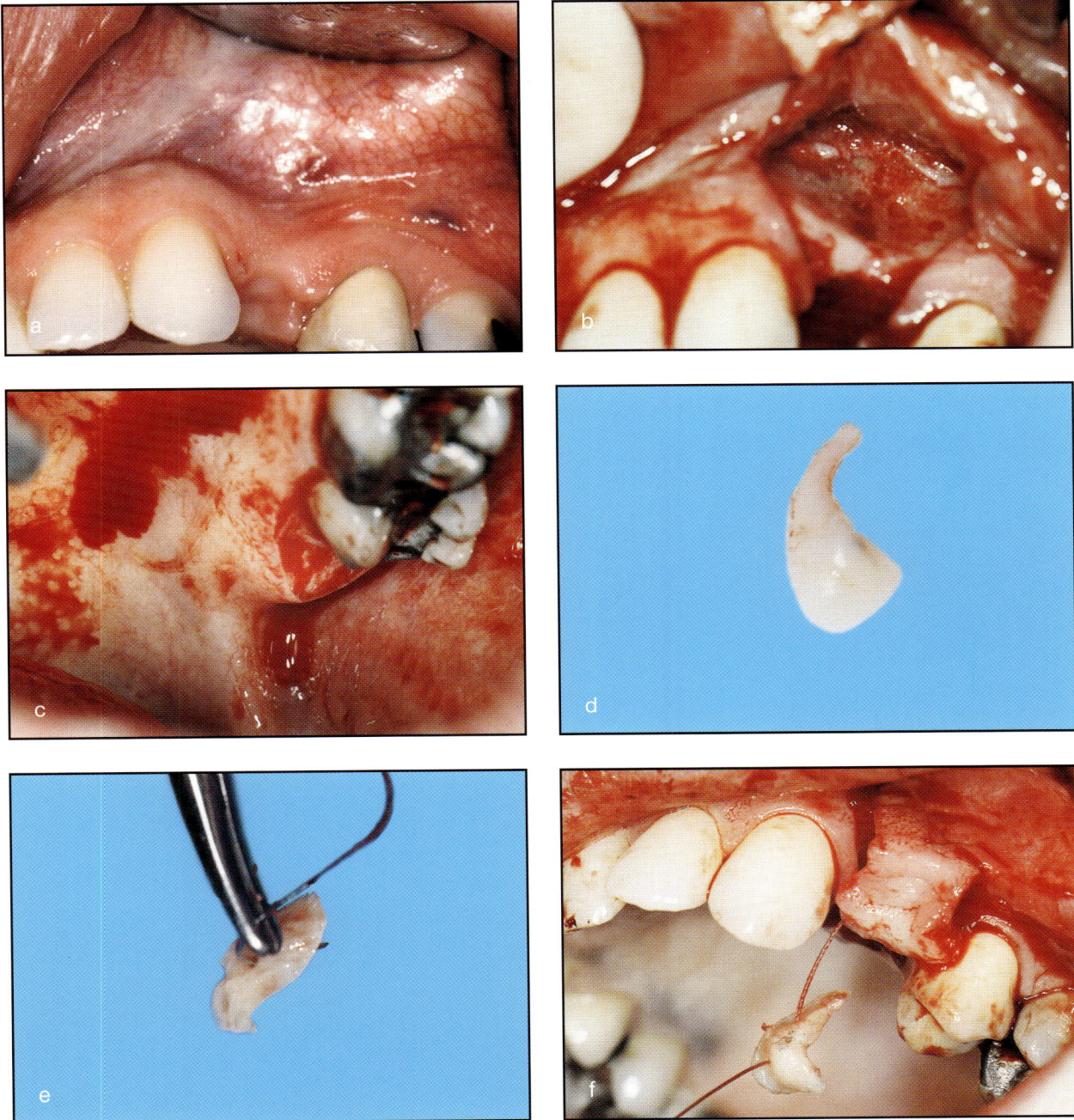

Fig 8-10 *(a)* Clinical case where a first maxillary premolar has to be replaced. Note the concavity resulting from the tooth loss. *(b)* A full-thickness flap is elevated. There is sufficient bone quantity to place an implant in adequate position; however the ridge has to be corrected to obtain an optimal esthetic result. *(c)* Clinical view of the tuber area. The connective tissue is harvested distal from the second molar. *(d)* The grafting material is prepared by removing the surface epithelium. *(e)* A 4.0 vicryl suture is used to hold the graft. *(f)* The connective tissue is stabilized in the desired position in the internal side of the flap.

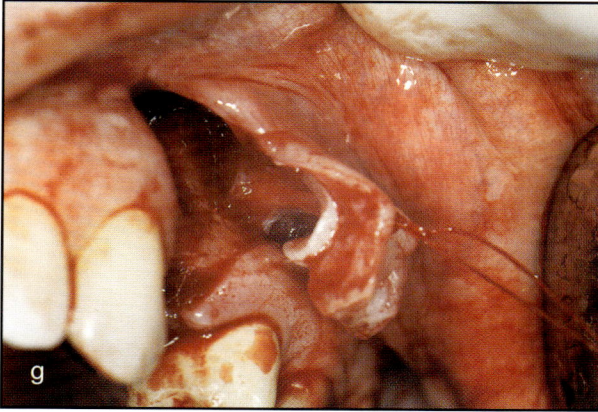

Fig 8-10 *(g)* Clinical view 2 months postoperative illustrating a significant gain of soft tissue and adequate ridge anatomy. *(h)* A full-thickness flap is elevated at second-stage surgery. Note the amount of connective tissue available. *(i)* A papilla regeneration technique can then be performed.

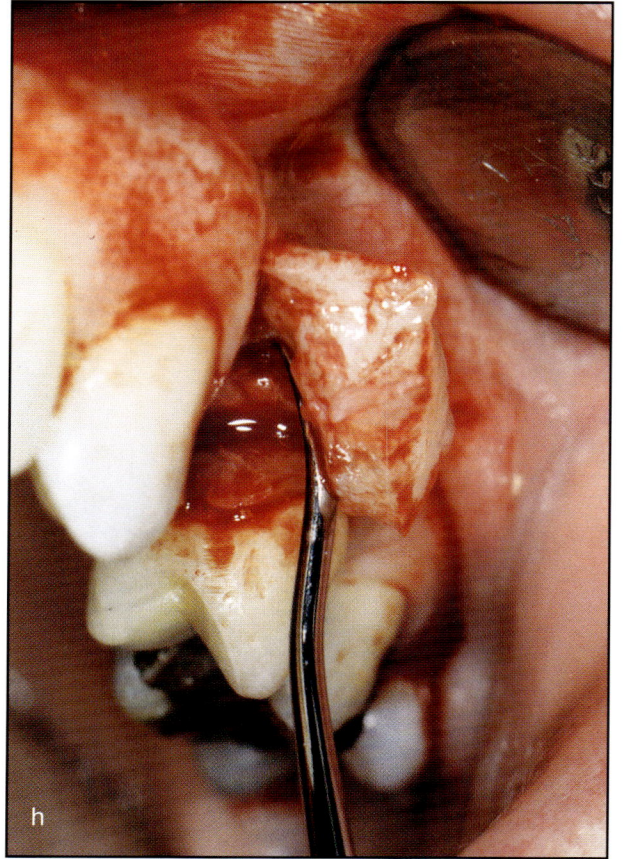

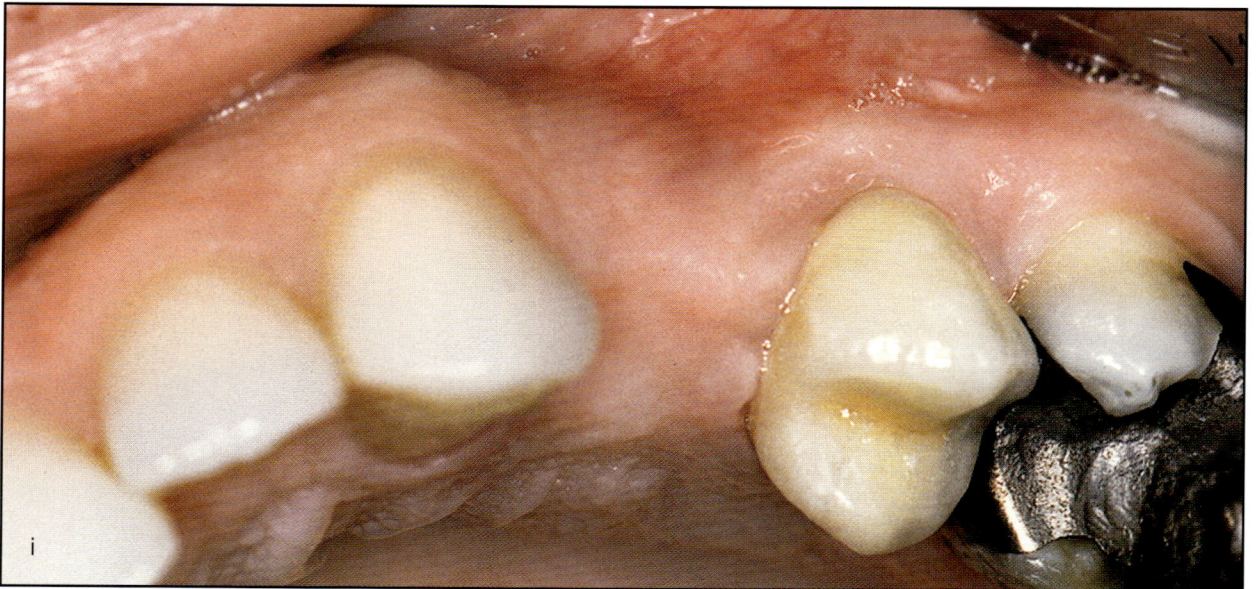

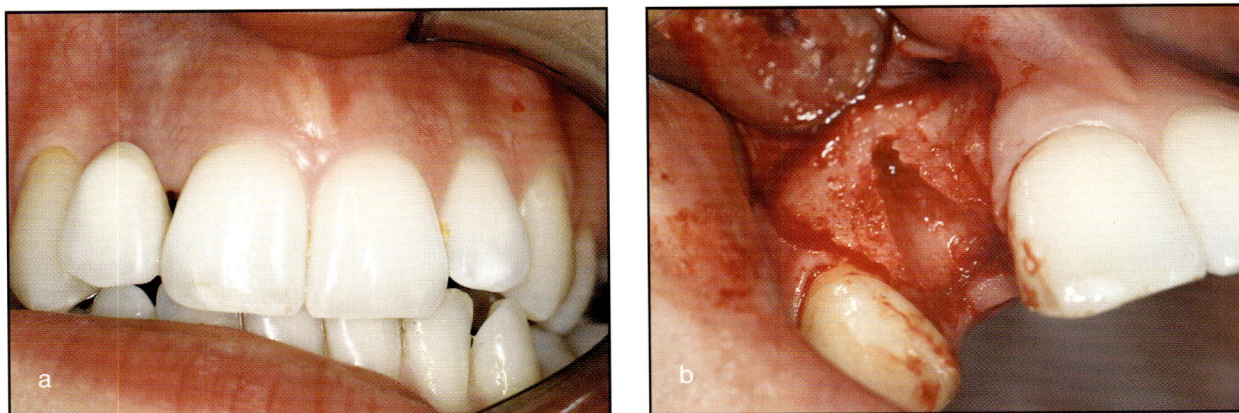

Fig 8-11 *(a)* Clinical situation where a maxillary right lateral incisor has to be replaced. A temporary crown is bonded to the adjacent teeth. Ridge collapse and loss of mesial papilla are the consequences of the tooth loss. *(b)* A flap is elevated. No hard tissue augmentation is needed.

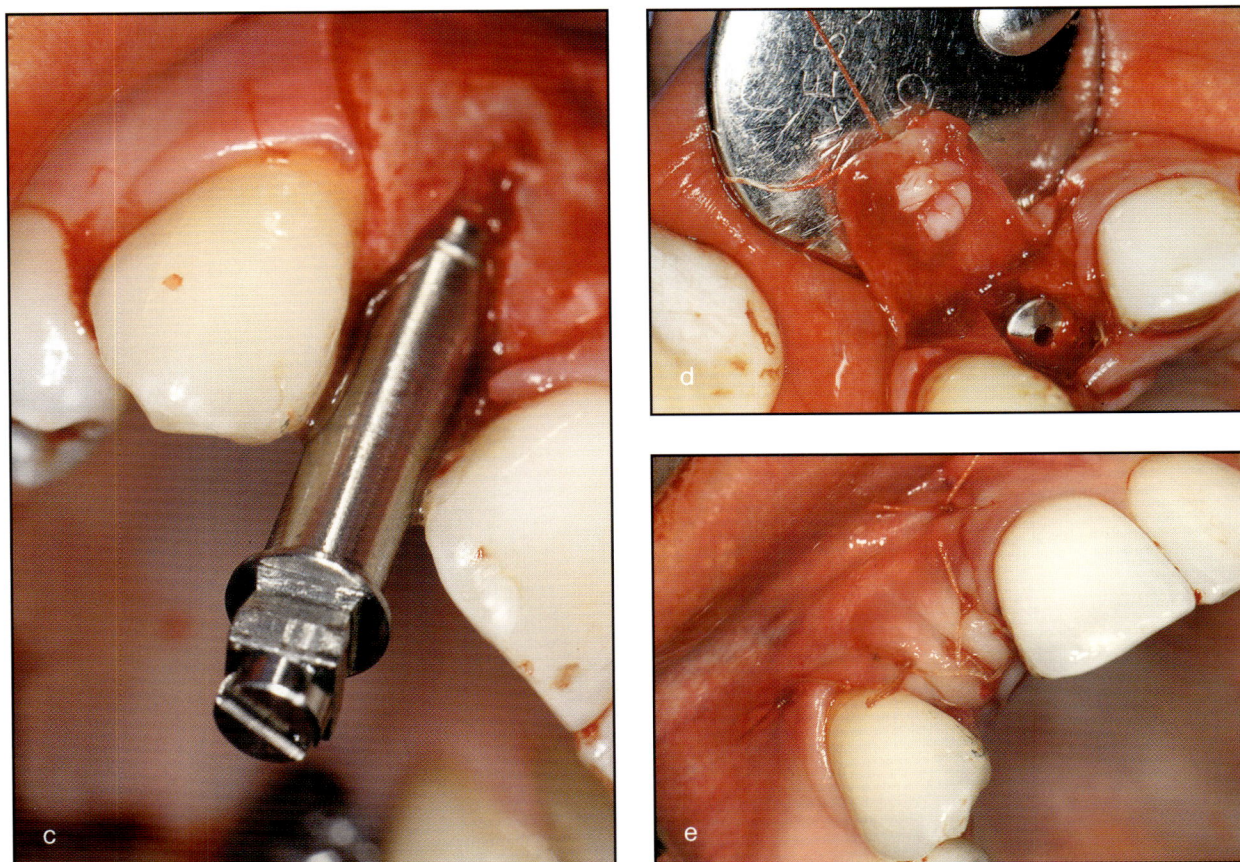

Fig 8-11 *(c)* A 13-mm regular-platform implant is placed 3 mm apical from the cementoenamel junction of the adjacent teeth. *(d)* The implant being placed, connective tissue harvested from the palatal area is sutured into position. A splitting of the flap in its apical portion will give more freedom and avoid any tension when suturing. *(e)* Clinical view of the site at the end of surgery. Note the amount of tissue gained, as well as the shape of the ridge, creating a more favorable situation for second-stage surgery.

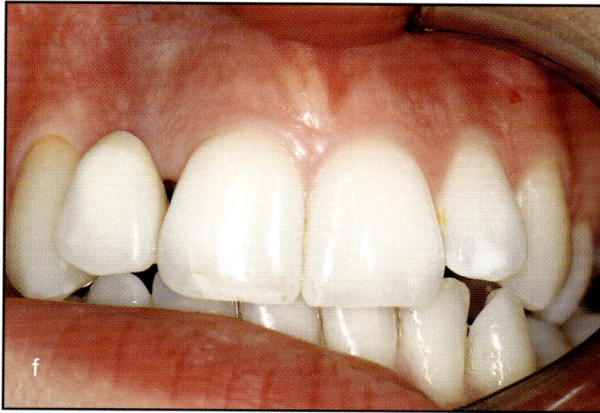

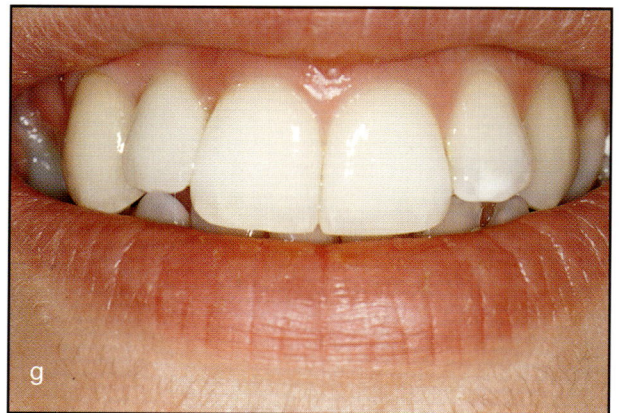

Fig 8-11 *(f and g)* Clinical views before and after treatment. Note the color, shape, and texture of the soft tissues surrounding the prosthetic restoration. This lateral incisor has been made using a CerAdapt abutment. *(h)* Same case 3 years later. (Prosthetic reconstruction: Dr Ph. Peruchetti.)

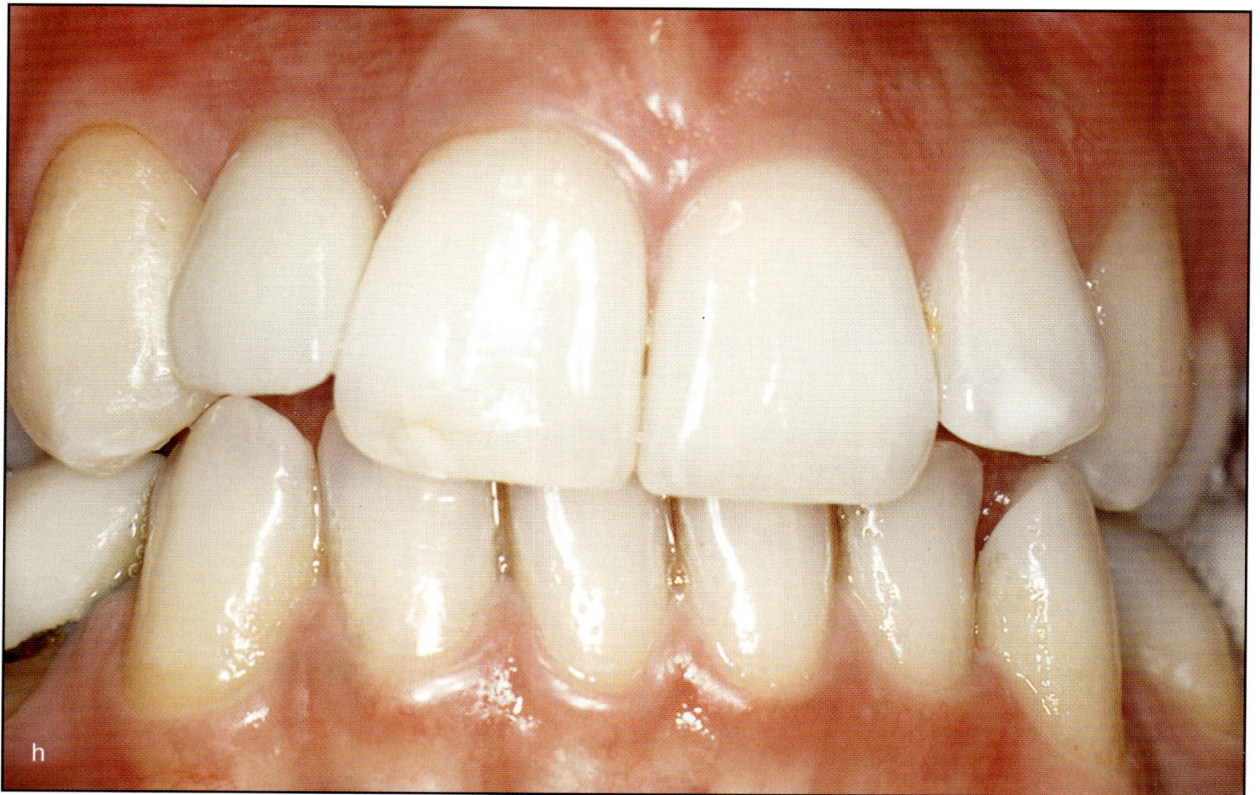

Papilla Regeneration Technique

Abutment connection has historically been performed using the tissue-punch technique (Fig 8-12) or full-thickness flaps (Adell et al 1985). These techniques are still useful in abutment connection procedures in specific situations, such as the treatment of edentulous mandibles with fixed supraconstructions or overdentures. Kenney et al (1989) described crestal incision and full-thickness flaps for abutment connection. This proce-

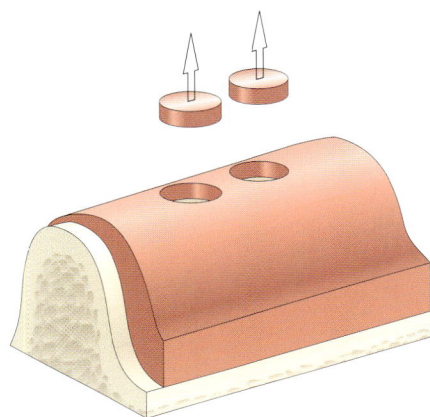

Fig 8-12 Identification of the implant heads and the amount of soft tissue to be punched.

dure allows better access to the cover screws and the anchoring bone but induces some tension in the mucosa around the abutments following adaptation and suturing. Furthermore, this approach results in a reversed soft tissue architecture (Fig 8-13). Moy and coworkers (1989) reported on a scalloping adjustment of the flaps that resulted in a better soft tissue adaptation to the titanium abutments but also in an almost linear soft tissue architecture (Fig 8-14). Several other techniques have been described (for example, Israelsson and Plemons 1993; Hertel et al 1994). However, none of these techniques

results in a papillalike formation of the peri-implant mucosa. Practitioners have claimed that "while the ability to regenerate lost contour has improved during the past 10 years, the unpredictability of the final result has led to the need, in many cases, for multiple surgical procedures to reach an esthetic result. Each procedure adds to the time and expense of the final result and significantly increases the risk of undesirable complications." Also, "the ability to regenerate or augment tissue in a coronal direction is more difficult to perform successfully than in other directions. Unfortunately, there is usually a need to replace lost tissue in that coronal dimension. Improved surgical procedures to recreate the appearance of an interdental papilla are needed to address this common shortcoming" (Sullivan et al 1994).

It is often recommended that clinicians evaluate the ridge mucosa prior to implant placement to judge whether surgical augmentation of the covering mucosa is needed. From studies on patients, Liljenberg et al (1996) reported on the height of the ridge and peri-implant mucosa. The authors observed that the mean height of the ridge mucosa was close to 2 mm and the mean height of peri-implant mucosa, 3 mm. This observation is in agreement with findings reported from a dog study by Berglundh and Lindhe (1996), who concluded that "a minimum width of peri-implant mucosa (approximately 3 mm) is required" and that, without sufficient mucosal width, "bone resorption will take place to allow a stable soft tissue attachment to form." However, when Wennström et al (1994) discussed the importance of an attached portion of masticatory mucosa as a border tissue around implants, they reported that their clinical study "failed to support the concept that the lack of an attached portion of masticatory mucosa may jeopardize the maintenance of soft tissue health around dental implants." These observations are in agreement with

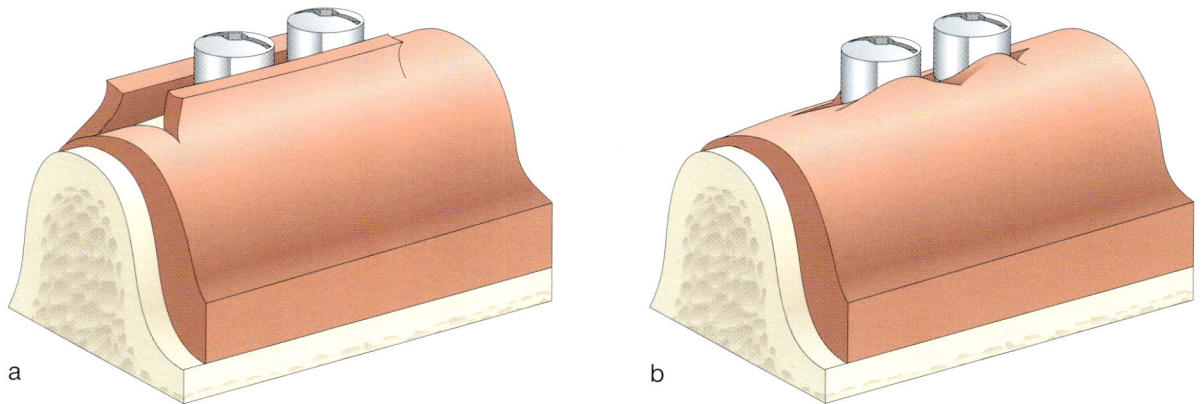

Fig 8-13 *(a)* Full-thickness flap technique. *(b)* Final result.

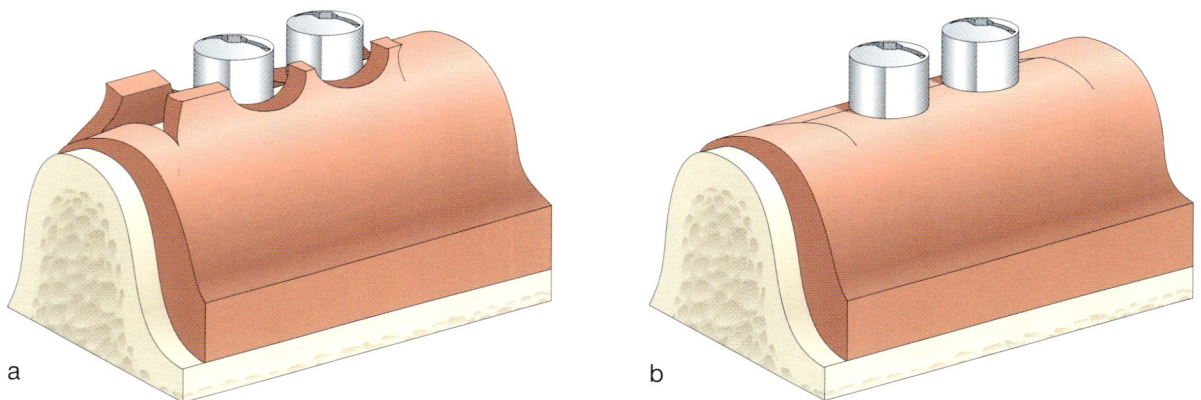

Fig 8-14 *(a)* Scalloping technique. *(b)* Final result.

findings presented by Strub et al (1991) from an experimental study in the dog. Furthermore, Bengazi et al (1996) performed a 2-year longitudinal prospective study on 163 Brånemark system implants. The authors reported that the observed recession of the peri-implant soft tissue margin over time was mainly the result of rebuilding of soft tissue "to establish appropriate biological dimensions of the soft tissue barrier, ie, the required dimension of epithelial-connective tissue attachment in relation to the faciolingual thickness of the supracrestal soft tissue."

Second-stage surgery

Second-stage surgery has two goals: *(1)* to allow the implant to pierce the mucosa and *(2)* to create a favorable soft tissue anatomy resulting in a perimucosal contour matching healthy gingival architecture (Fig 8-15). To reach these goals, the surgical technique should be based on biological principles—that is, the blood supply to the involved hard and soft tissue should be maintained to allow the formation of a proper soft tissue barrier. For example, in the creation of a papilla, manipu-

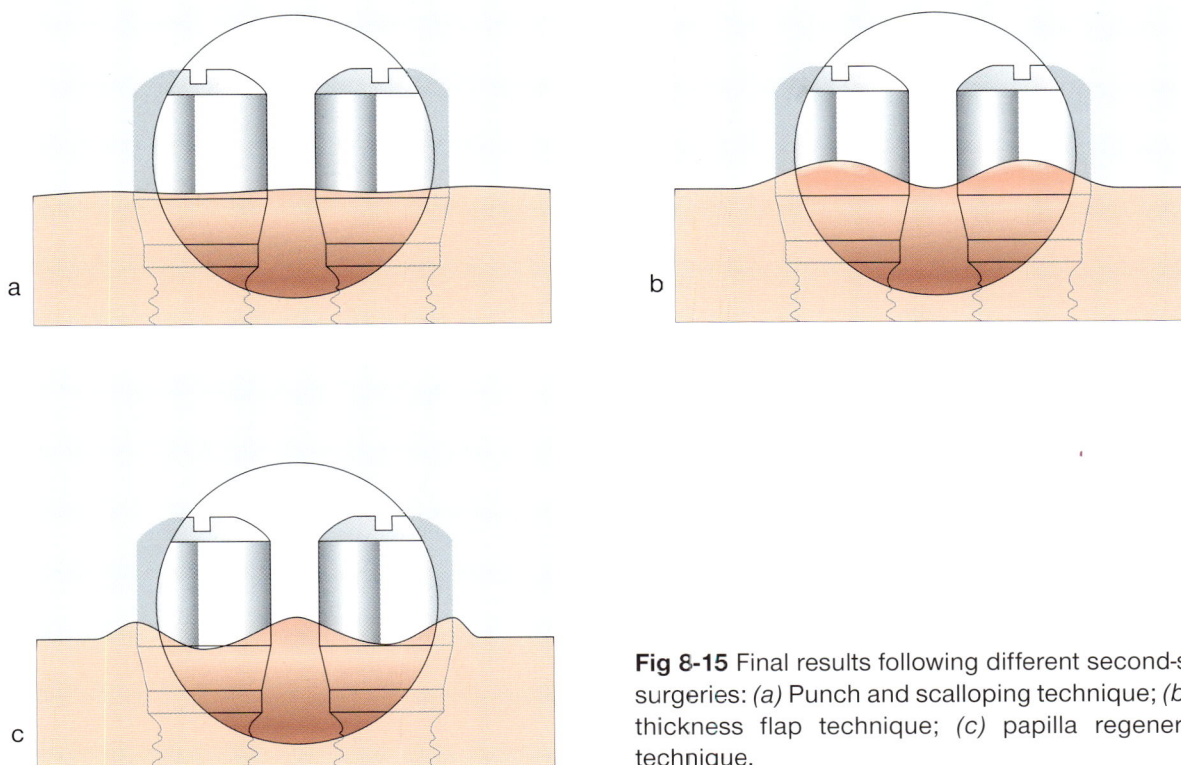

Fig 8-15 Final results following different second-stage surgeries: *(a)* Punch and scalloping technique; *(b)* full-thickness flap technique; *(c)* papilla regeneration technique.

lation of the soft tissue adjacent to the implant allows proper peri-implant tissue healing, thus resulting in a soft tissue architecture similar to the healthy gingival anatomy around teeth.

A surgical technique has been developed to optimize the esthetic outcome of soft tissue healing after the second-stage surgery to obtain papillalike formations (Palacci 1992, 1996; Andreasen et al 1994). This technique pushes the attached mucosa at the top of the ridge in the buccal direction, thus increasing the tissue volume at the buccal aspect of the implant. This larger tissue portion is kept in

place by the connected abutment. The excess soft tissue in the buccal position allows for dissection and rotation of pedicles, thus filling the spaces between implants replacing adjacent teeth. This technique results in a harmonious soft tissue architecture adjacent to implant-supported prostheses, provided that the implants are properly positioned. This, in turn, results in a better outcome in terms of esthetics, phonetics, and oral hygiene.

The papilla regeneration technique is performed as follows:

Papilla Regeneration Technique (see Figs 8-16 to 8-32)

1. Identify the location of the cover screws through the covering mucosa.
2. Make an incision at the palatal-lingual aspect of the cover screws, followed by vertical releasing incisions in a buccal and divergent direction to allow better blood supply to the flap. It is important to preserve the gingival cuffs at neighboring teeth.
3. Elevate a full-thickness flap in the buccal direction.
4. Remove the cover screws.
5. Select the proper abutments, and connect them to the implants.
6. Make semilunar bevel incisions in the buccal flap toward each abutment. Start at the distal aspect of the most mesially located implant.
7. Disengage the pedicle, then rotate it 90 degrees toward the palatal side to fill in the interimplant space.
8. Suture the tissues, allowing no tension within the pedicles.

Figs 8-16 to 8-32 Step-by-step illustrations of papilla regeneration technique.

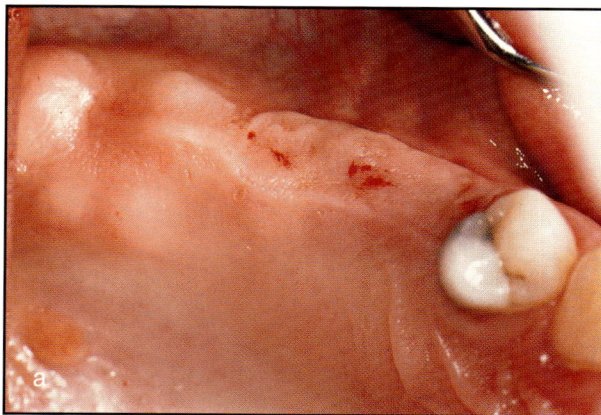

Fig 8-16 *(a)* Edentulous area distal to the first premolar in the first quadrant, in which implants have already been placed. The abutment connection procedure has not yet been performed.

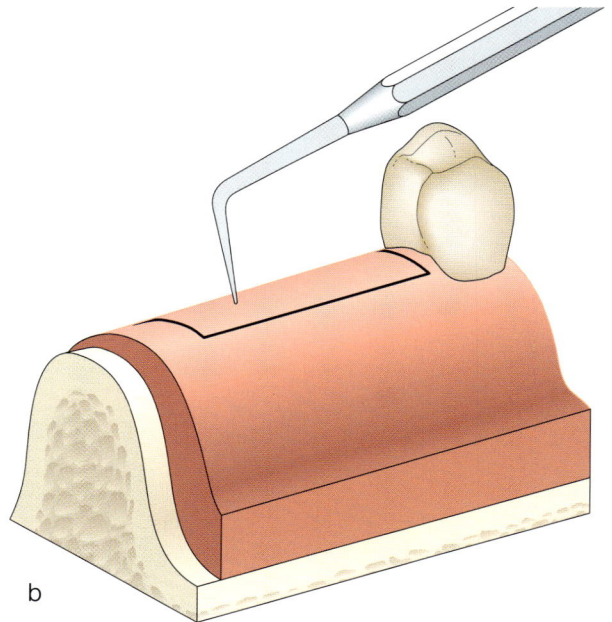

Fig 8-16 *(b)* Technique for identifying the cover screws by use of the probe tip. The horizontal incision must be made at the palatal aspect of the cover screws and the vertical releasing incisions made in the buccal direction. The gingival cuff at the distal aspect of the first premolar must be preserved according to the clinical situation and the final objective.

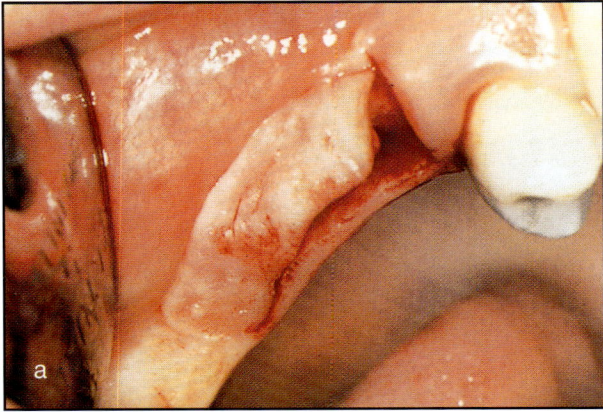

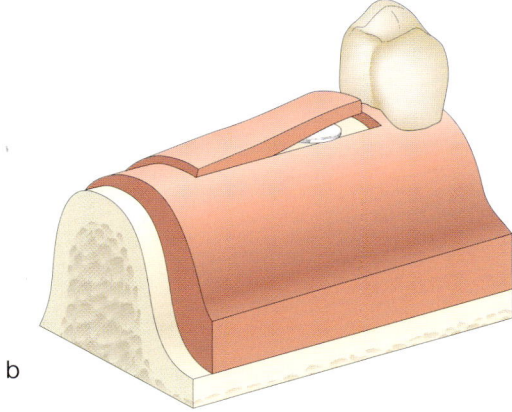

Fig 8-17 *(a)* The situation after the incisions. *(b)* Beginning of flap elevation.

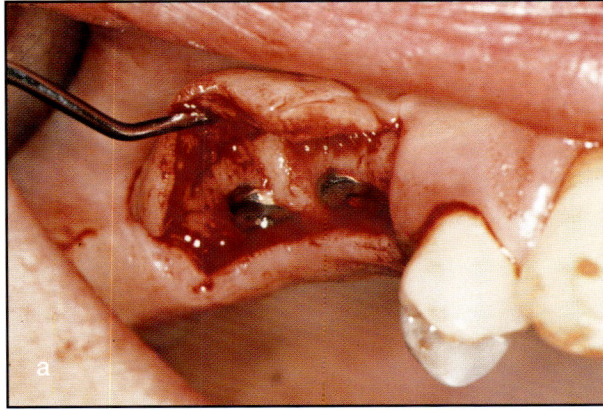

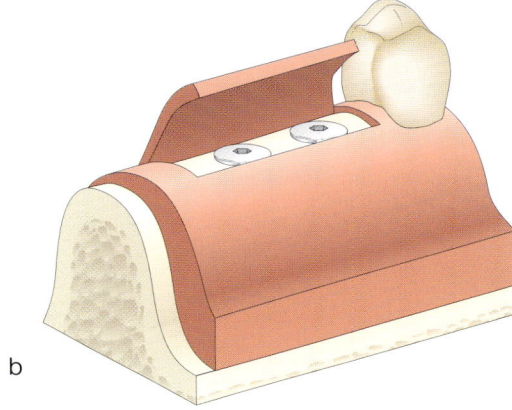

Fig 8-18 *(a and b)* Elevated full-thickness flap with cover screws exposed.

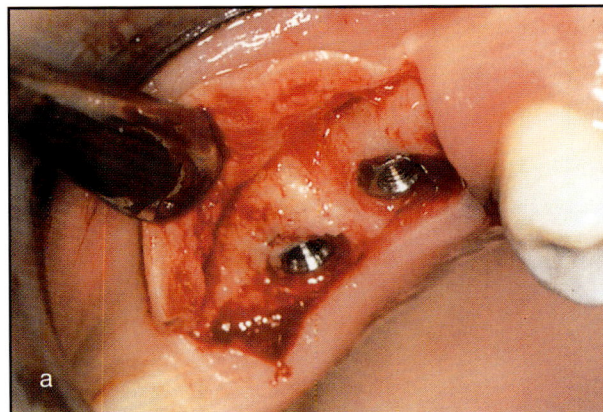

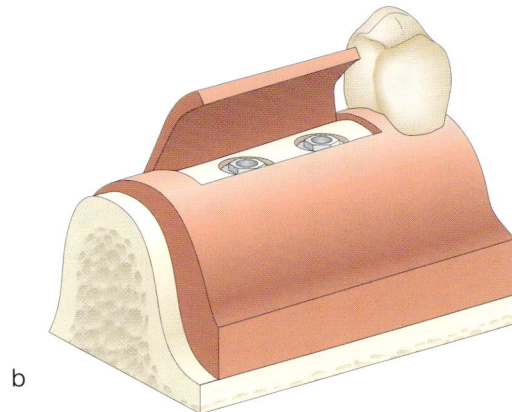

Fig 8-19 *(a and b)* Cover screws removed and implant heads exposed.

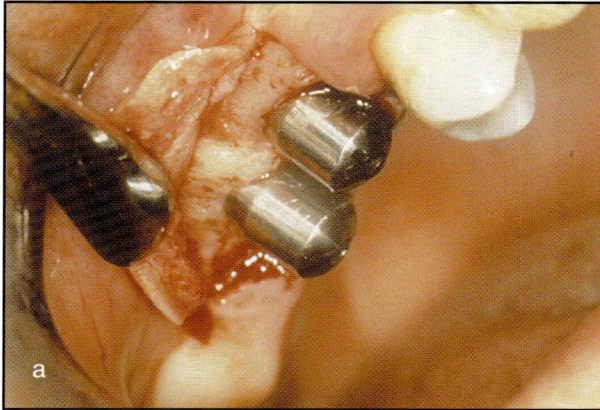

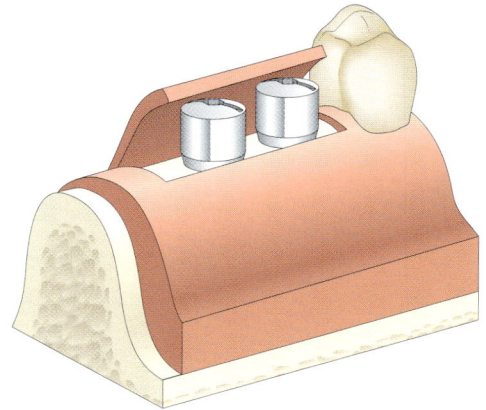

Fig 8-20 *(a and b)* Healing abutments have been selected and connected to the implants.

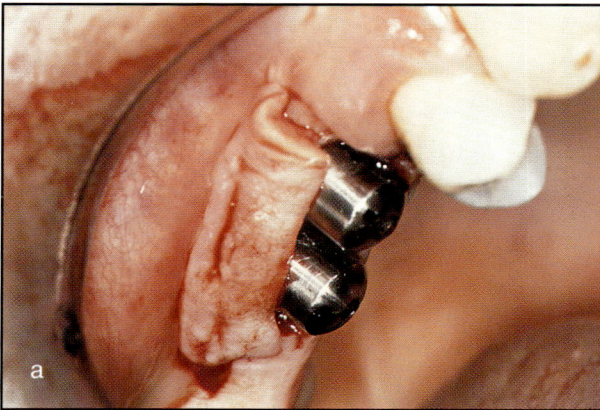

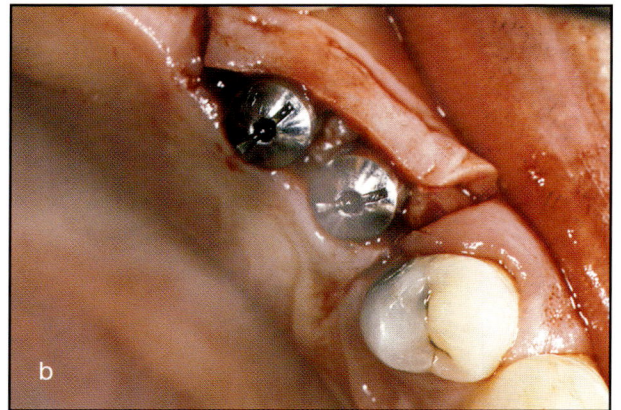

Fig 8-21 *(a and b)* Selected healing abutments should have sufficient length to support the flap. The increased soft tissue volume at the buccal aspect of the implants is clearly shown.

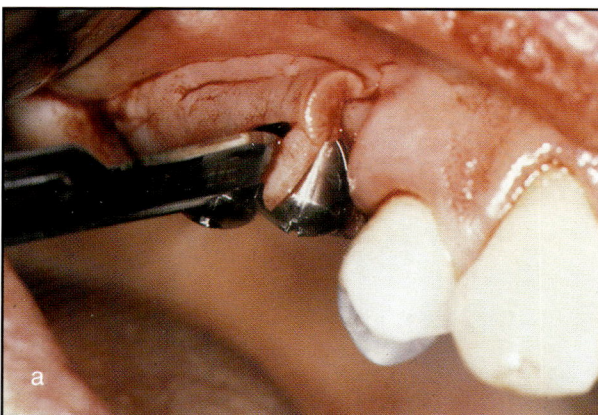

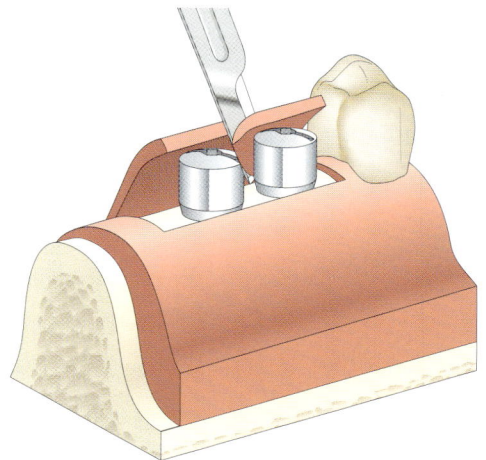

Fig 8-22 *(a and b)* Semilunar bevel incision made in the flap in relation to each implant. The first incision is made starting at the distal aspect of the most mesial implant.

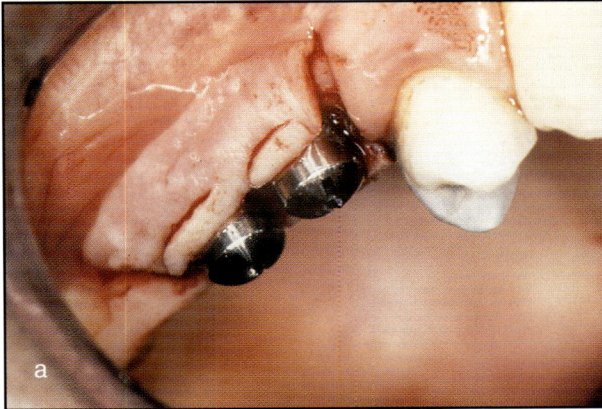

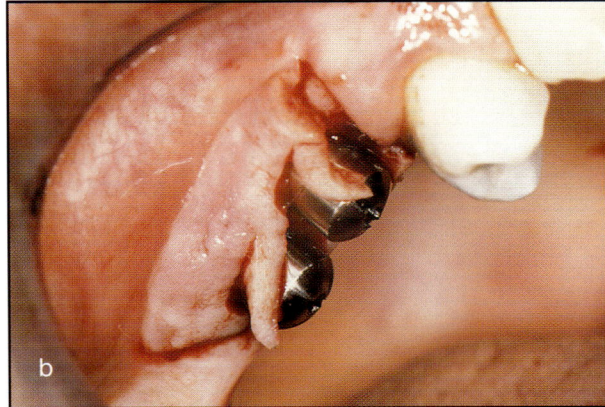

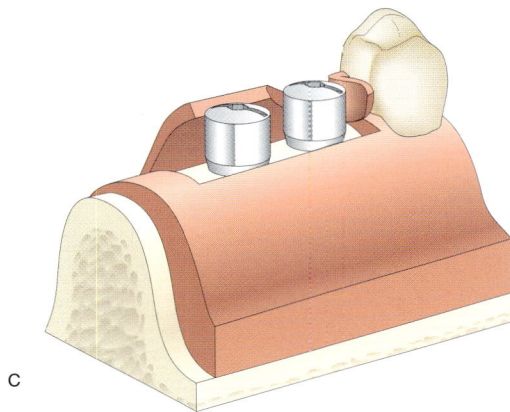

Fig 8-23 *(a to c)* The incision creates a pedicle that is rotated 90 degrees toward the mesial aspect of the abutment. The semilunar bevel incision must be extended far enough to allow the pedicle to be rotated and placed in the interproximal area without tension. According to the specific case, the semilunar bevel incision may vary in terms of shape and bevel. The thickness of the pedicle graft will vary depending on whether the need is to augment tissues in a more vertical or horizontal direction.

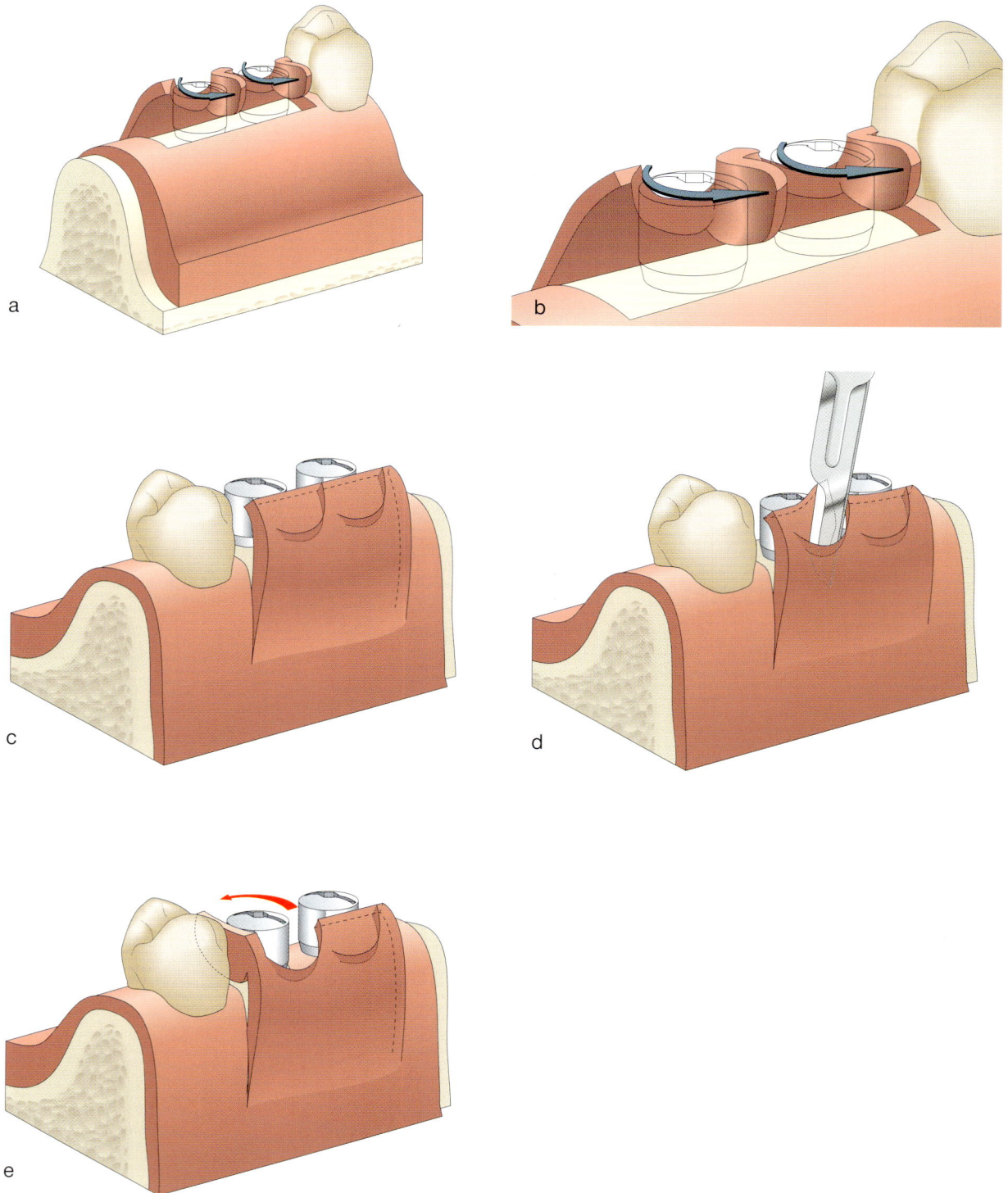

Fig 8-24 *(a and b)* Semilunar bevel incision and rotation of the pedicle repeated for each implant. *(c to e)* Labial view of the pedicle grafts, the semilunar bevel incisions, and the 90-degree rotation of pedicles, leaving a harmonious contour of the mucosa around the abutment as well as the future crown restoration.

a

b

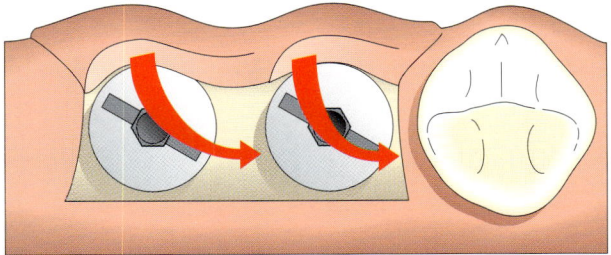

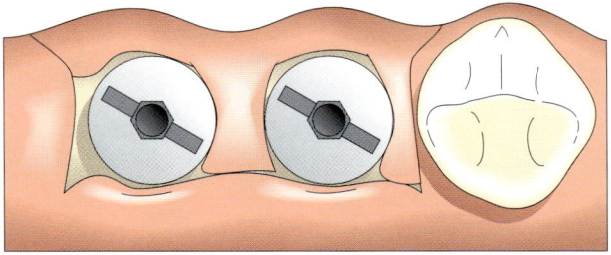

Fig 8-25 *(a and b)* Occlusal view of pedicle rotation.

a

b

c

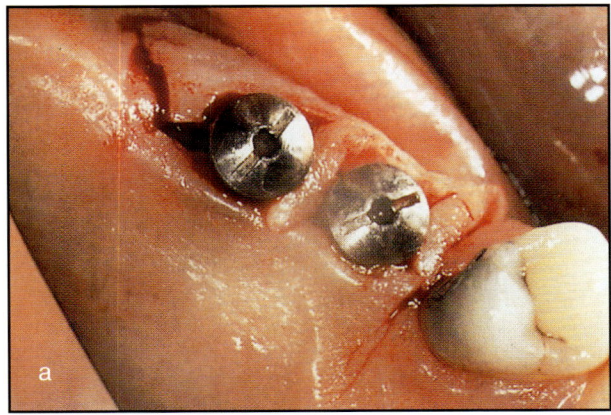

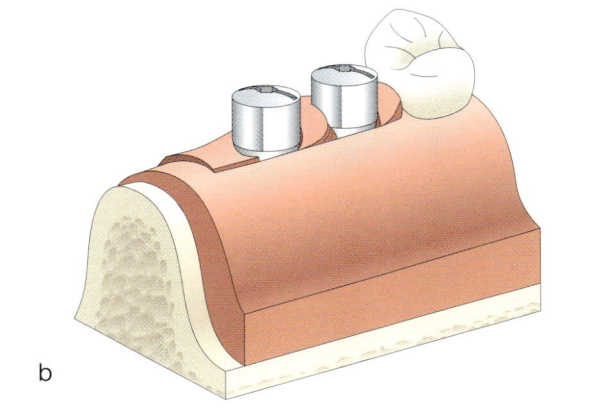

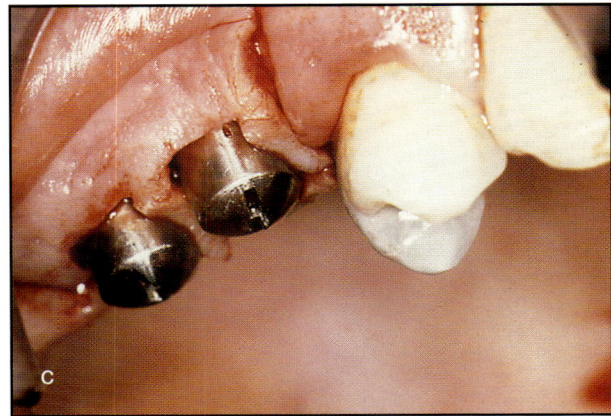

Fig 8-26 *(a to c)* The rotated pedicles occupy the interproximal areas, resulting in gain of soft tissue height. This soft tissue portion will become a papillalike formation.

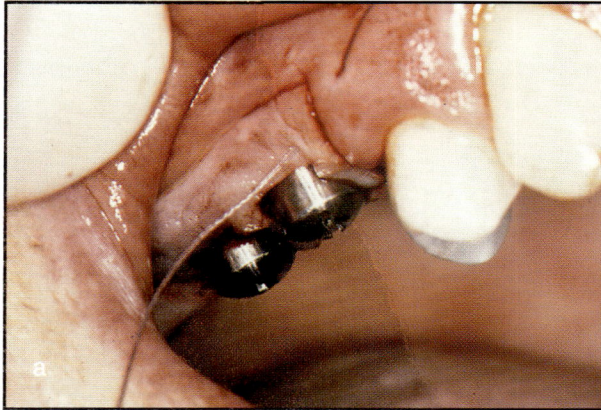

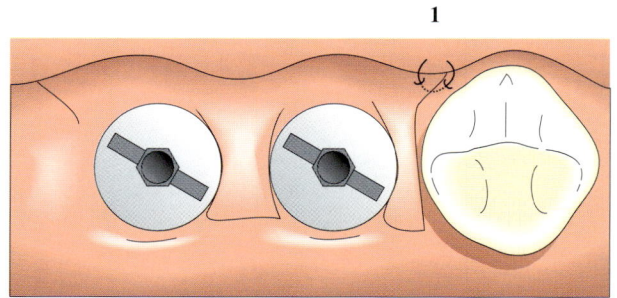

Fig 8-27 *(a and b)* The suturing procedure starts at the mesial aspect of the flap, with a single suture at the releasing incision (step 1).

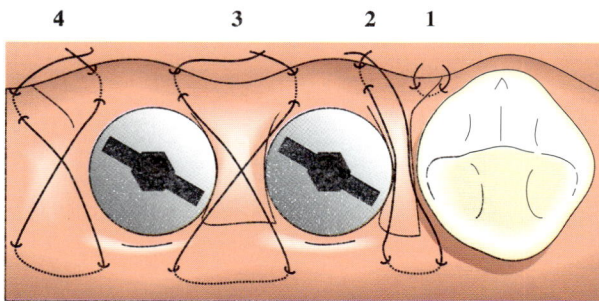

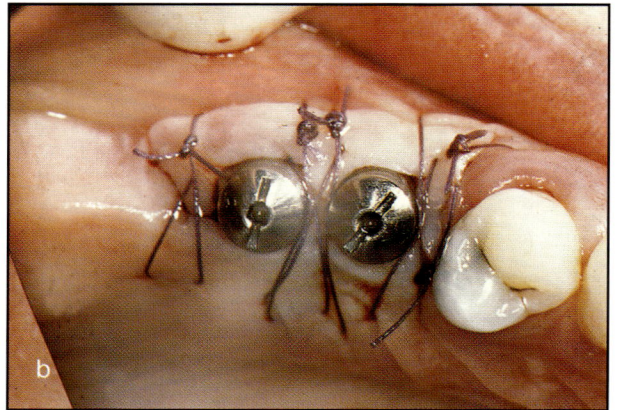

Fig 8-28 *(a)* The first suture is made labially at the releasing incision level, then a mattress suture is made starting buccally and running to the palatal aspect and back (steps 2, 3, and 4). This suture design stabilizes the pedicle in the interproximal area and adapts this tissue portion to the underlying bone. *(b and c)* Furthermore, this suture technique minimizes the risk of rupturing the pedicle.

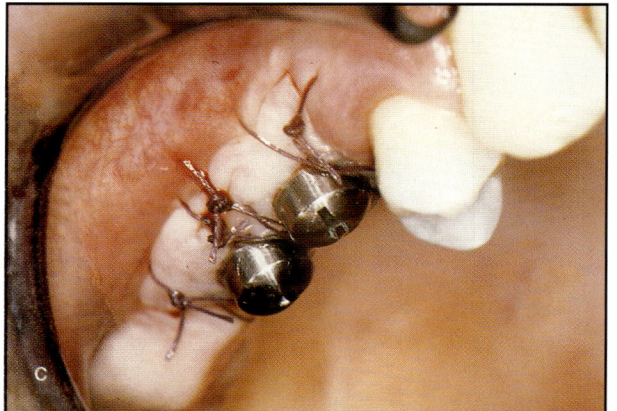

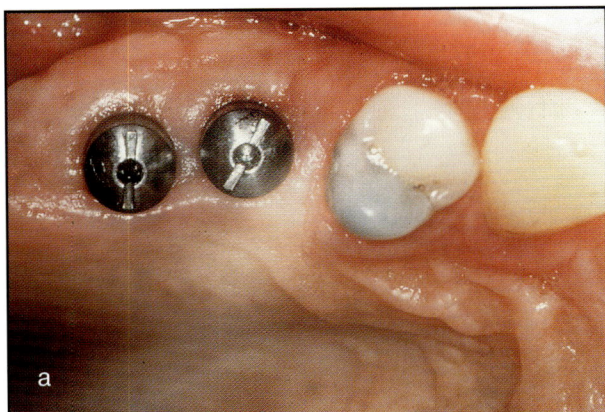

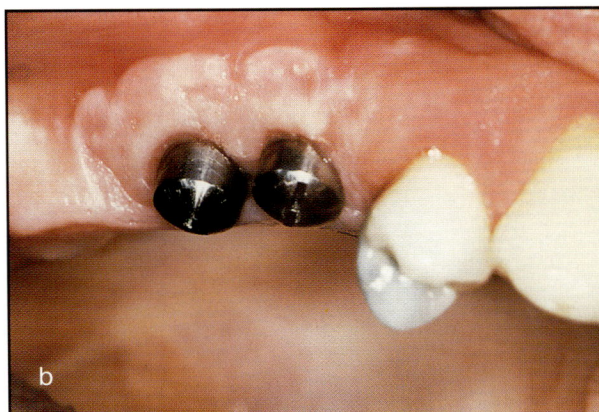

Fig 8-29 *(a and b)* Healing seen from an occlusal aspect 6 weeks after abutment connection. Note the increased tissue volume obtained at the buccal aspect.

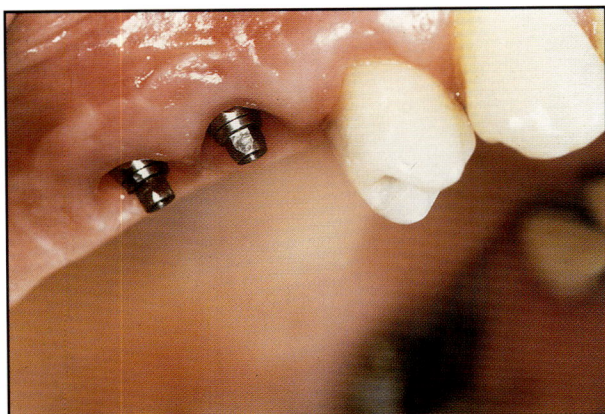

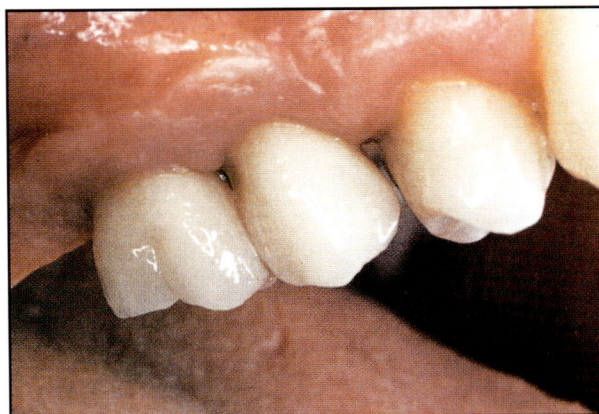

Fig 8-30 Healing abutments replaced by final abutments (EsthetiCone) 2 to 6 weeks following second-stage surgery. At this stage of treatment, it is obvious that the surgical soft tissue manipulation created a perimucosal soft tissue contour matching the gingival architecture.

Fig 8-31 Prosthesis in place.

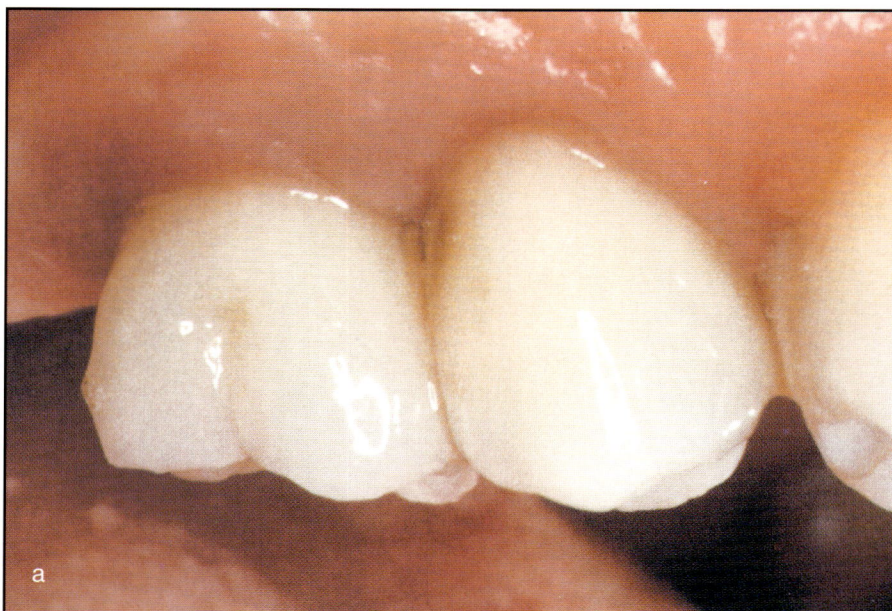

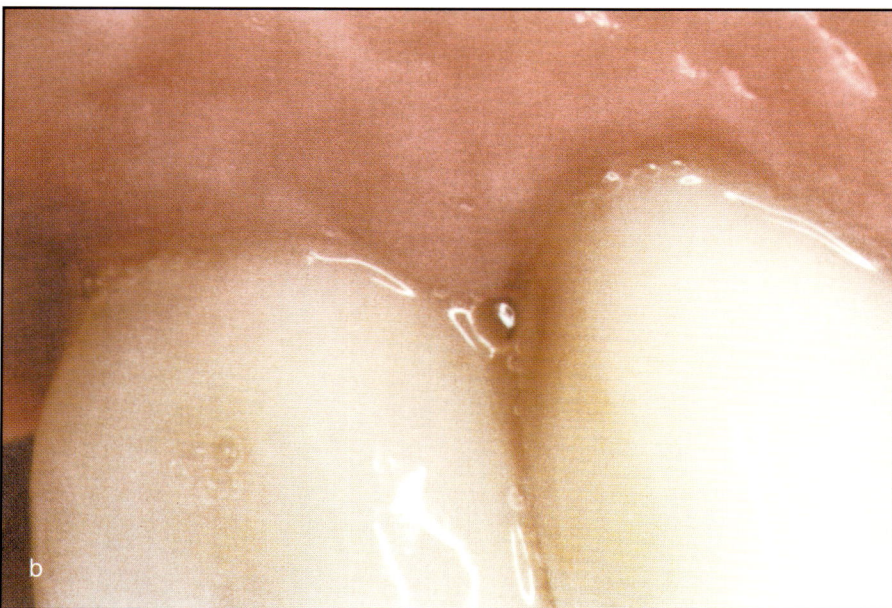

Fig 8-32 *(a and b)* Condition and architecture of perimucosal soft tissue, as seen 2 years after placement of the fixed prosthesis.

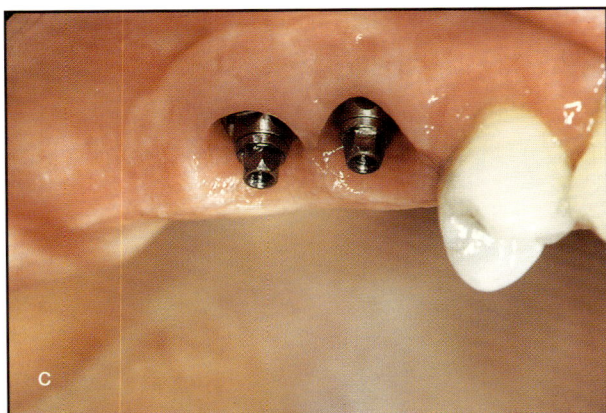

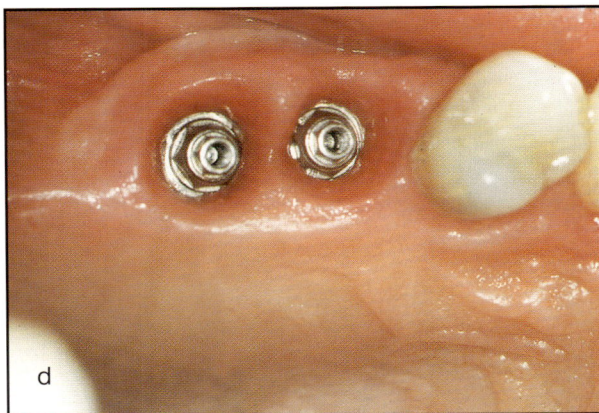

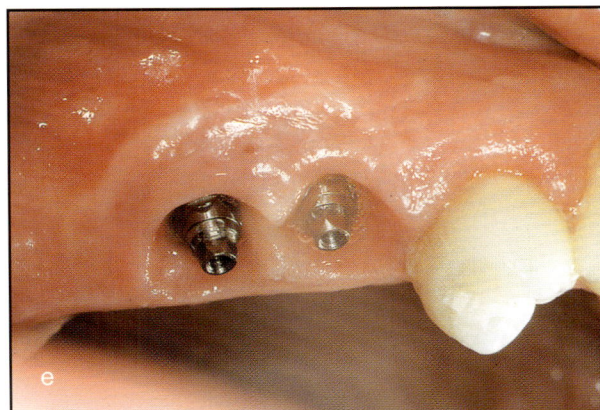

Fig 8-32 Four years (c) and 7 years (d and e) after placement of the fixed prosthesis. The fixed partial denture has just been removed to control soft tissue health and anatomy.

Remarks on the surgical technique

The technique described for second-stage surgery will vary according to several factors. They include the edentulous zones, the space between the implants, the cylindrical abutments, the increase in the alveolar ridge in the buccal direction from pushing of soft tissues, and the geometric displacement of the pedicles.

The apparent simplicity of the technique should not mask its sensitivity. Accordingly, the clinician should keep the following in mind:

1. The tissues should be handled in such a way as to avoid trauma, including minimal disturbance of vascularization.
2. The bevel incisions in the mobile flap are delicate and should vary according to patient's needs (thickness, height, or both).
3. The rotated pedicles should stay in place without any tension.
4. The suturing technique should allow a tight and firm connection of the pedicles to the supporting bone and abutments.

Single-tooth restoration

The papilla regeneration technique is modified for single-tooth restorations. Because of the need to restore mesial and distal papillae, the lack of sufficient tissue, and the possibility of inducing tension in the flaps, the first incision is more palatal in order to increase the amount of available tissue to be pushed buccally and to decrease the risk of failure. Furthermore, the releasing incisions are made more mesial and distal in the apical portion of the elevated mucoperiosteal flap, thus allowing reflection of a thick, wide flap from which two pedicles can be disengaged (Fig 8-33). The mesial papilla is created with a pedicle rotated 90 degrees mesially, and the distally rotated pedicle creates the distal papilla (Figs 8-34 to 8-36). Mesial and distal papillae can also be created according to the technique illustrated in Fig 8-37. Although the spaces between the implant and the adjacent teeth are limited in the anterior maxilla, this technique allows an adequate quantity of tissue in the buccal, as well as coronal, direction. As in the standard papilla regeneration technique, horizontal mattress sutures are used here to stabilize the flap in an optimal position without tension (Fig 8-38).

Figures 8-39 to 8-44 are case presentations that demonstrate the good results obtained using the papilla regeneration technique.

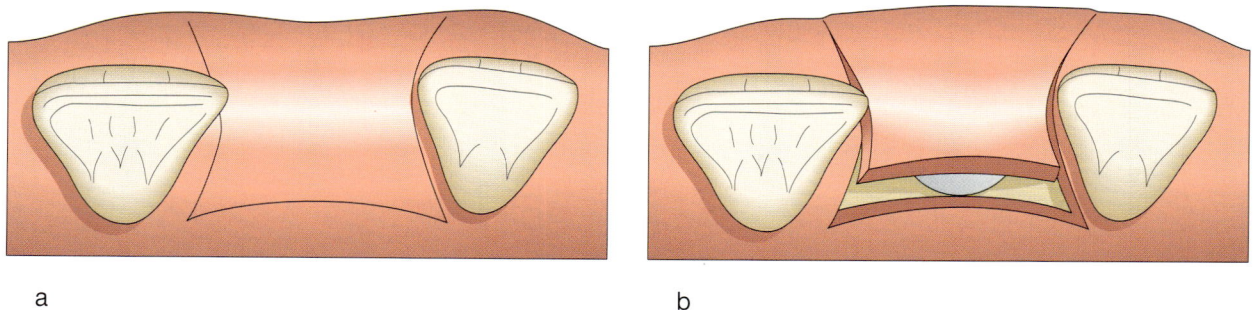

a   b

Fig 8-33 *(a and b)* When dealing with single-tooth restorations, one should notice that there is generally minimal soft tissue available and more risk for tension, ischemy, and failure. The concept is the same as the basic technique but the horizontal incision is made more palatally in order to gain more tissue buccally. If the mesial and distal papillae are present (Class I or Class II) they should be preserved. If they need to be augmented (Class III) they should be included in the flap design.

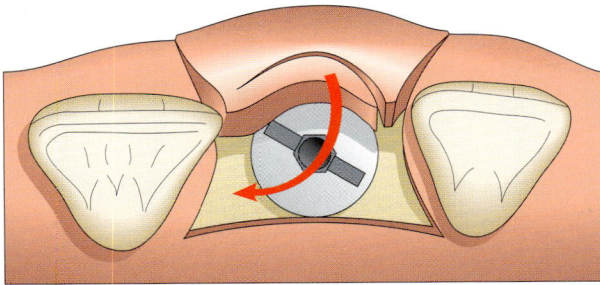

Fig 8-34 Schematic drawing illustrating the semilunar bevel incision made distal to mesial and the 90-degree rotation of the pedicle.

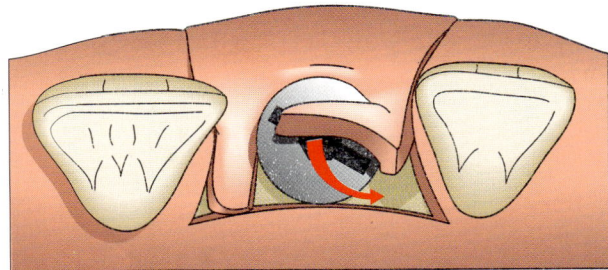

Fig 8-35 Once the first pedicle is in place, a second semilunar bevel incision is made mesial to distal. The pedicle is then rotated 90 degrees to fill the space between the abutment and the distal teeth.

Fig 8-36 Occlusal view of the sliding of the two pedicles from each side of the abutment creating newly formed papillae.

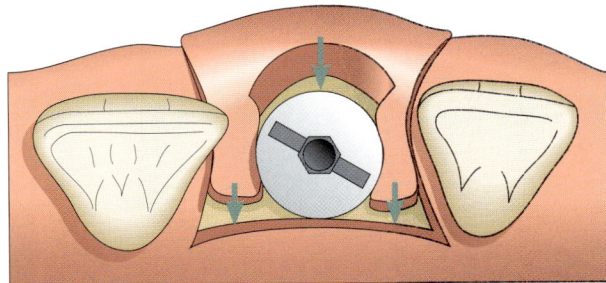

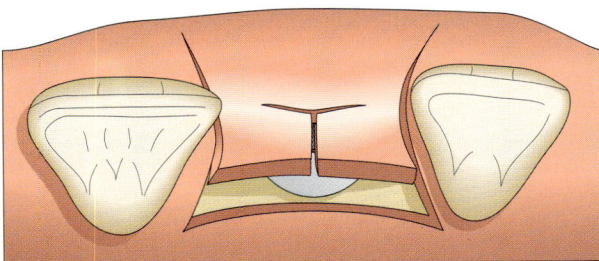

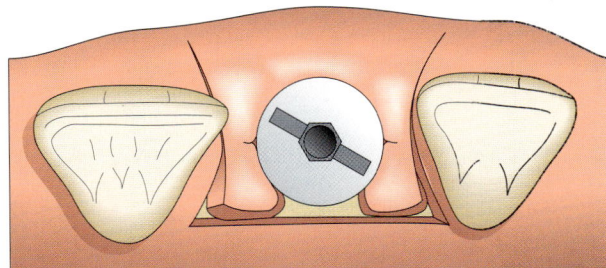

Figs 8-37 and 8-38 In some situations, a T shape incision can be made and both sides of the flap can slide laterally to fill the spaces between the abutment and the adjacent teeth as illustrated in Fig 8-38.

Peri-implant Soft Tissue Augmentation Procedures

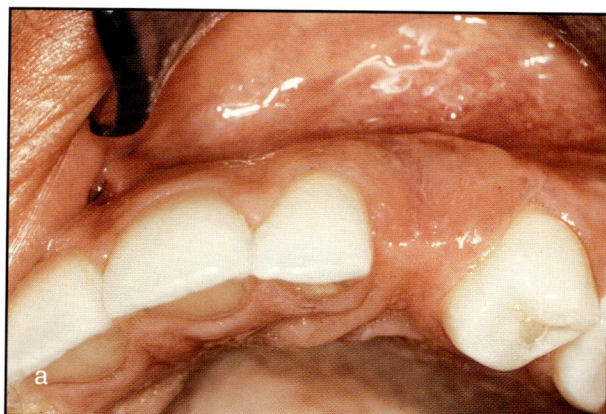

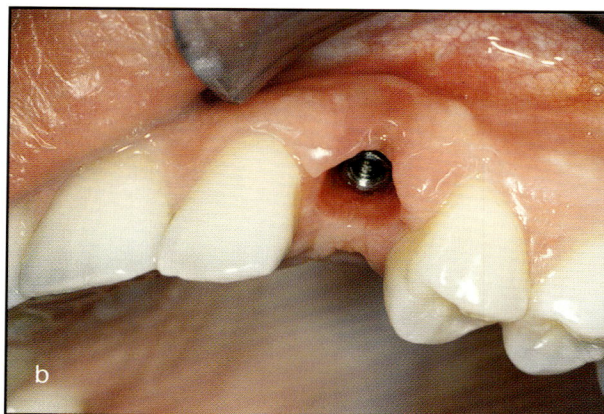

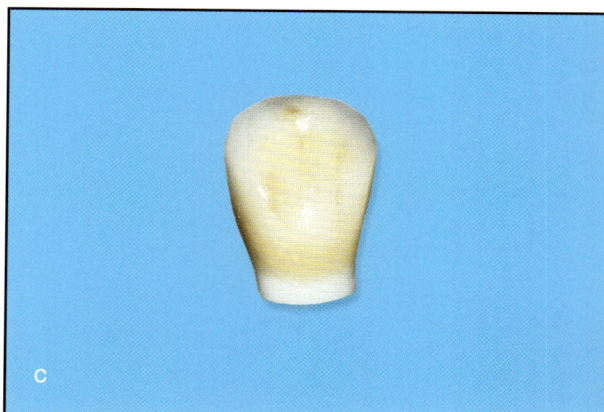

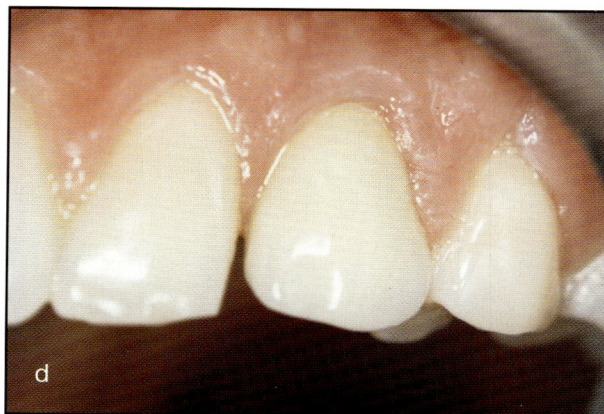

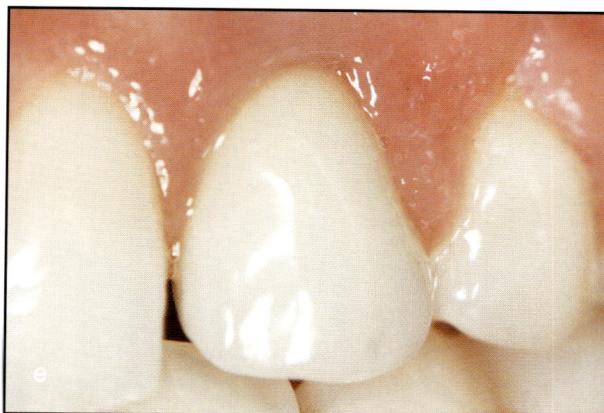

Fig 8-39 *(a and b)* Placement of implant to restore a missing maxillary left canine. *(c)* Implant-supported single-tooth restoration fabricated using a CeraOne abutment and ceramic cap. *(d)* Clinical appearance 3 years after restoration placement. The papilla regeneration technique has been used to created harmonious soft tissue architecture. *(e)* Clinical view 6 years later. Note the harmonious contour around the crown and the cleft on the labial of the first premolar due to traumatic hygiene (aggressive use of dental floss).

184

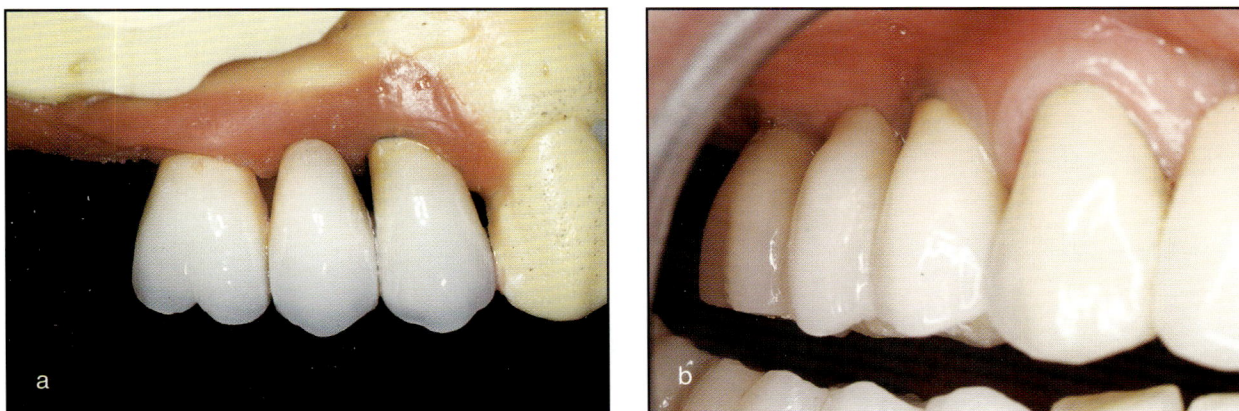

Fig 8-40 *(a)* Clinical case where two 13-mm regular-platform implants have been used to replace three teeth. Adequate implant placement helps the lab technician to build a fixed partial denture with physiologic embrasures. *(b)* Clinical view at the time of placement. Note the papilla created between the first premolar and canine and soft tissue contour around the abutments. *(c)* Clinical view 10 years later, the tissue is stable and healthy. The patient can adequately maintain the soft tissues around the prosthetic crowns.

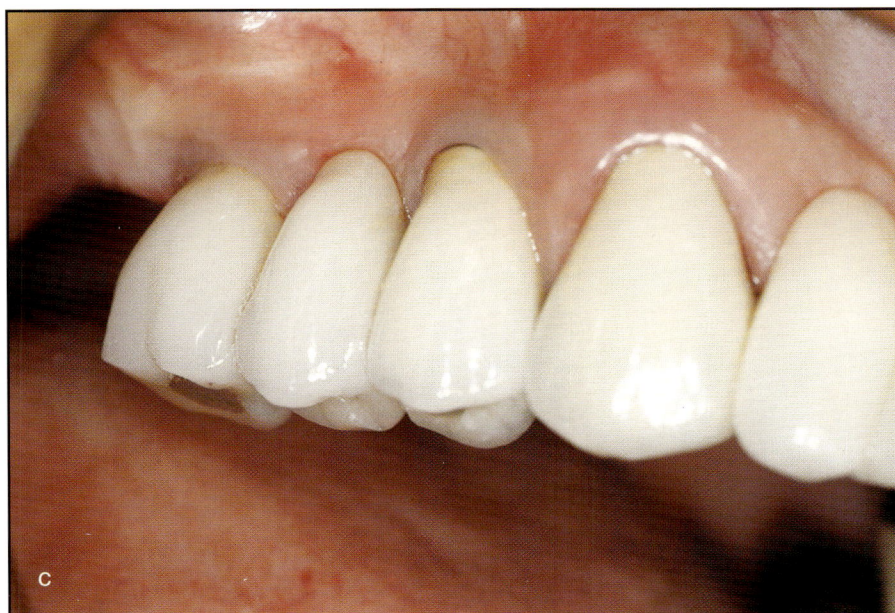

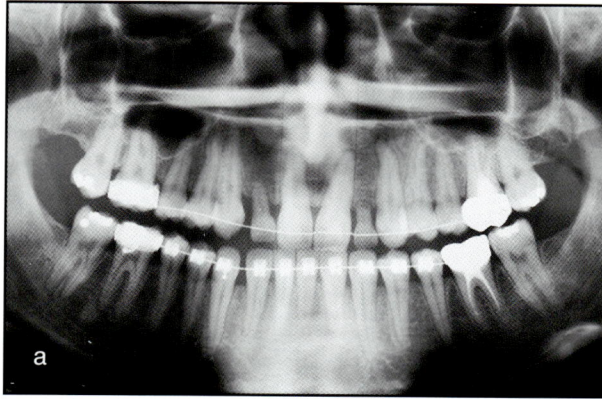

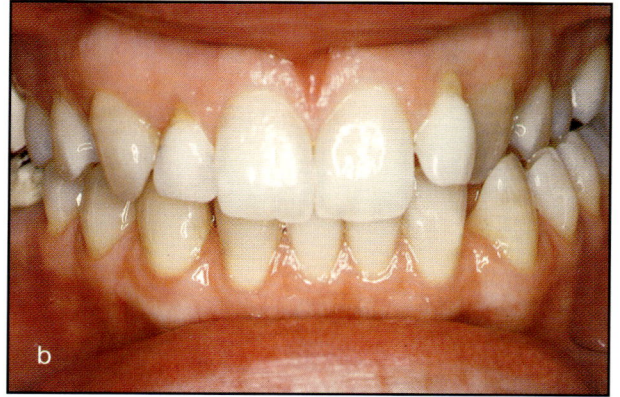

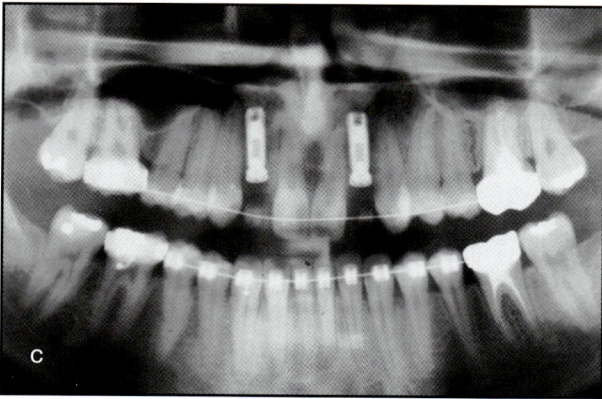

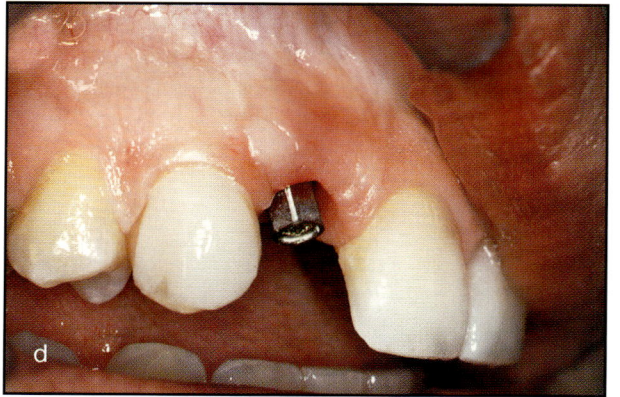

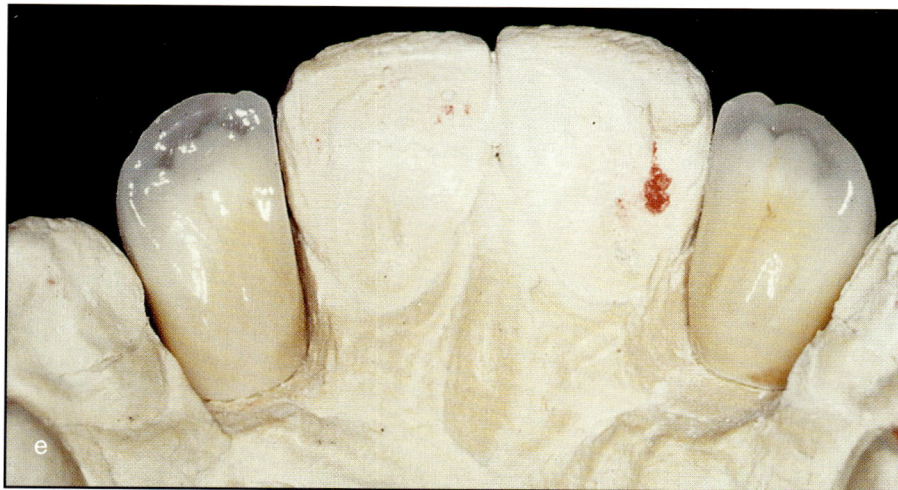

Fig 8-41 *(a to k)* A 25-year-old woman with congenital aplasia of the permanent maxillary lateral incisors. The remaining deciduous lateral incisors, showing signs of severe root resorption, were extracted and replaced with implant-supported single restorations. Following healing, CeraOne abutments were connected to fixtures, and ceramic crowns were fabricated and placed.

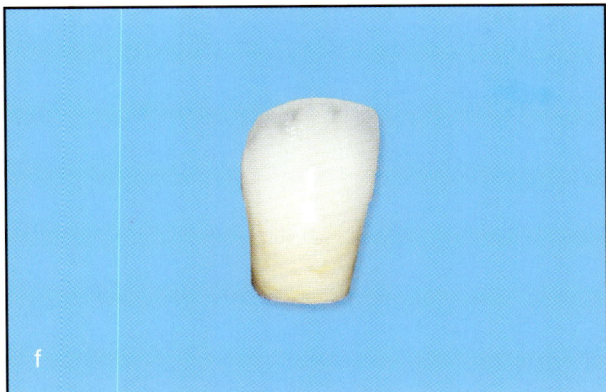

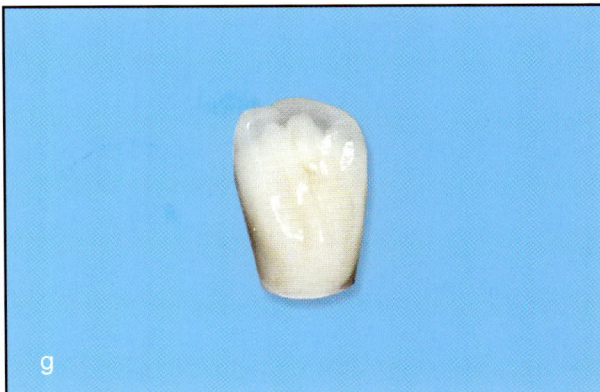

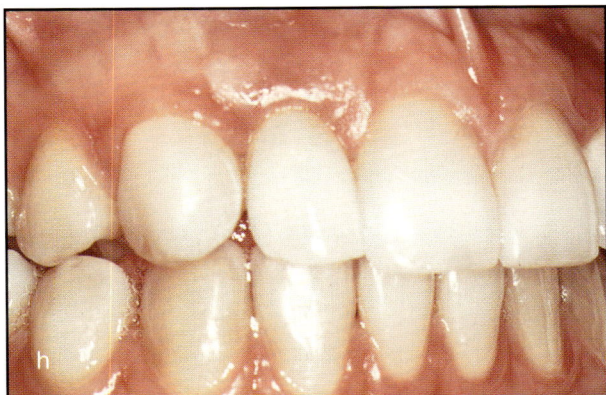

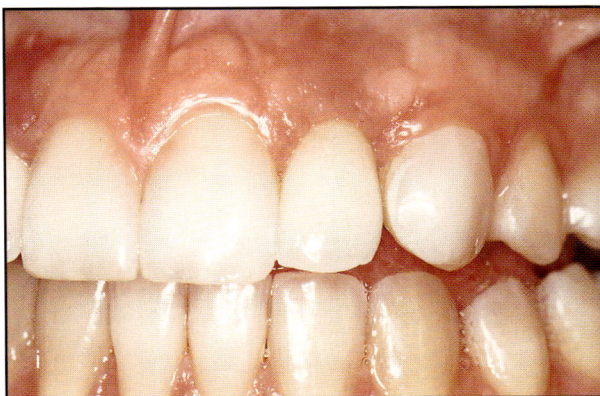

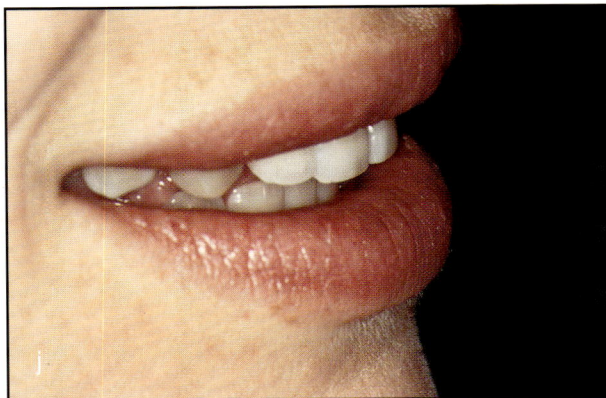

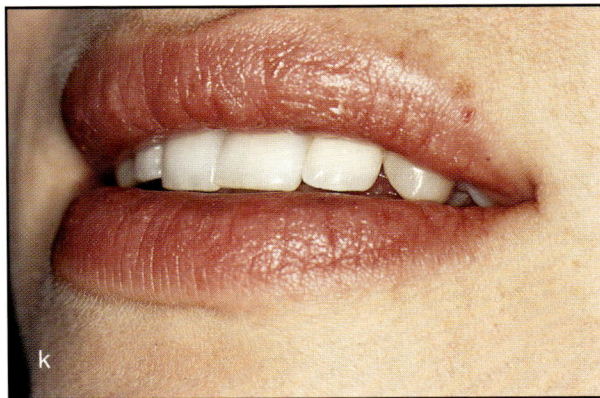

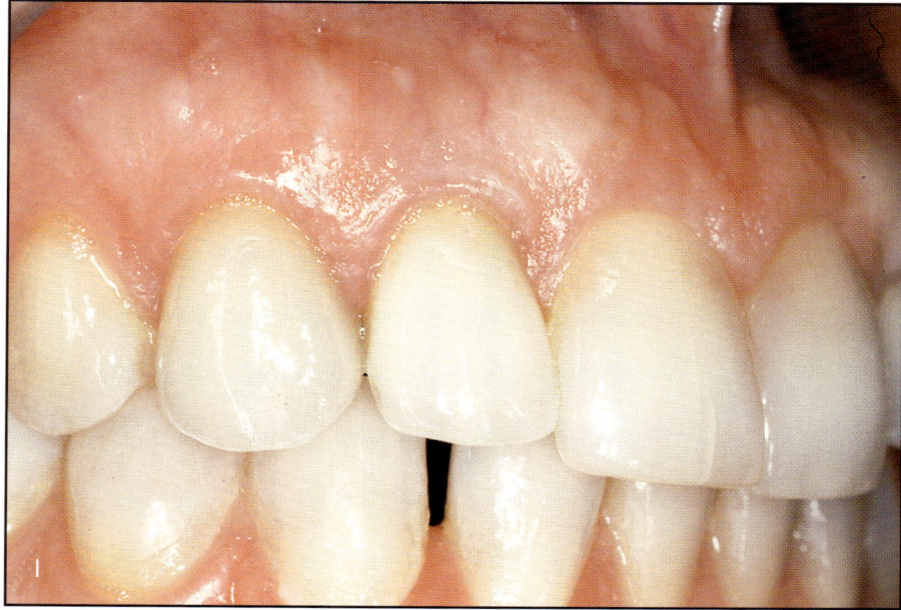

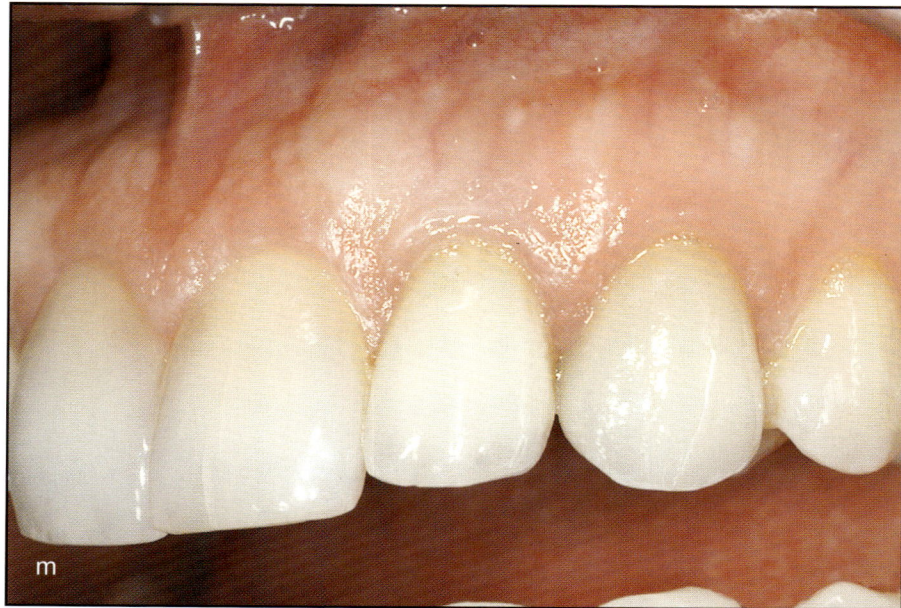

Fig 8-41 *(l and m)* Clinical view 9 years later. Note good adaptation of the peri-implant tissues around the CeraOne crowns as well as the maintenance of the created papillae between the implants and teeth using the papilla regeneration technique.

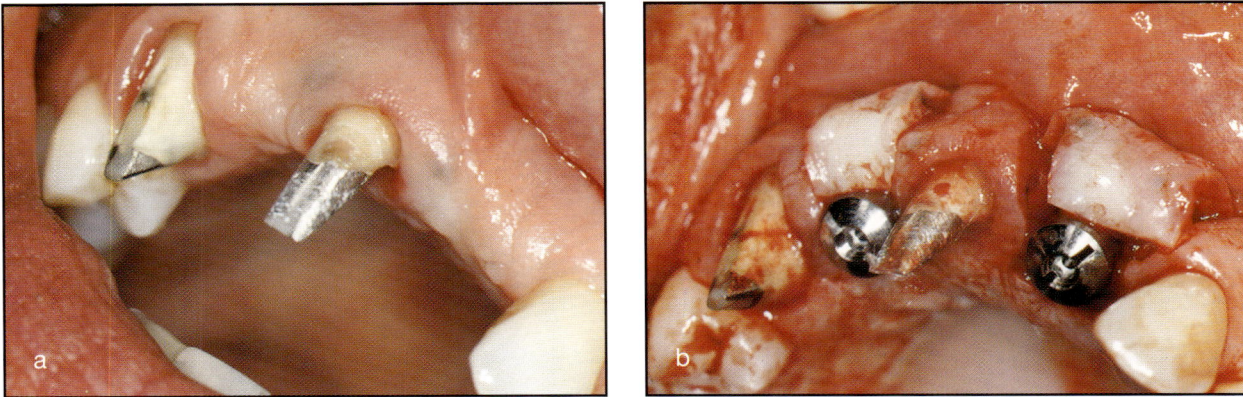

Fig 8-42 *(a)* Anterior maxilla edentation. Note the resorption of the alveolar ridge. Two implants are planned to replace lateral and central incisors. *(b)* Second-stage surgery is performed 6 months after implant placement. The design of the flap as well as the placement of the healing abutments will promote an adequate contour of the alveolar ridge.

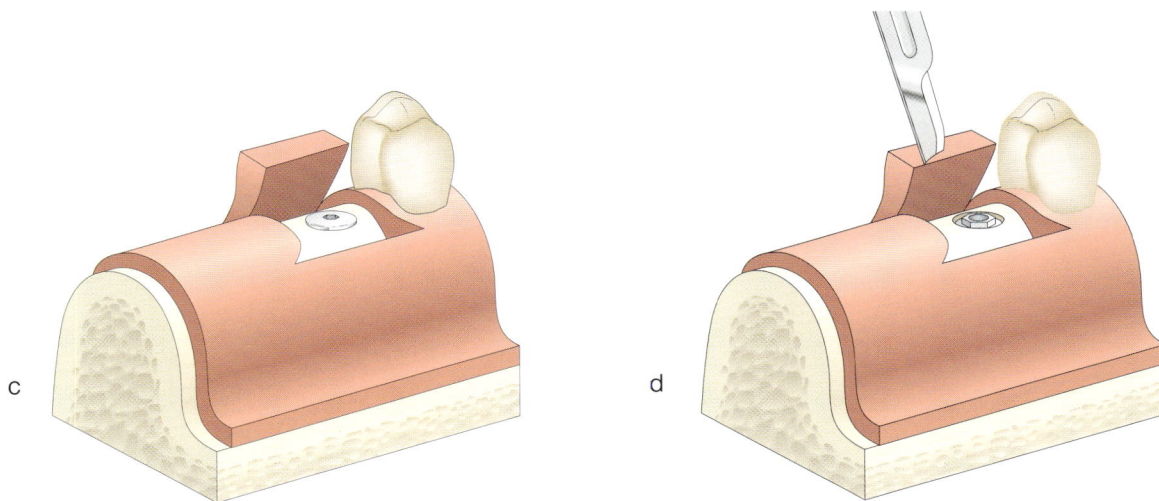

Fig 8-42 *(c to f)* Different steps of papilla regeneration technique for a single-tooth restoration. The basic concept is used with slight modifications due to the specific situation:
- A full-thickness flap is elevated for the basic technique, but the horizontal incision is made in a more palatal position to gain more soft tissue.
- The flap being elevated, a semilunar bevel incision is made distal to mesial. Then another semilunar bevel incision is made mesial to distal.
- The double papillae will then be created by a 90-degree rotation. Each side of the abutment will then be filled by these pedicle grafts.

This technique is very sensitive to the risks of tension and ischemy when placing and suturing the papillae due to the lack of tissue. In some situations a narrower healing abutment should be used instead of a regular healing abutment. In any case, wide abutments should never be used.

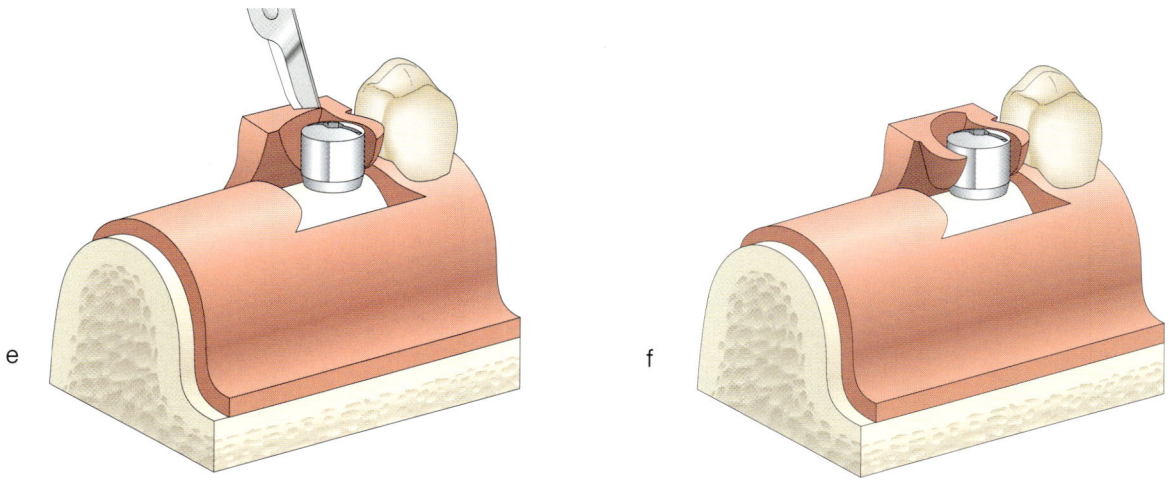

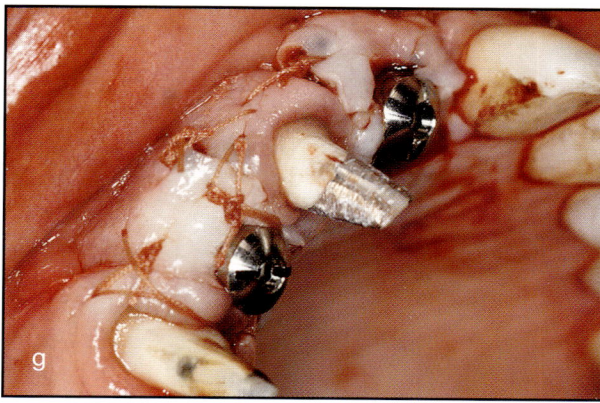

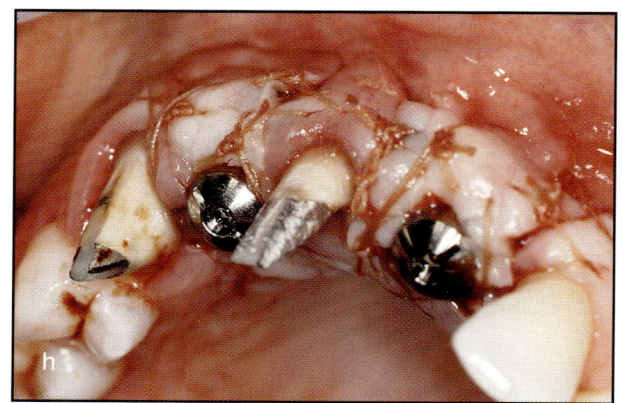

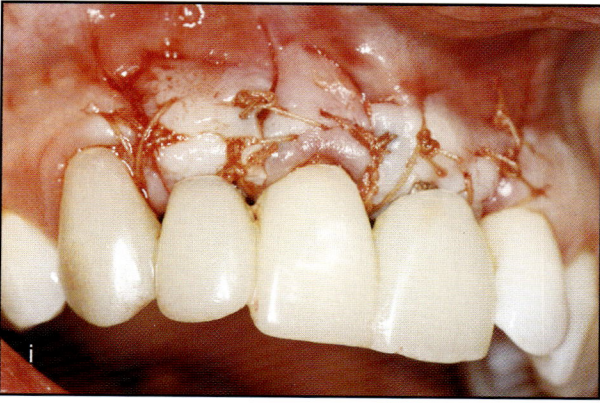

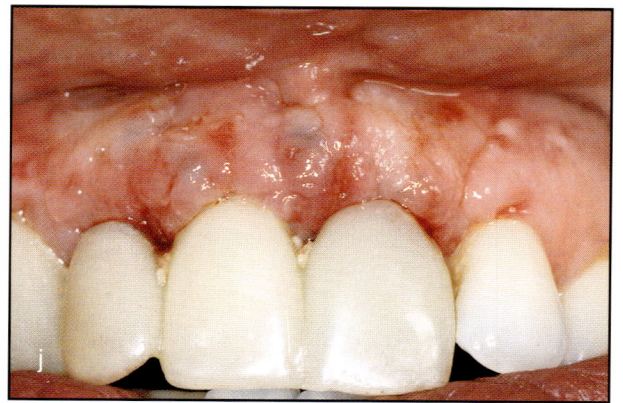

Fig 8-42 *(g to i)* Papillae sutured in place and the modification of the ridge in the edentulous areas. Note the coaptation of the soft tissues around the abutments as well as the re-establishment of the natural contours of the peri-implant mucosa. *(j)* Removal of the sutures 8 days after surgery. Tissue looks healthy and well vascularized.

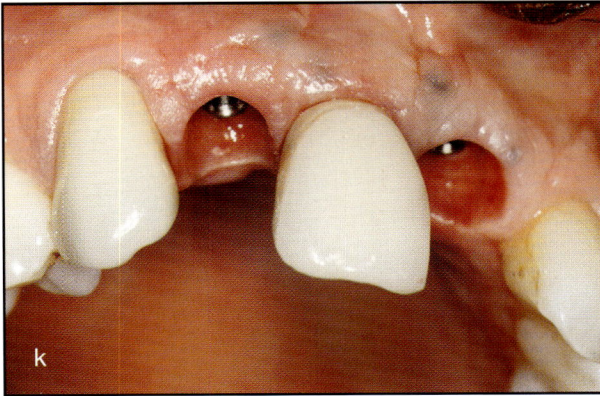

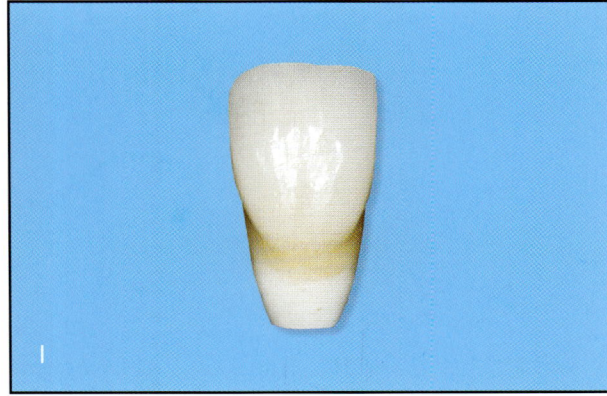

Fig 8-42 *(k)* The impression is taken at the fixture level 4 to 6 weeks later. Crowns are placed on the natural teeth. *(l)* CerAdapt restoration. Note the emergent profile from 4 to 6 mm at the cementoenamel junction.

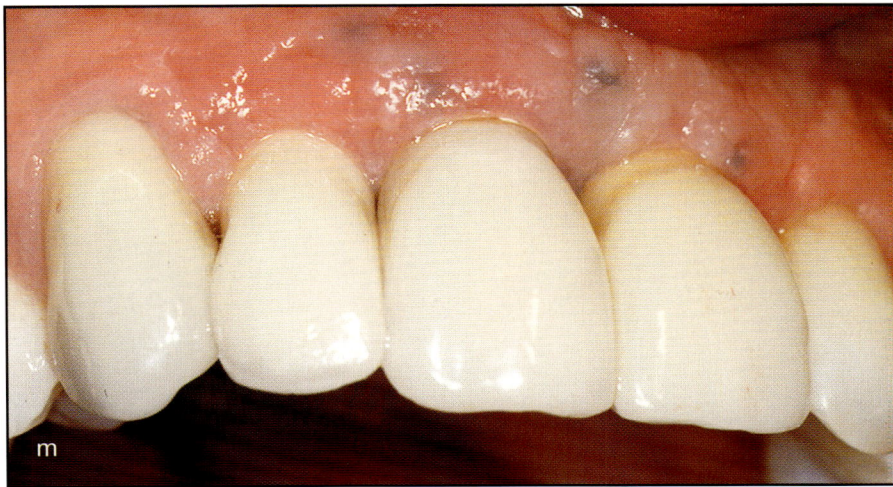

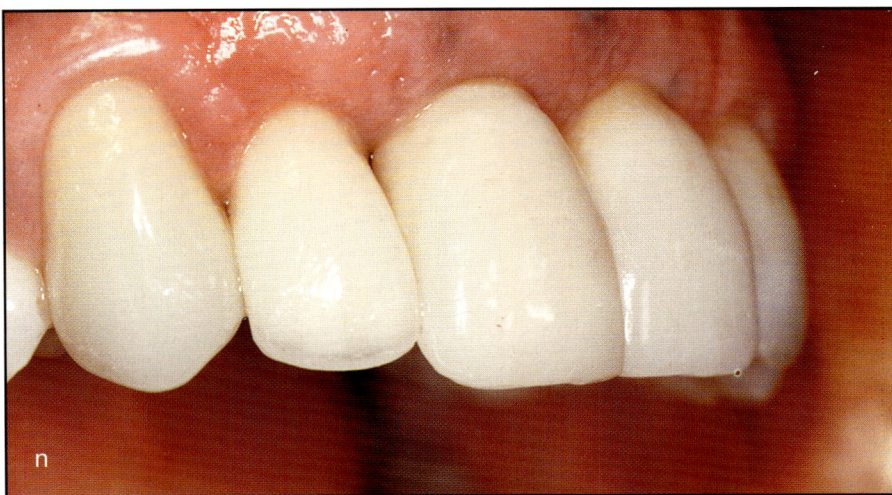

Fig 8-42 Clinical situation 6 months *(m)* and 3 years *(n)* after prosthetic insertion. (Prosthetic restoration: Prof A. J. Faucher, prosthodontist.)

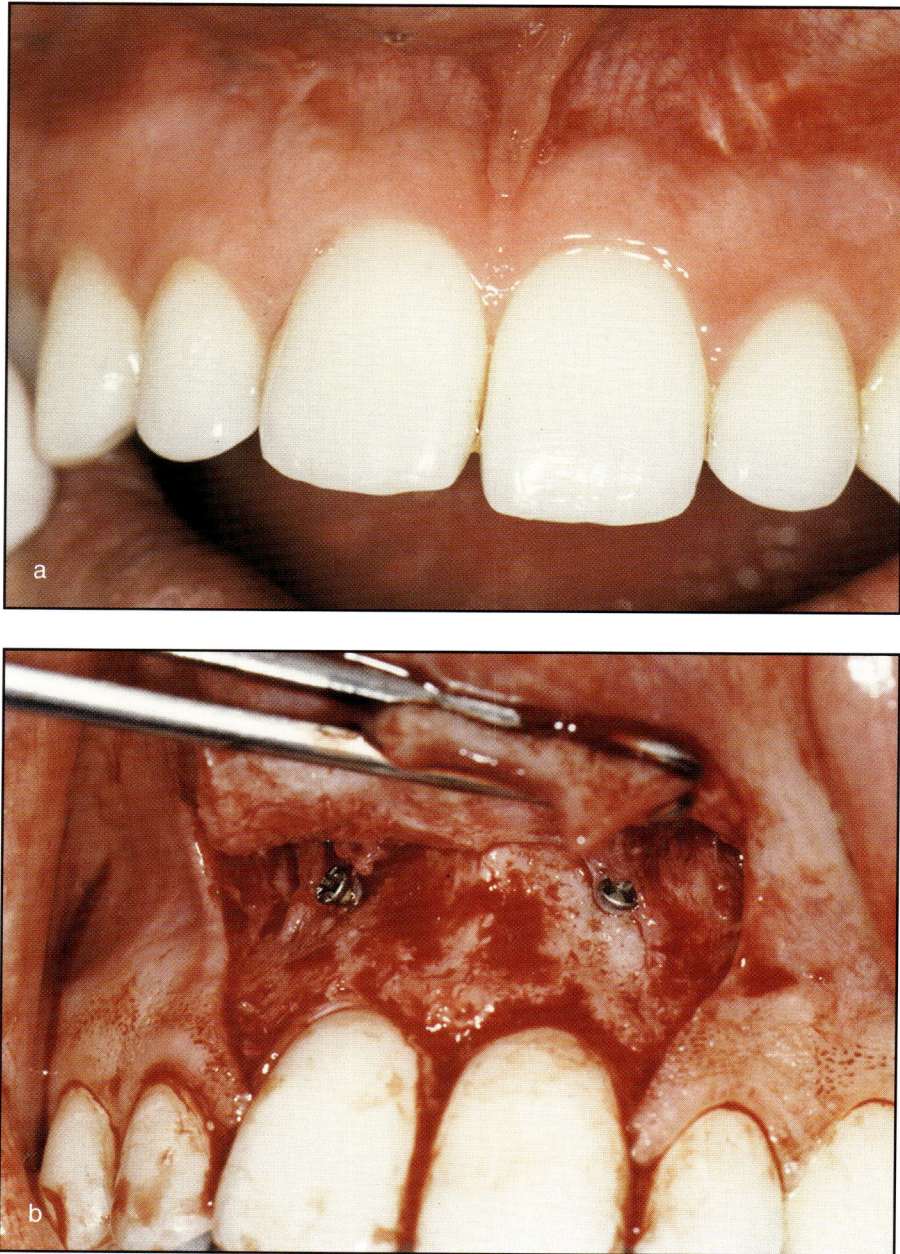

Fig 8-43 *(a)* Patient, a 20-year-old female, presenting with high mobility of the two maxillary central incisors due to root resorption after hiatrogenic orthodontic treatment. *(b)* A bone graft has been performed to correct the significant concavity of the alveolar ridge 4 months prior to tooth extraction and implant installation. The graft has been taken from the ramus area.

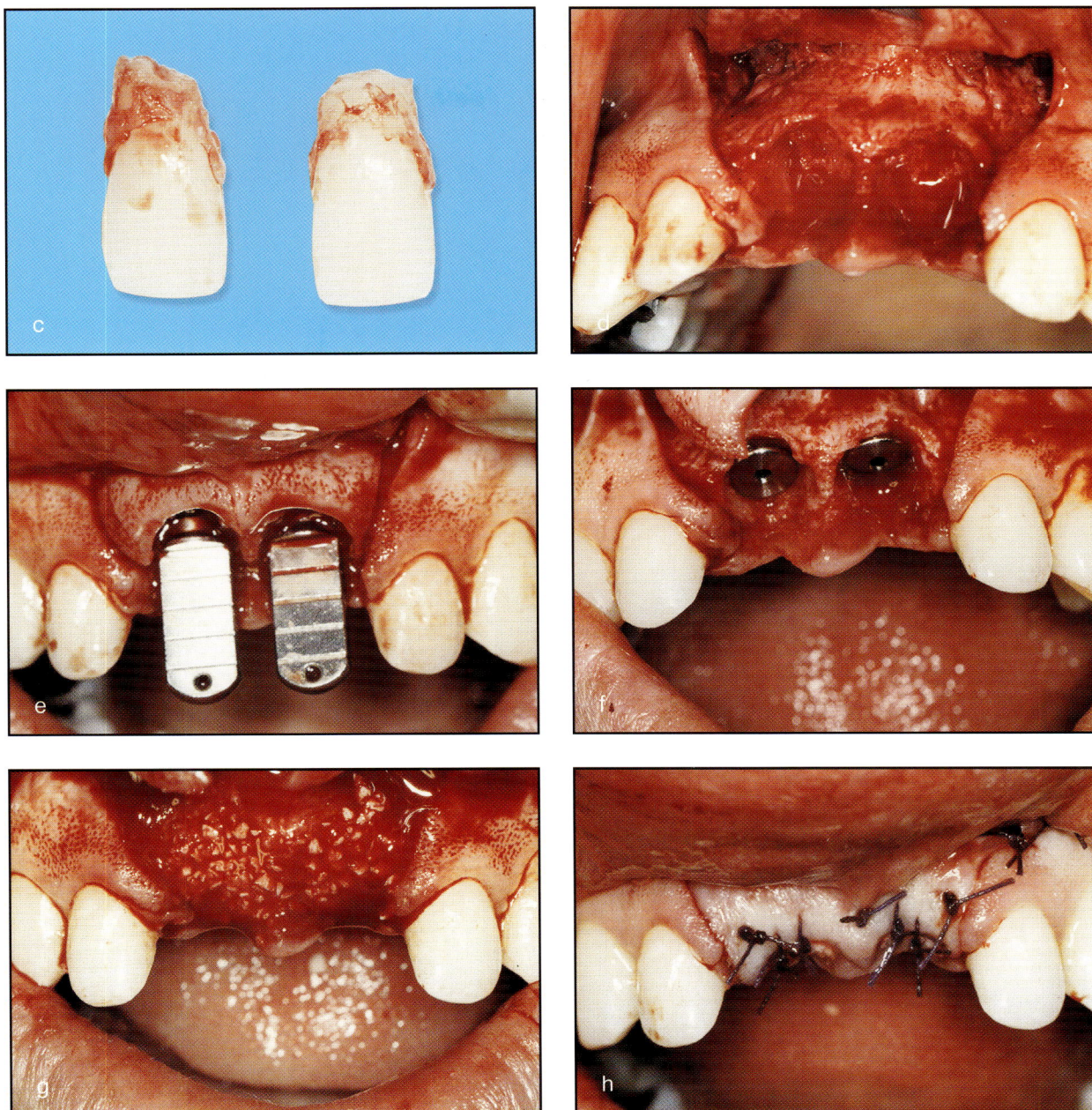

Fig 8-43 *(c)* Extracted teeth. Note the amount of root resorption. *(d)* Clinical situation of the ridge after extraction. The bone graft has created a more favorable situation for implant placement. *(e)* Fixture positioning guides in place representing the implant's position and its relationship with the future prosthetic restorations. *(f)* Implants in place. Note their apical position to the cementoenamel junction of the adjacent teeth and the preservation of the bone pick between the implants. *(g)* The alveolar ridge as well as the cover screws are covered with a mixture of collected bone and Bio-oss (Geistlich Biomaterials), thus adding support to the overlaying soft tissues.

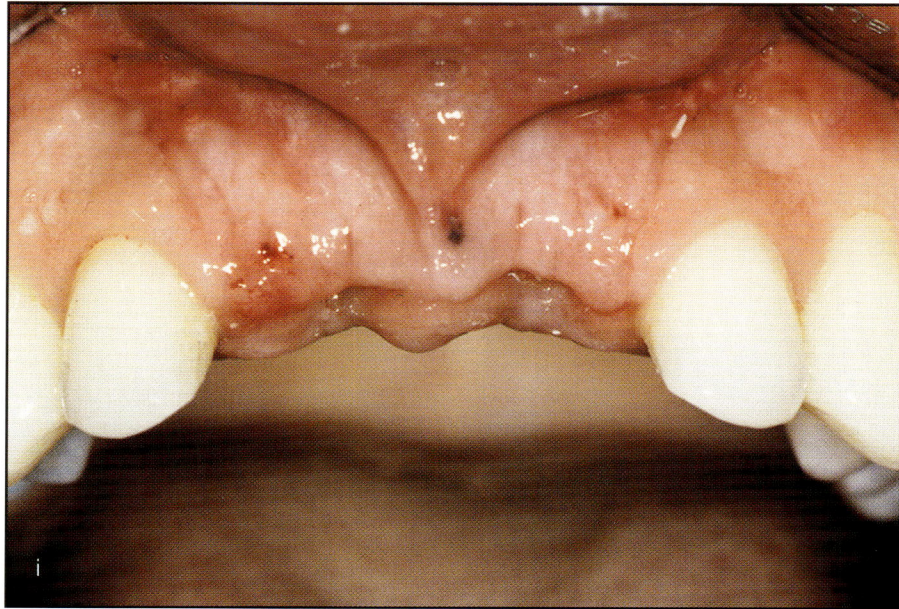

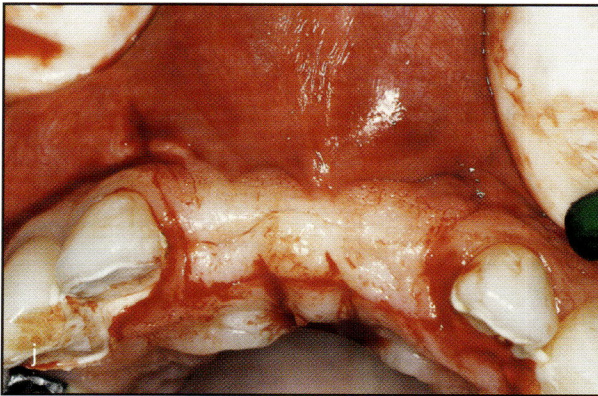

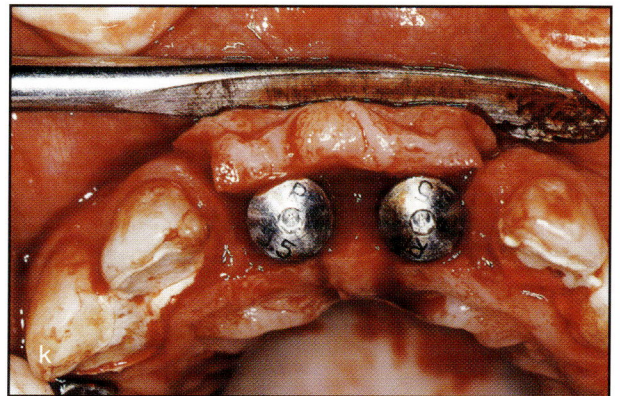

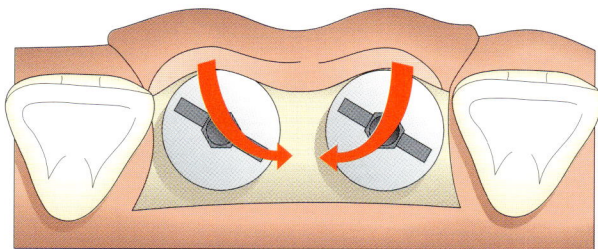

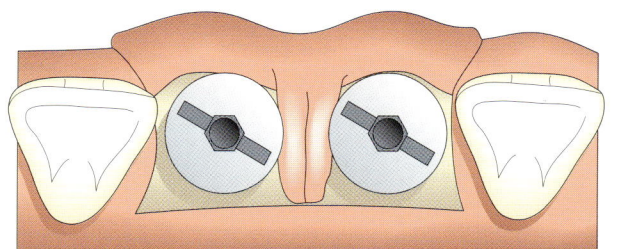

Fig 8-43 *(i)* Clinical situation 6 months after implant placement. *(j)* At second-stage surgery, a palatal horizontal incision as well as two vertical releasing incisions are made, preserving the existing papillae at the level of the lateral incisors. *(k)* The healing abutment will maintain the soft tissue in a more labial position, thus creating an adequate ridge contour. *(l)* Flaps used to create a central papilla between two implants. Semilunar bevel incisions distal to mesial will allow two pedicles to rotate with a 90-degree angulation. *(m)* The two pedicles in place after a 90-degree rotation creating a central papillalike formation.

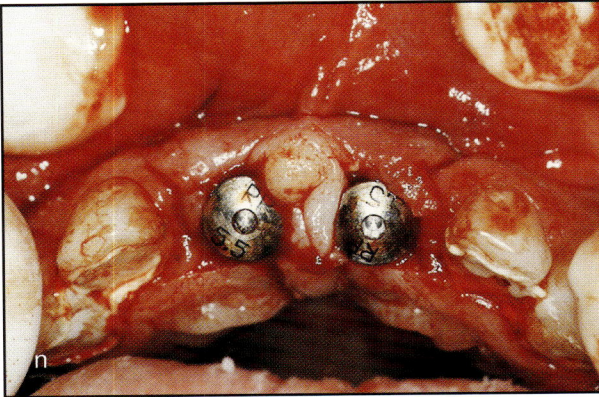

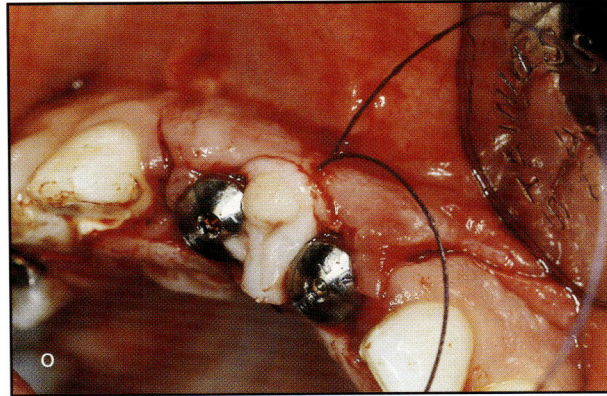

Fig 8-43 *(n to p)* Clinical situation with the two pedicles in place. A through-and-through suture from the labial to the palatal will hold the tissues in place. Then a periosteal mattress suture, as shown previously in Fig 8-28, is performed.

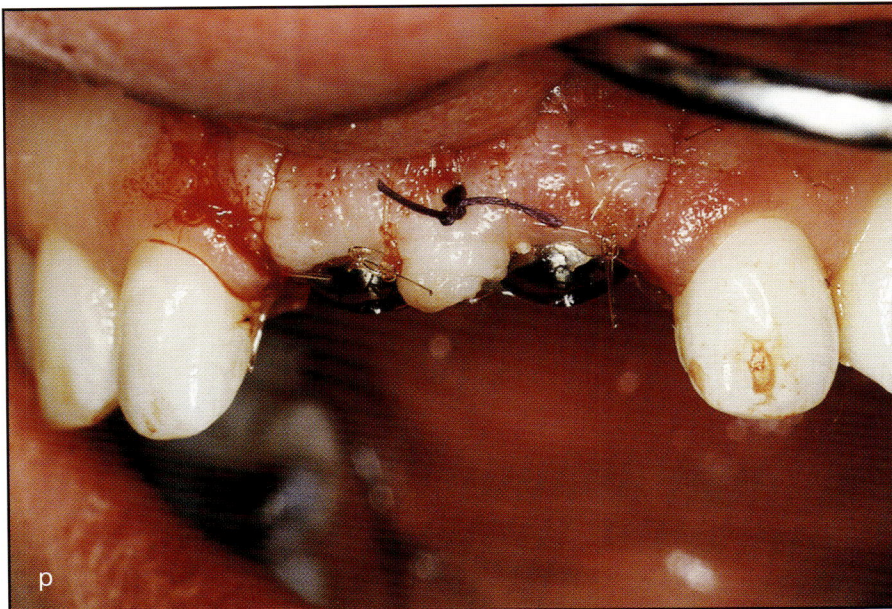

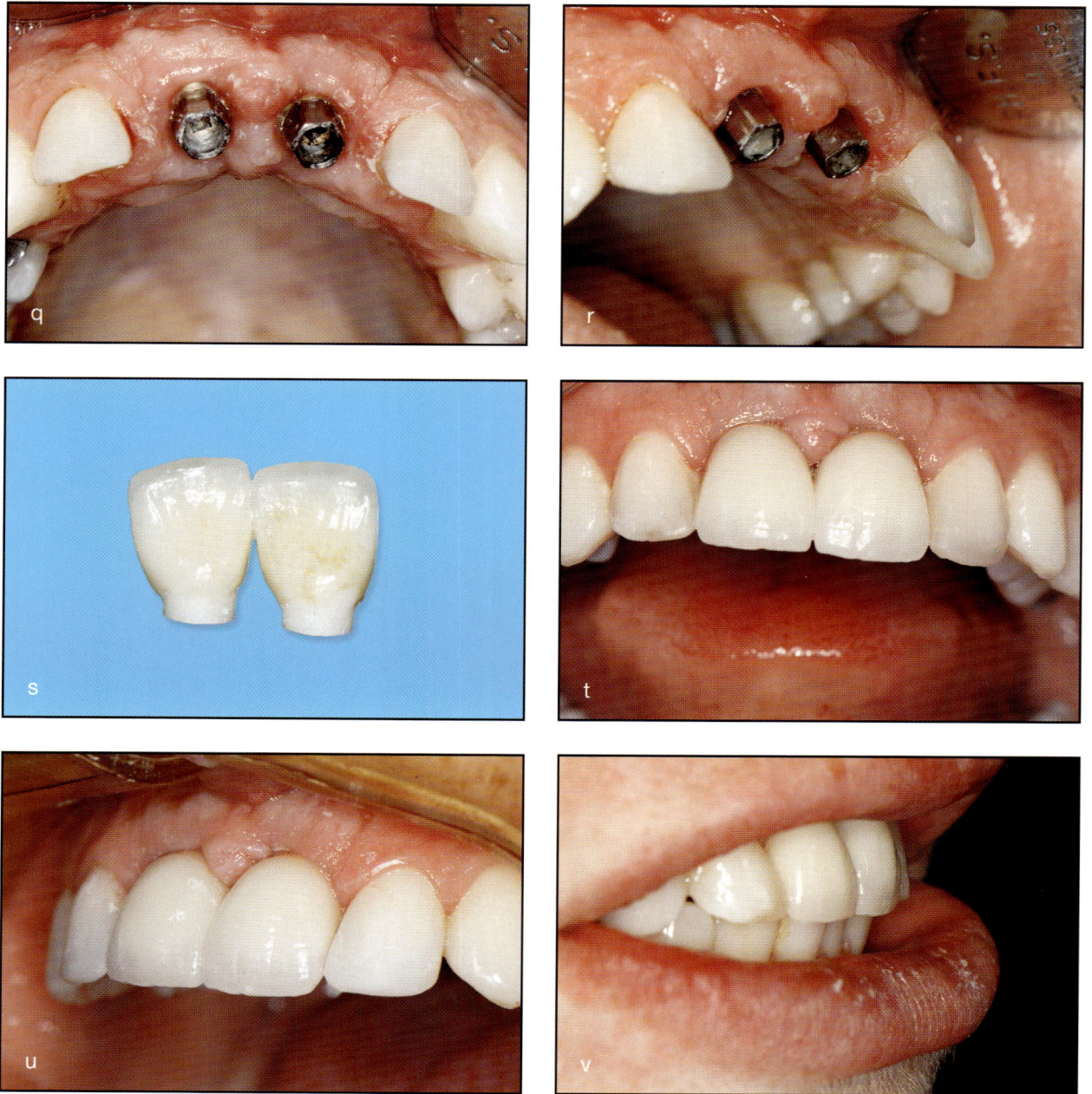

Fig 8-43 *(q and r)* Healing abutments are removed 4 weeks later and two CeraOne abutments are placed. The impression can then be taken. Note the re-creation of an adequate ridge contour as well as the central papilla between the two implants. *(s)* Palatal view of the porcelain crowns. *(t to v)* Tissue maturation takes place after the two crowns are placed. One can expect an optimal result 4 to 6 months later in terms of form, texture, and color.

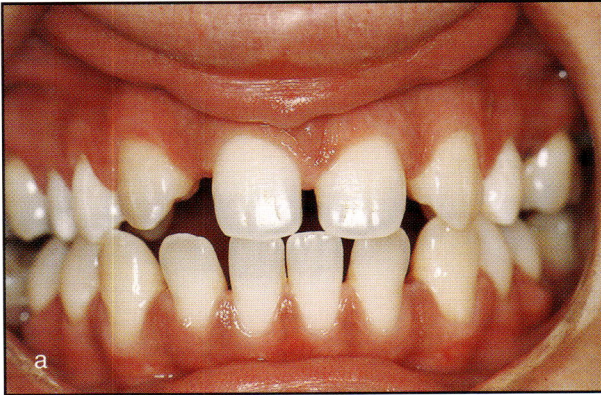

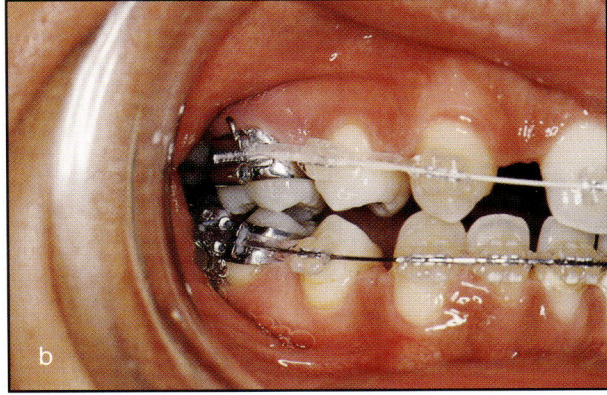

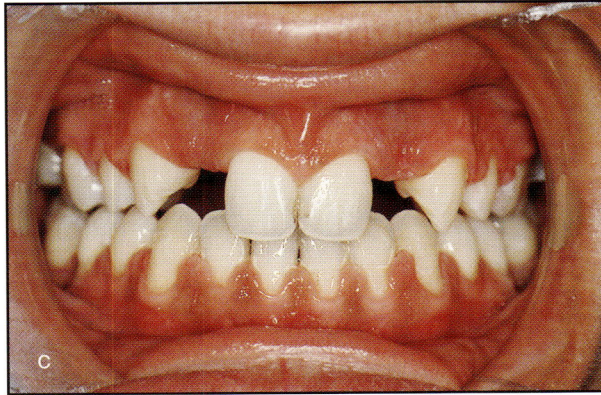

Fig 8-44 *(a)* Female patient, 24 years old, presenting with lateral incisor anodontia resulting in a malposition of the anterior teeth. *(b)* Orthodontic treatment will allow the creation of a more favorable situation for implant placement. (Orthodontic treatment: Drs J. Lacout and D. Deroze.) *(c)* Clinical view after orthodontic treatment. *(d to f)* Implant placement. At the right side, the ridge is adequate. A concavity on the opposite side results in the implant being placed with exposed threads. Autogenous bone is packed on the labial site to cover the threads and optimize ridge anatomy.

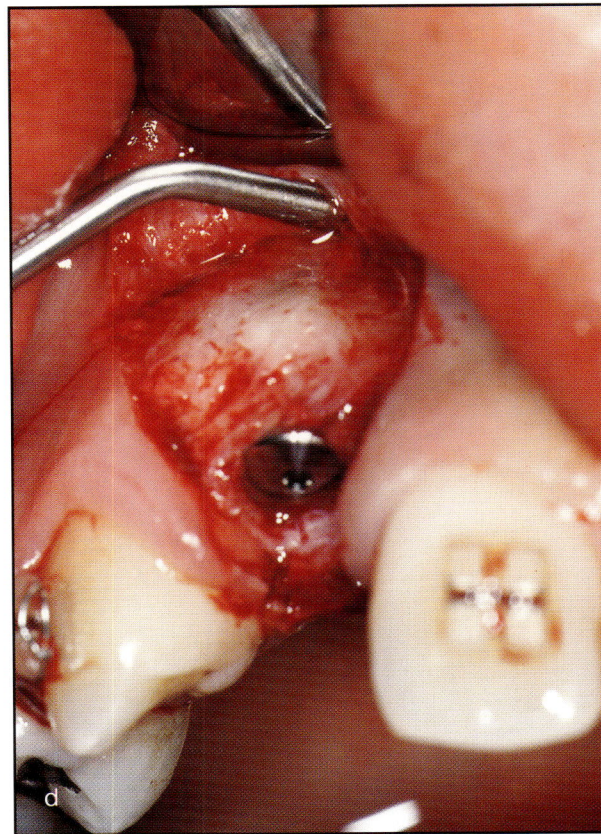

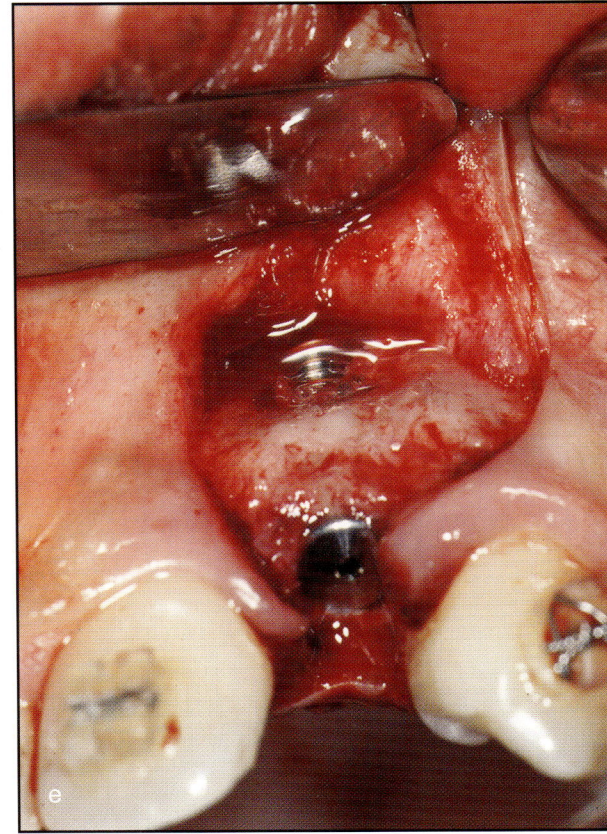

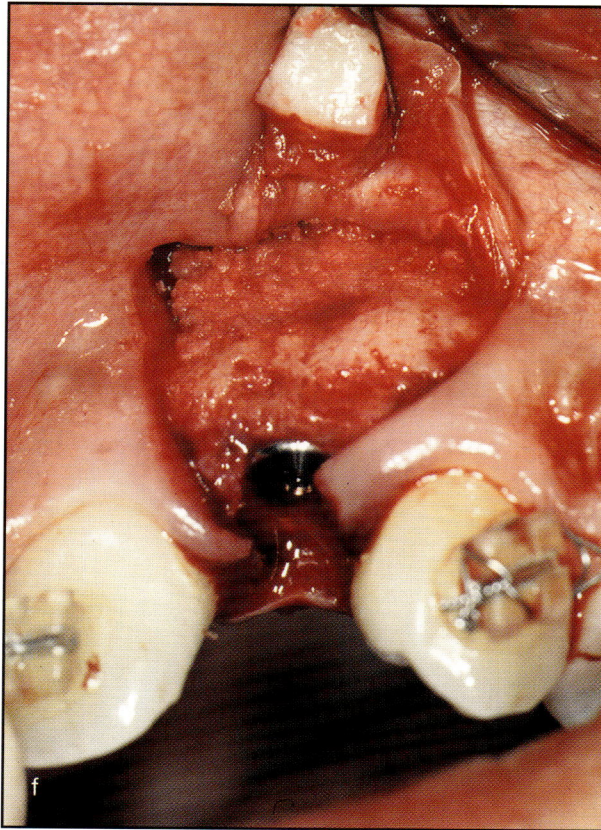

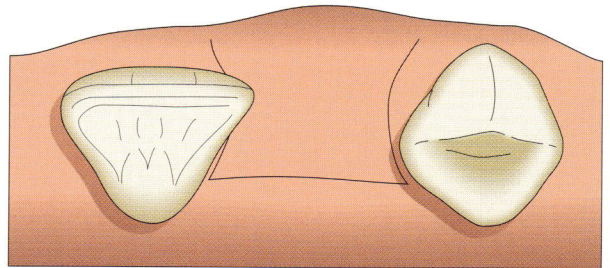

g

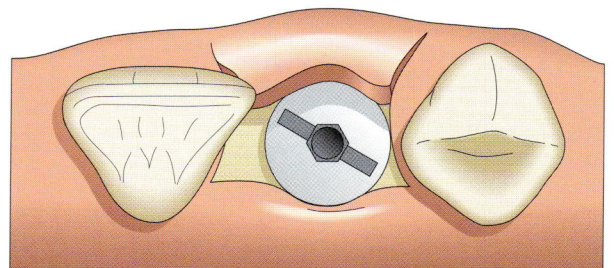

h

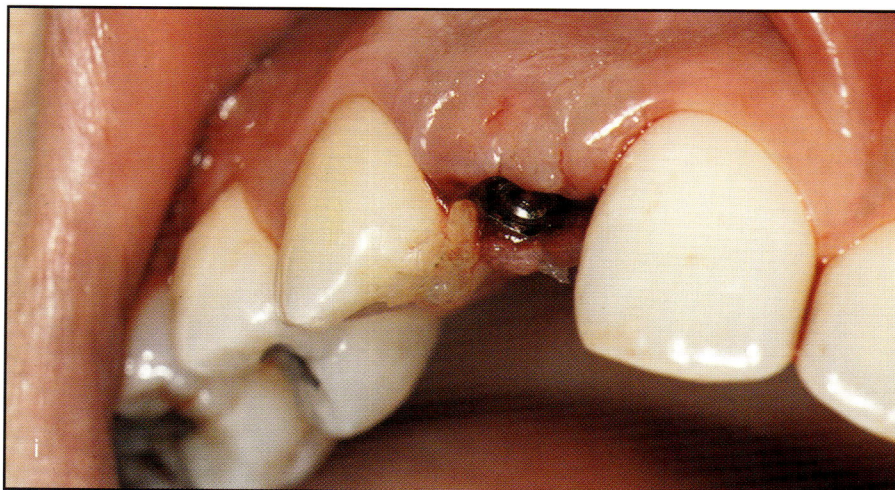

Fig 8-44 *(g and h)* Papilla technique for an anterior single-tooth restoration with a moderate ridge resorption. A palatal incision and two releasing incisions (if necessary) will allow a full-thickness flap to be labially pushed by the abutment. The ridge loss being moderate, the horizontal incision should not be extended too palatally. *(i and j)* In this clinical situation, releasing incisions were not necessary because the semilunar bevel incision creates an adequate soft tissue contour, while the rotated pedicle will fill the space between the healing abutment and the central incision, thus creating a papilla. In such situations where limited amounts of space and tissue are available, a 4-mm-diameter healing abutment is used to avoid any tension on the flap.

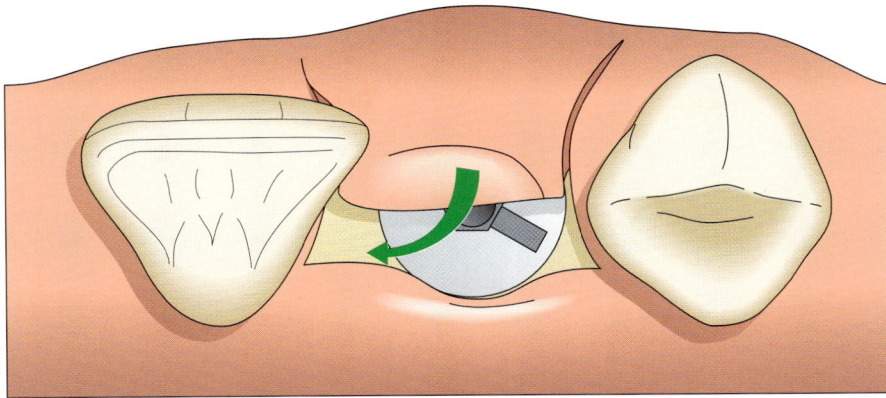

j

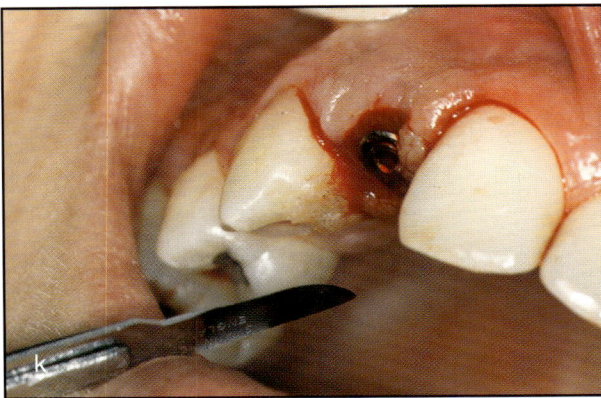

k

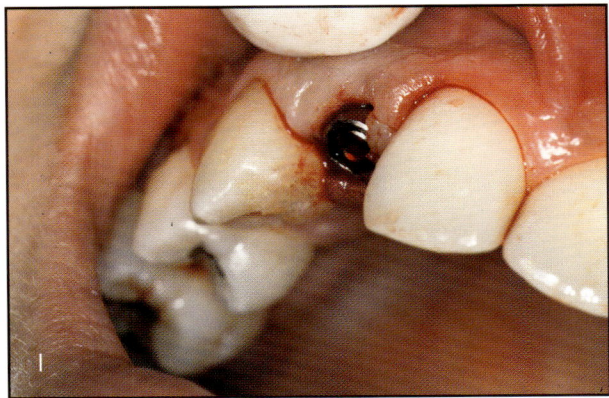

l

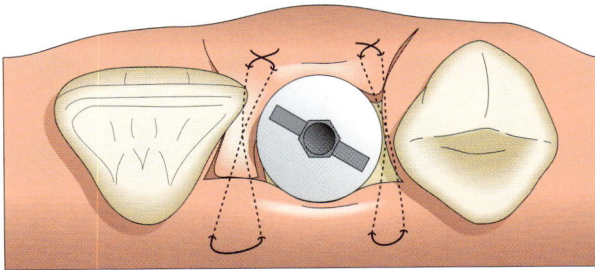

m

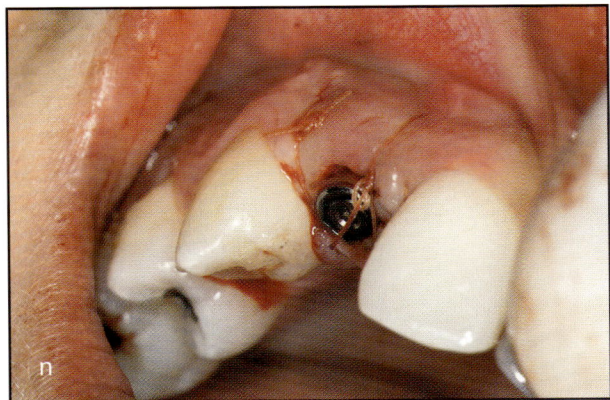

n

Fig 8-44 *(k and l)* Rotation of the pedicle and the resulting soft tissue anatomy. *(m and n)* Suturing technique (as mentioned earlier).

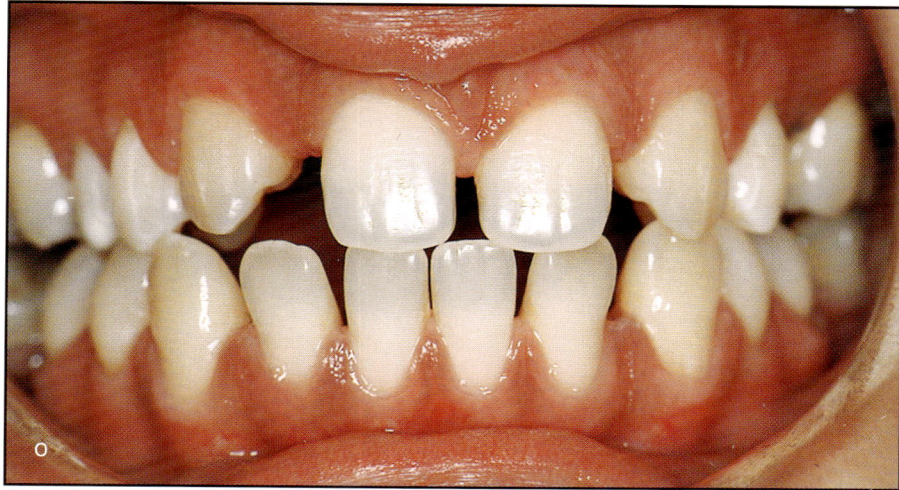

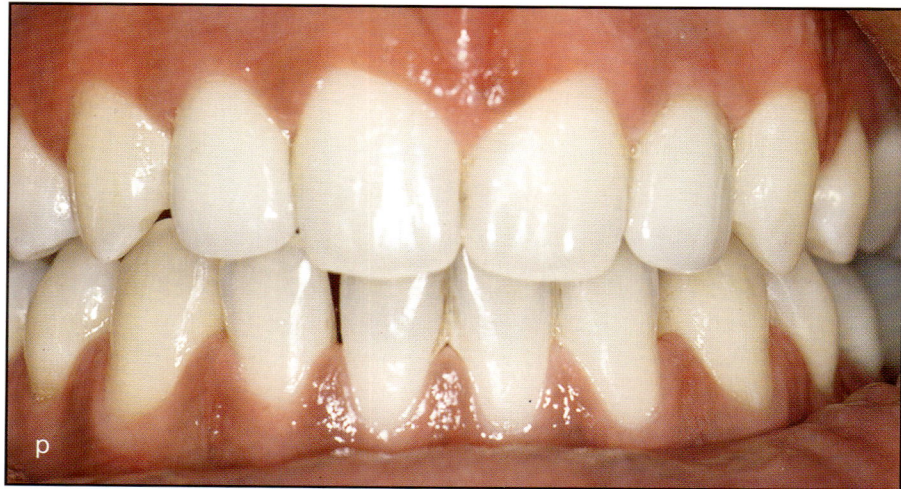

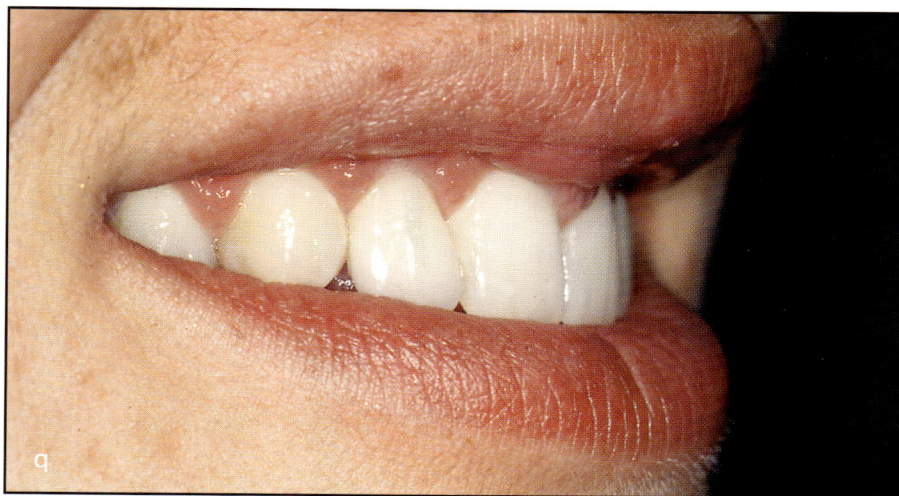

Fig 8-44 *(o to q)* Before and after treatment, clinical result illustrating that an optimal result relies not only on implant placement, gingival scaffold, and prosthetic restoration, but also on the lip framework.

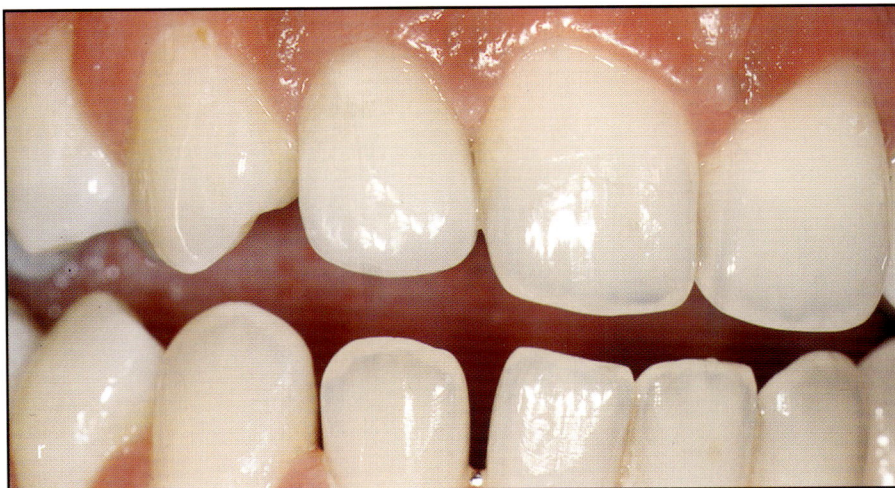
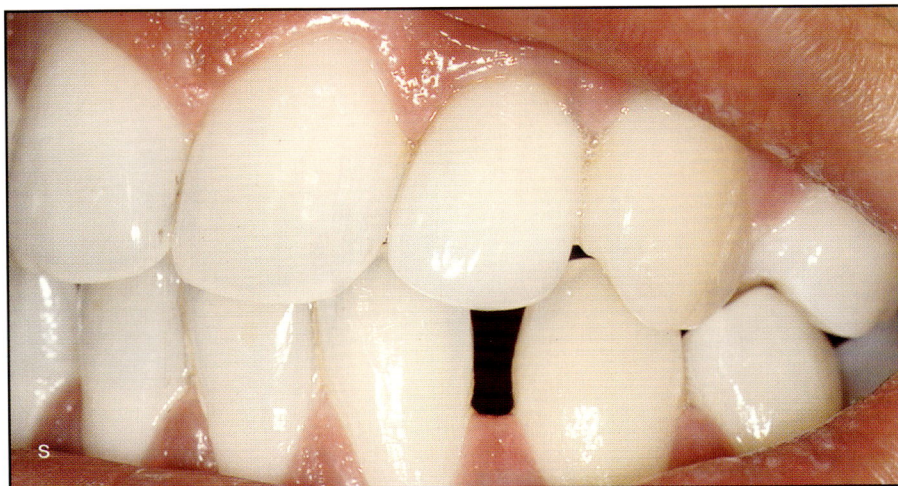
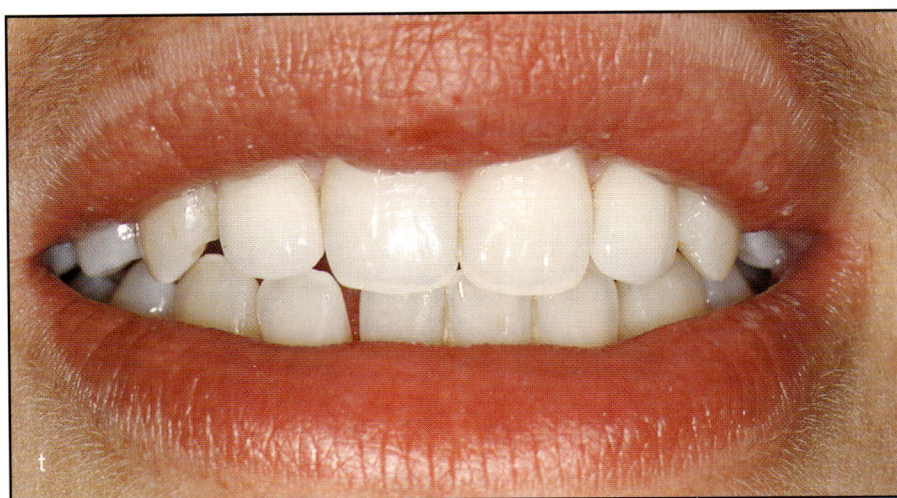

Fig 8-44 *(r to t)* Clinical result 4 years later.

Conclusions

The surgical papilla regeneration technique described in the chapter predictably creates better initial conditions for mucosal soft tissue to form a perimucosal contour matching healthy gingival architecture. However, peri-implant soft tissue, as well as gingival tissue, needs to be supported by hard tissue. A predictable treatment outcome, then, depends not only on proper hard tissue support of the perimucosal soft tissue but also on proper implant positioning. Improper implant placement jeopardizes the ability to create papillae.

References

Adell R, Lekholm U, Brånemark P-I. Surgical procedures. In: Brånemark P-I, Zarb GA, Albrektsson T (eds). Tissue-integrated Prostheses: Osseointegration in Clinical Dentistry. Chicago: Quintessence, 1985:211–232.

Andreasen JO, Kristerson L, Nilson H, Dahlin K, Schwartz O, Palacci P, et al. Implants in the anterior region. In: Andreasen JO, Andreasen FM (eds). Textbook and Color Atlas of Traumatic Injuries to the Teeth, ed 3. Copenhagen: Munksgaard, 1994.

Bengazi F, Wennström JL, Lekholm U. Recession of the soft tissue margin at oral implants: A 2-year longitudinal prospective study. Clin Oral Implants Res 1996;7:303–310.

Berglundh T, Lindhe J. Dimension of the periimplant mucosa: Biological width revisited. J Clin Periodontol 1996;23:971–973.

Hertel RC, Blijdorp PA, Kalk W, Baker DL. Stage 2 surgical techniques in endosseous implantation. Int J Oral Maxillofac Implants 1994;9:273–278.

Israelsson H, Plemons JM. Dental implants, regenerative techniques, and periodontal plastic surgery to restore maxillary anterior esthetics. Int J Oral Maxillofac Implants 1993;8:555–561.

Kenney EB, Weinlander M, Moy PK. Uncovering implants: A review of the UCLA modification of second stage surgical technique for uncovering implants. J Calif Dent Assoc 1989;3:18–22.

Liljenberg B, Gualini F, Berglundh T, Tonetti T, Lindhe J. Some characteristics of the ridge mucosa before and after implant installation: A prospective study in humans. J Clin Periodontol 1996;23:1008–1013.

Moy PK, Weinlaender M, Kenney EB. Soft tissue modifications of surgical techniques for placement and uncovering of osseointegrated implants. Dent Clin North Am 1989;33:665–681.

Palacci P. Amenagement des tissus peri-implantaires interet de la regeneration des papilles. Real Clin 1992;3:381–387.

Palacci P. Optimal implant positioning and soft-tissue considerations. Oral Maxillofac Surg Clin North Am 1996;8:445–452.

Seibert J, Lindhe J. Esthetics in periodontal therapy. In: Lindhe J, Karring T, Lang NP (eds). Clinical Periodontology and Implant Dentistry, ed 3. Copenhagen: Munksgaard, 1997:647–681.

Strub JP, Garberthuel TW, Grunder U. The role of attached gingiva in the health of peri-implant tissues in dogs. Int J Periodontics Restorative Dent 1991;11:317–333.

Sullivan D, Kay H, Schwartz M, Gelb D. Esthetic problems in the anterior maxilla. Int J Oral Maxillofac Implants 1994;9(suppl):64–74.

Wennström JL, Bengazi F, Lekholm U. The influence of the masticatory mucosa on the peri-implant soft tissue condition. Clin Oral Implants Res 1994;5:1–8.

Chapter 9

Rationale for the Use of Different Prosthetic Components

Hans Nilson, LDS, Ingvar Ericsson, LDS, Odont Dr, and Patrick Palacci, DDS

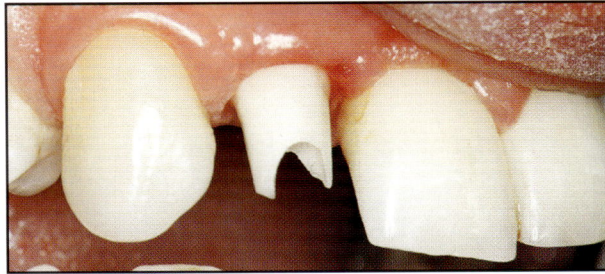

The variety of prosthetic components used in implant dentistry has increased tremendously in recent years. One of the main reasons is the increasing number of patients with implant-supported reconstructions in the last 2 decades. These patients represent a wide variety of demands, especially regarding esthetics and function. In addition, an increasing number of dentists with differing demands and knowledge are engaged in this type of oral rehabilitation. Another important factor in the development of prosthetic component types is the increase in the number of implant companies in the market and the fact that variation in implant components is an important part of the marketing process.

The availability and stocking of a wide variety of components—for example, different abutments (type and length), impression copings, connecting screws, and so on—helps fulfill the demands of most patients and dentists. However, it also results in increased costs and the need for increased knowledge by the treating team. This situation has resulted in a trend to minimize the number of components and in a change to components with wide application, thus facilitating the treatment procedure. In other words, the goal today is to be able to treat a majority (90% to 95%) of patients using a "standard assortment" of prosthetic components. A very limited number of patients with Brånemark system implants require so-called custom-designed components to fulfill acceptable esthetic and functional demands.

Proper patient selection and treatment planning are the keys to success in all implant-supported reconstructions. Inappropriate patient selection and treatment planning can compromise treatment outcome and jeopardize the osseointegration process. In other words, optimal positioning of the implant is the main criterion for success in implant-supported oral rehabilitation in regard to esthetics, function, and phonetics (see Chapter 4).

The existence of a variety of prosthetic components has only limited value with improper implant placement.

Treatment of the Patient with Single-Tooth Loss

Platforms

The introduction of different platforms—that is, different diameters of implants and abutments—has helped optimize restoration in patients with single-tooth losses. For example, the narrow platform (diameter = 3.3 mm) has facilitated the replacement of lateral maxillary incisors and mandibular incisors. The wide platform (diameter = 5.0 mm) is used for molars and sometimes premolars when bone volume is sufficient to anchor such an implant. The regular platform (diameter = 3.75 or 4.0 mm) is the most commonly used of the three available platforms.

The appropriate selection of components (implant plus abutment) to match the tooth or teeth to be replaced depends on which segment of the arch is to be restored. For detailed information, see Chapters 3 and 4.

CeraOne abutment

The most frequently used abutment for single-tooth restorations is the CeraOne abutment (Fig 9-1). The gold abutment screw must be tightened using the torque control set at 20, 32, or 45 Ncm. The lightest torque (20 Ncm) is used with the narrow platform, whereas 45 Ncm is used with the wide platform. Clinicians have found that the CeraOne abutment yields nice esthetic results and has safe, fast, and easy handling. Long-term use of this abutment has shown good treatment outcome (Jemt and Pettersson 1993; Andersson et al 1995; Henry et al 1996).

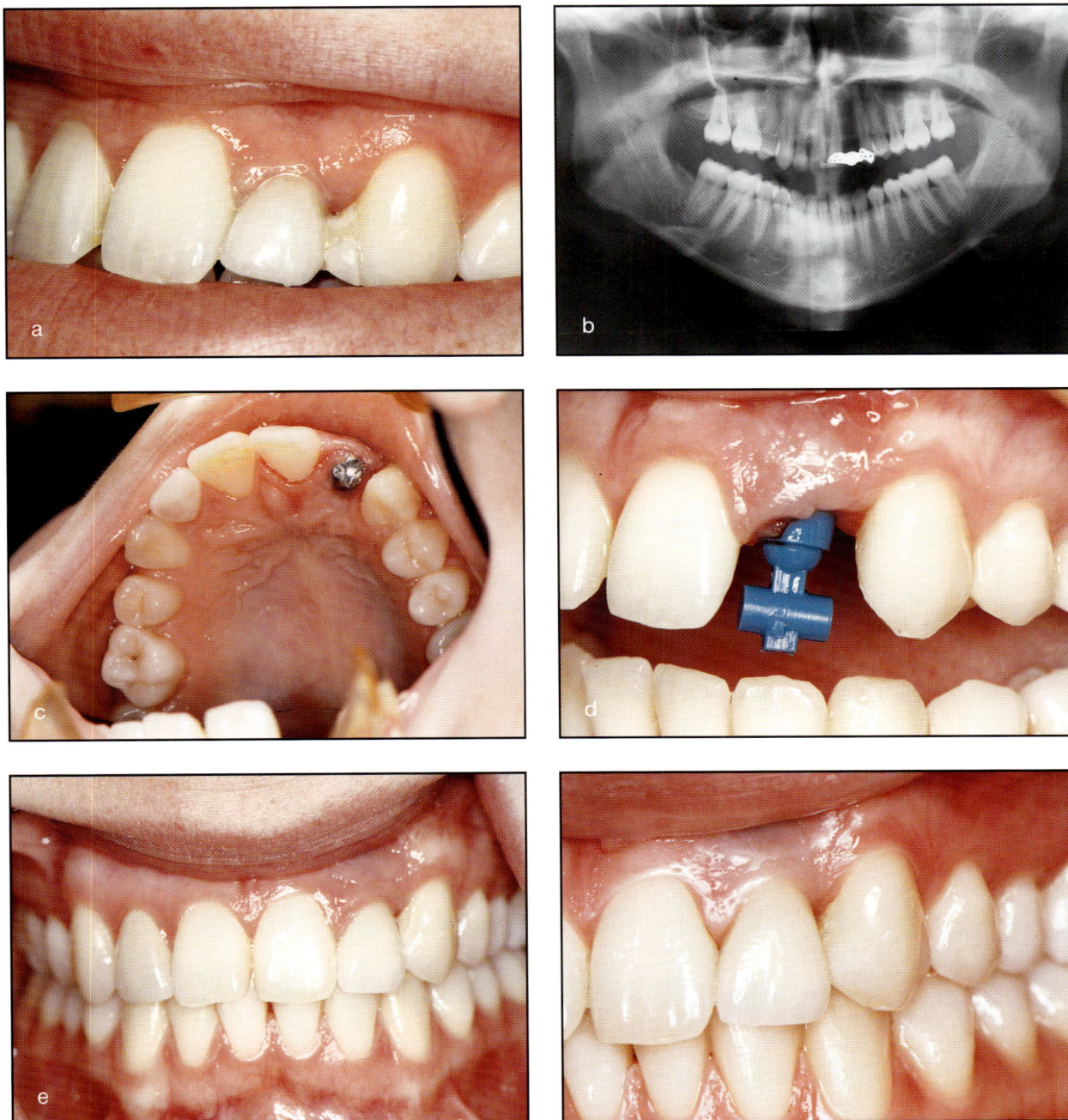

Fig 9-1 *(a)* Missing lateral incisor caused by aplasia. *(b)* Panoramic view. *(c)* CeraOne abutment connected to the implant with a gold screw. *(d)* Impression coping in position. *(e)* One-year follow-up. *(f)* Three-year follow-up.

Using the CeraOne protocol, the abutment can be placed either during the surgical abutment connection procedure or following soft tissue healing during which a healing abutment has been used. The use of healing abutments is preferable in regions in which esthet-

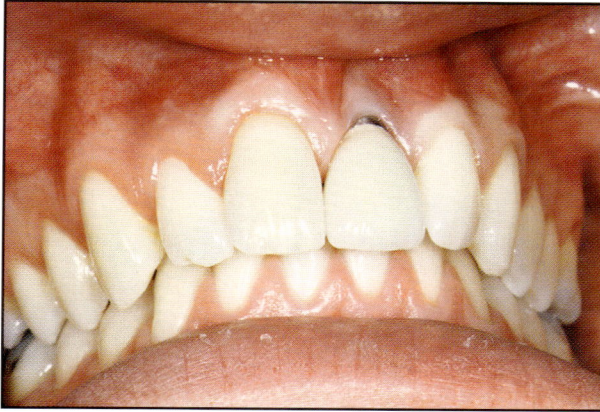

Fig 9-2 Part of the titanium abutment exposed at the buccal aspect because of excessively superficial placement of the implant.

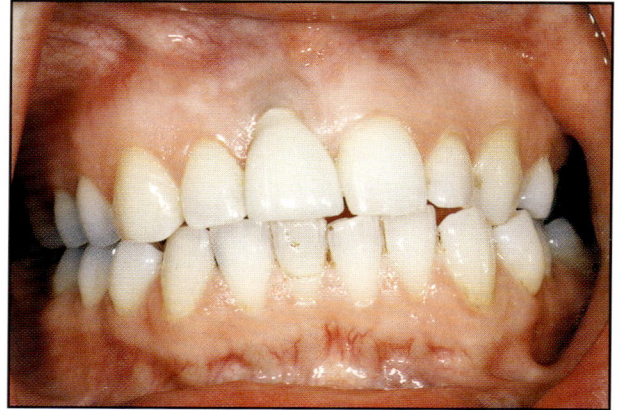

Fig 9-3 "Shining-through" effect of the titanium.

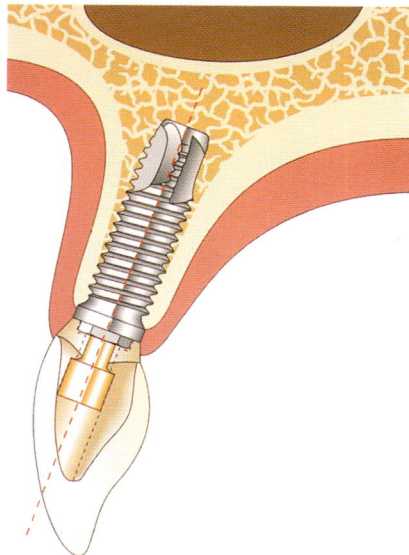

Fig 9-4 Implant placed with a buccal inclination, resulting in an undesired form of the crown restoration.

ic demands are higher. However, the fact that repeated abutment exchanges may result in downgrowth of junctional epithelium and subsequent bone resorption must be considered (Abrahamsson et al 1997).

CerAdapt abutment

The CerAdapt abutment is a ceramic abutment that has further improved the esthetic outcome for single-tooth restorations. The CerAdapt abutment is individually designed by grinding. The finishing line as well as the angulation can be altered, depending on individual needs. The crown can be cemented to this individually designed abutment, or porcelain can be baked directly onto the ceramic abutment. However, prerequisite for the approach using direct porcelain baking is proper angulation of the implant.

Use of the CerAdapt abutment is indicated in the following three situations in particular:
1. An implant that was placed too superficially, resulting in exposed titanium at the buccal aspect (Fig 9-2)
2. An implant with excessively buccal placement and thin peri-implant mucosa, resulting in a "shining-through" effect of the titanium abutment (Fig 9-3)
3. A slight disangulation of the implant, resulting in a need to correct the direction of the implant pillar to create a harmonious embrasure and anatomy of the crown restoration (Fig 9-4)

However, the use of the CerAdapt abutment is limited (Fig 9-5). Because of the limited strength of the material, this abutment should not be used in molar areas or in patients demonstrating excessive chewing and biting forces or bruxism. Furthermore, the CerAdapt abutment is available only in the regular platform. This fact eliminates the use of this abutment in situations where the narrow or wide platform must be used; however,

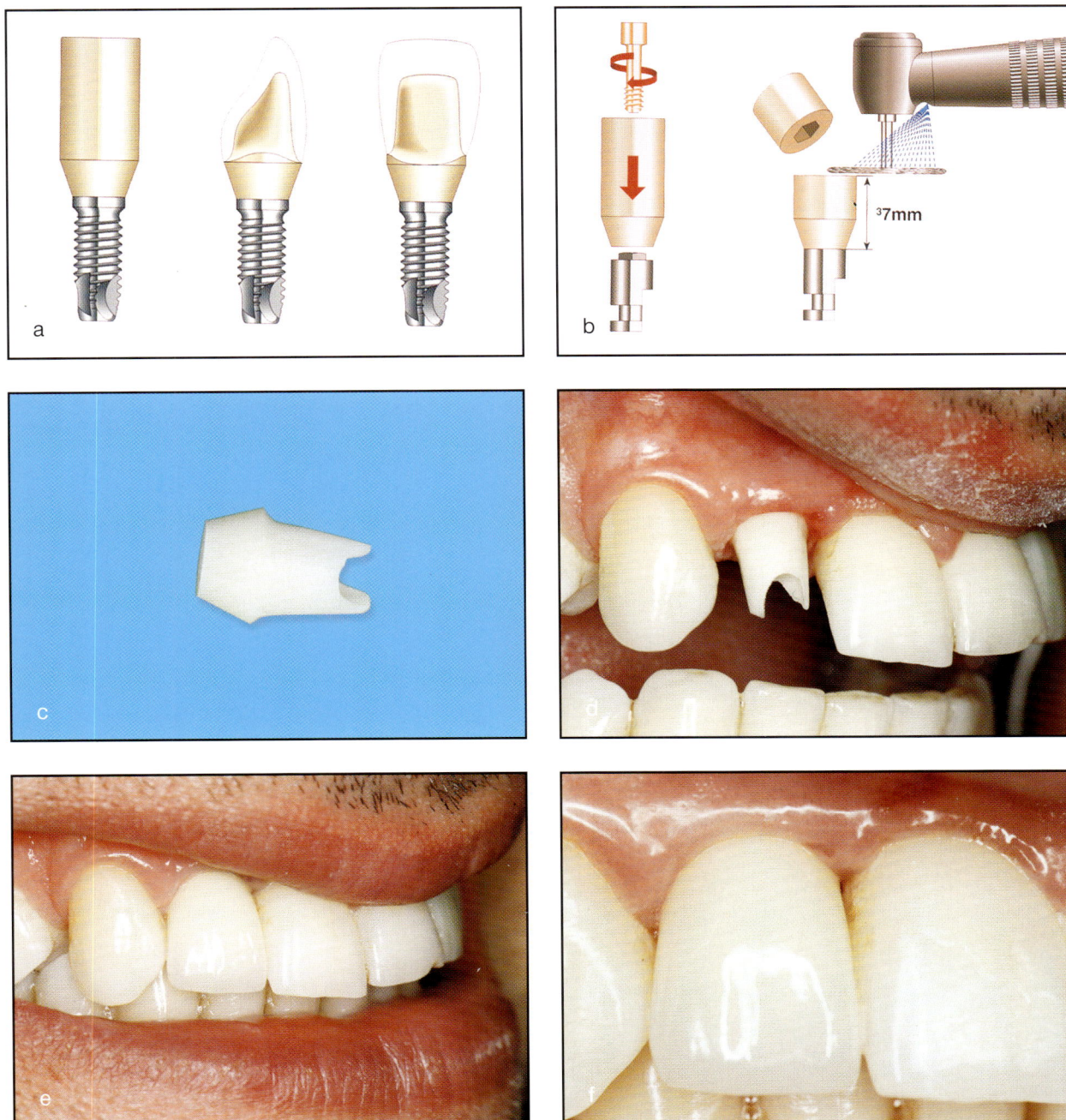

Fig 9-5 (a) CerAdapt abutment. (b) Minimum height of the CerAdapt abutment. (c) Prepared CerAdapt abutment. (d) Try-in of prepared CerAdapt abutment. (e) AllCeram crown cemented to the CerAdapt abutment. (f) Close-up view.

further development of both wide and narrow platforms is ongoing with the all-ceramic abutment. Finally, in order to preserve adequate strength, only a limited amount of material can be removed from the CerAdapt abutment. This characteristic has to be considered, especially where there is pronounced disangulation of the implant. The maximum disangulation in relation to the long axis of the implant is recommended not to exceed 30 degrees.

When the implant position is ideal, a screw can be used to retain a crown that is baked directly onto the abutment (Fig 9-6). This can be useful if there are uncertainties (for example, regarding esthetics). An impression is taken at the implant level, and the technician prepares the abutment. During the try-in procedure small adjustments can be performed in the clinical setting. When the adjustment is satisfactory, the abutment is sent back to the technician for fabrication of the crown. The

crown is then tried in and affixed to the implant with a screw. The access hole is covered with a composite resin filling on the palatal-lingual aspect of the crown restoration.

Alternatively, a ceramic crown can be cemented to the prepared abutment (see Figs 9-5d to 9-5f). An impression is taken at the implant level. The abutment is prepared and connected to the implant with a gold screw tightened at 32 Ncm. A conventional impression is then taken using an elastic impression material after the placement of retraction cords to get a proper impression of the prepared margins of the abutment.

Another technique is to send the abutment back to the technician, who will scan the form of the abutment and fabricate an AllCeram crown according to the Procera technique. The abutment is attached to the implant as described earlier. Finally, the permanent crown restoration is cemented to the abutment using an ordinary cement.

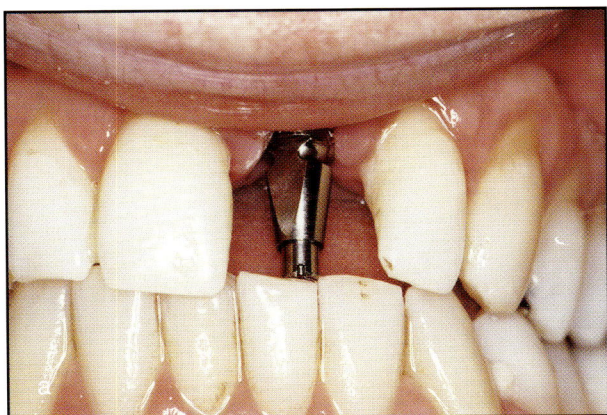

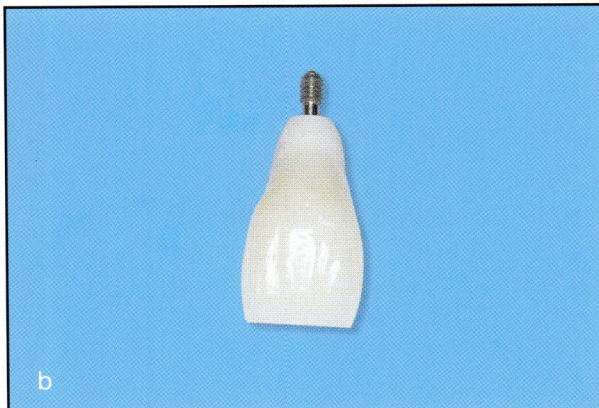

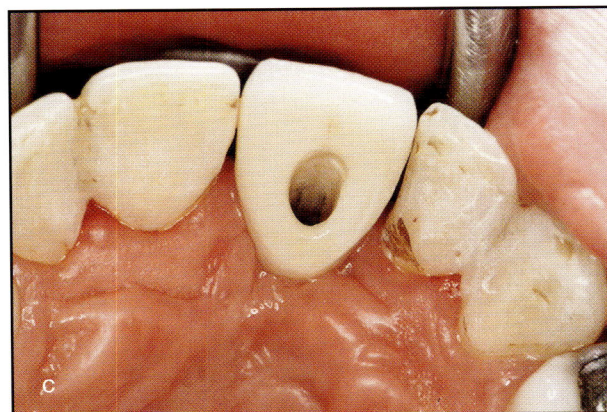

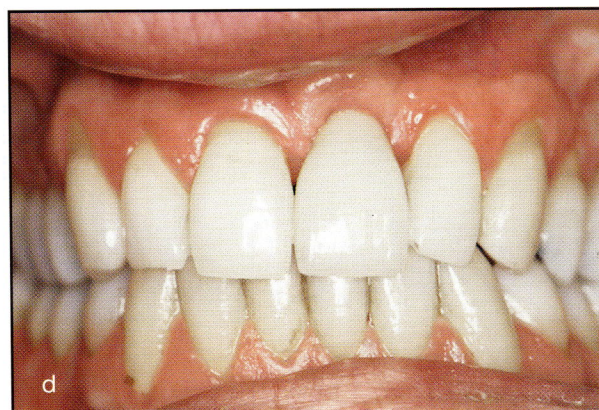

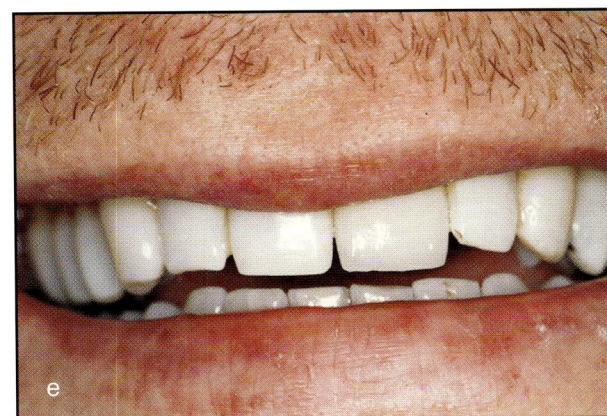

Fig 9-6 *(a)* Coping placed for an impression at the implant level. *(b)* Screw-retained CerAdapt abutment. *(c)* Palatal aspect. *(d)* Buccal aspect. *(e)* Facial aspect.

TiAdapt abutment

TiAdapt is another abutment that can be prepared extraorally, adjusted clinically, and affixed to the implant with a screw (Fig 9-7). The TiAdapt abutment is available for all three platforms. Following an impression, a crown restoration is fabricated and cemented to the abutment. One advantage of the TiAdapt abutment is its strength, compared with the CerAdapt, combined with the potential for individual design in shape and form. The increased strength implies that more material can be removed from the abutment, allowing more flexibility than the CerAdapt abutment.

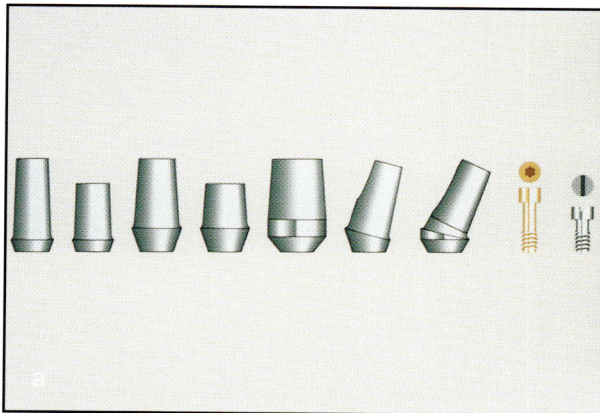

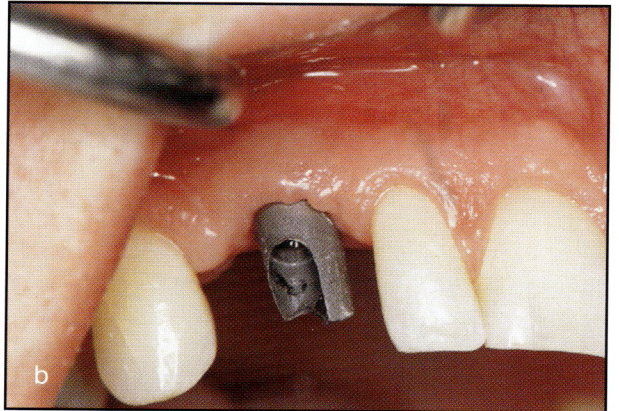

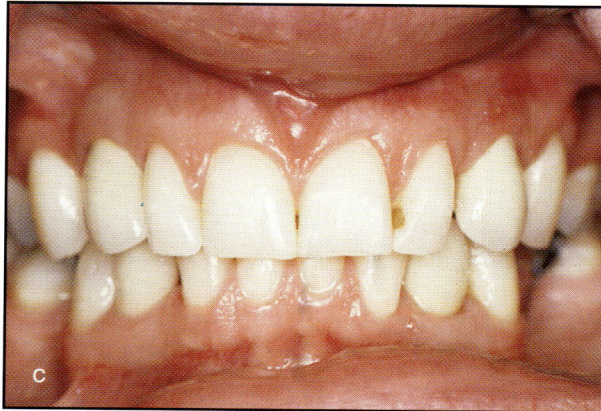

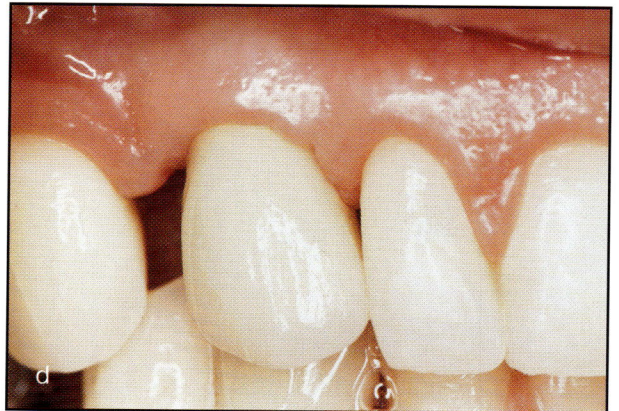

Fig 9-7 *(a)* TiAdapt abutment for the regular platform. *(b)* Try-in of the prepared TiAdapt abutment before impression taking. *(c)* AllCeram crown cemented to the TiAdapt abutment in position 13. *(d)* Close-up view.

Procera abutment

The concept of the Procera titanium abutment is similar to that of the TiAdapt. However, the Procera abutment is individually designed using the computer-assisted dental design (CADD) technique (Fig 9-8a) or a special waxup technique. With the CADD technique, an impression is taken at the implant level, and a cast is fabricated (Fig 9-8b). The position of the hex of the implant and the implant angulation are determined by means of a special T-bar. This information is transferred to a computer. The dental technician creates the abutment on a computer screen in a three-dimensional pattern, and the data are then sent to the factory for fabrication of the Procera abutment using a milling machine. This technique allows the fabrication of abutment profiles adapted to specific clinical situations. After try-in of the abutment, a crown restoration is created (Fig 9-8c).

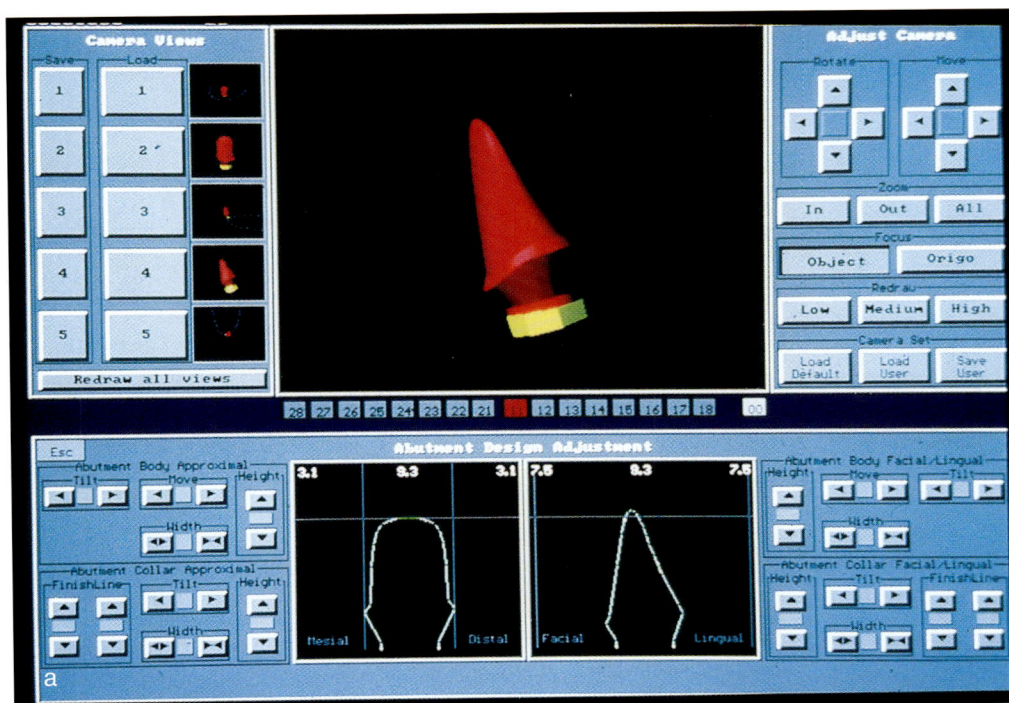

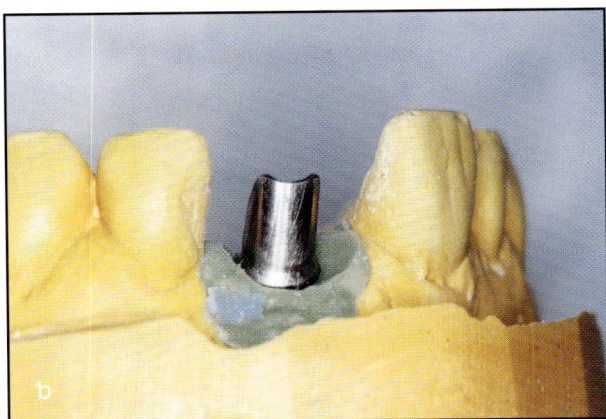

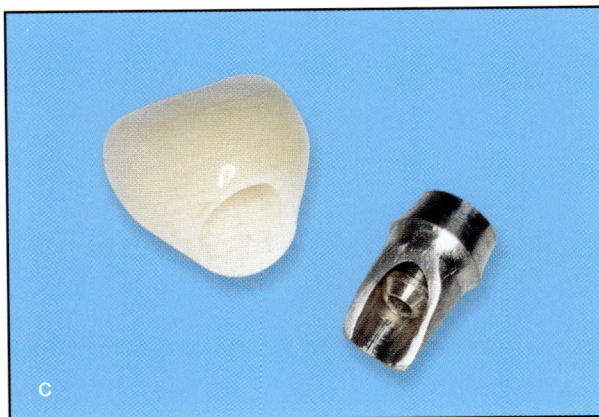

Fig 9-8 (a) Procera abutment designed using the computer-assisted dental design technique. (b) Procera abutment on a working cast. (c) Procera abutment and AllCeram crown.

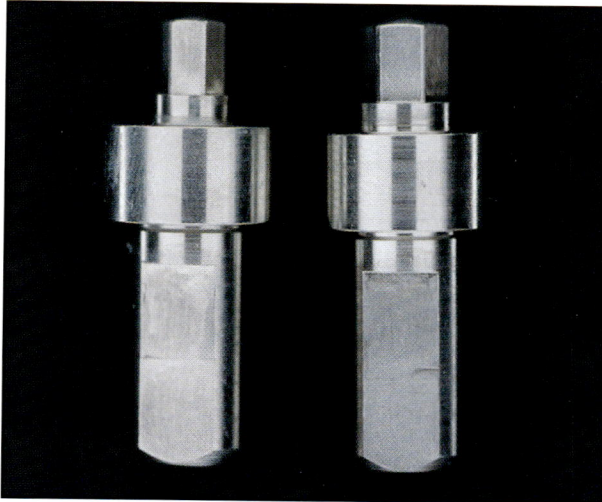

Fig 9-9 CeraOne replicas for the waxup technique.

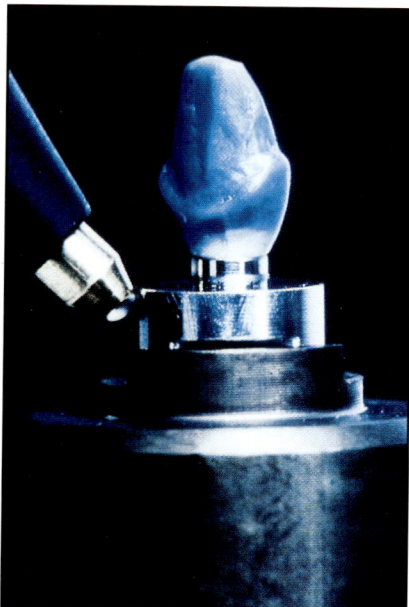

Fig 9-10 Completed waxup of an abutment before use of the Procera scanner.

The waxup technique uses a special abutment holder (Figs 9-9 and 9-10) and exchangeable platforms, which facilitate the procedure. The Procera abutment is individualized, so an inventory of abutments is not needed.

AurAdapt abutment

Another option is the AurAdapt abutment, an abutment fabricated of a gold alloy. Using this abutment as a base, a waxup is made and cast. Finally, porcelain is baked on the gold alloy abutment. The crown restoration is then affixed to the implant by a screw, using the appropriate tightening force. A disadvantage with the AurAdapt abutment is that gold is brought down to the implant level, thus interfering with the soft and hard tissue. Abrahamsson et al (1998), in experimental studies, demonstrated that such a treatment protocol frequently results in soft tissue recession and subsequent bone resorption.

Other methods using a waxup technique similar to the one used with the AurAdapt abutment are especially popular among dental technicians. Some use plastic waxup cylinders to fabricate the abutment. It must be emphasized, however, that a premachined surface on the abutment demonstrates a better fit compared with a waxup and cast surface. These factors must be evaluated when selecting the type of abutment and technique to be used.

In conclusion, the CeraOne abutment offers an easy, fast, and safe technique with good esthetic results. However, in especially demanding and challenging clinical situations, the Brånemark system offers several abutment alternatives to satisfy esthetic and functional needs.

Treatment of Partially and Totally Edentulous Patients

The Brånemark system offers various treatment protocols in the treatment of partially and totally edentulous patients. The question is whether to use cemented or screw-retained supraconstructions. Historically, the restorations have been retained by screws, but a trend toward cemented supraconstructions has become obvious. Another trend is a decrease in the number of components used. The latest development, the Multi-Unit abutment, radically improves the restorative protocol and decreases the number of abutments. The use of a titanium framework (that is, a framework milled from a piece of titanium) has further facilitated the technical restorative procedure. The so-called All-in-One technique, which has been recently developed, is a further step toward simplicity and reliability in the Brånemark system.

Screw-retained supraconstructions have proved to be successful over the years. All the reported good long-term results using the Brånemark system have been achieved with screw-retained restorations. The overall advantage of a screw-retained restoration is its retrievability. However, the cementation of fixed partial dentures to teeth has a long tradition and history and is a well-known technique. The technique to cement prosthetic restorations on implants was originally designed to compensate for a misfit of the framework. Furthermore, the cementation of implant-supported supraconstructions can be justified by the need to avoid screw-access holes on occlusal surfaces. In short, the demands of the patient and the treatment planning must determine whether a screw-retained or cemented restoration is the best choice.

Screw-retained fixed partial dentures

The majority of implant-supported reconstructions in both partially and totally edentulous patients undergoing oral rehabilitation use screws. Beginning with the cylindrical Standard abutment originally used, over the years several abutments have been developed and introduced in the market to optimize the final esthetic outcome of treatment. A major improvement has been the EsthetiCone abutment. The submarginal placement of the titanium collar and the slim design of the abutment make the EsthetiCone attractive. The MirusCone abutment, developed a few years later, has a similar design and a gain of 2.2 mm in total height. It was originally designed to be used in situations with limited vertical space. Angulated abutments (17 or 30 degrees) are more of a rescue type and are mainly used in cases of implant disangulation.

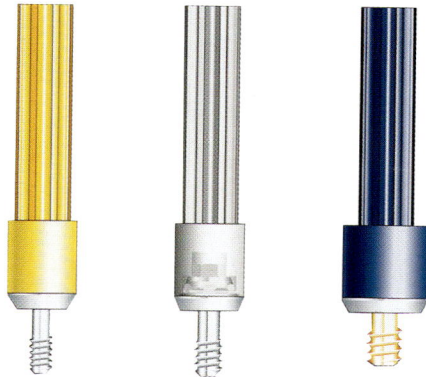

Fig 9-11 Multi-Unit abutments with premounted holders for all three platforms. Yellow indicates narrow platform; white, regular platform; and blue, wide platform.

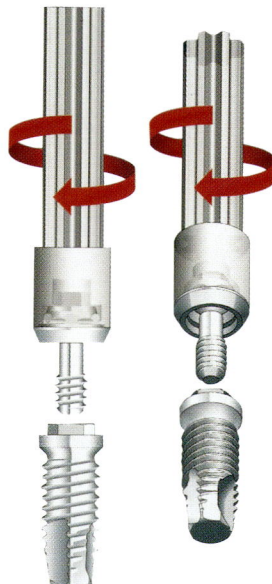

Fig 9-12 Multi-Unit abutment attached to the implant using a premounted plastic holder. Note that there is no internal hex in the abutment.

The increasing number of abutments has led to more complex treatment protocols and the need for a large inventory of components. The recently introduced Multi-Unit abutment (available for all three platforms) is a solution to these problems and facilitates abutment selection (Fig 9-11). The Multi-Unit abutment can be used in most clinical situations and replaces the Standard, EsthetiCone, and MirusCone abutments.

Another feature of the Multi-Unit abutment is simplified connection of abutment to implant hex; the Multi-Unit abutment does not have an internal hex that must match the hex of the implant. The Multi-Unit abutment also has a premounted plastic abutment holder to facilitate proper placement of the abutment to the implant head (Fig 9-12). The premounted holder allows the abutment to serve as a one-piece abutment. The abutment is positioned at the implant head, and the abutment holder serves as a manual screwdriver. When the abutment is seated, the plastic holder is removed by a bending movement before final tightening using the torque control (Fig 9-13).

The abutment screw of the Multi-Unit abutment is made of a titanium alloy, which imparts increased screw joint stability and pillar strength. It also yields lower screw friction and higher screw strength, leading to an increase in preload of 15% to 20% compared with that obtained with the MirusCone abutment.

The Multi-Unit abutment is available in seven lengths for each platform, from a 1- to 9-mm collar (Fig 9-14). The total height of the 1-mm Multi-Unit abutment, including the gold cylinder and the UniGrip prosthetic screw, is 5.05 mm. The Multi-Unit abutment allows for a disangulation of as much as 40 degrees between the long axis of the implants. In situations with greater disangulation, the Angulated abutment is used. Figure 9-15 illustrates a clinical case of a patient with a two-unit fixed partial denture on a Multi-Unit abutment in the mandibular right quadrant.

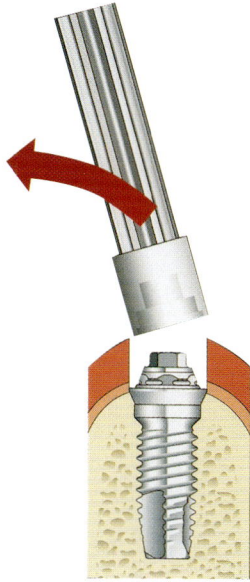

Fig 9-13 The plastic holder can be removed easily with a bending movement.

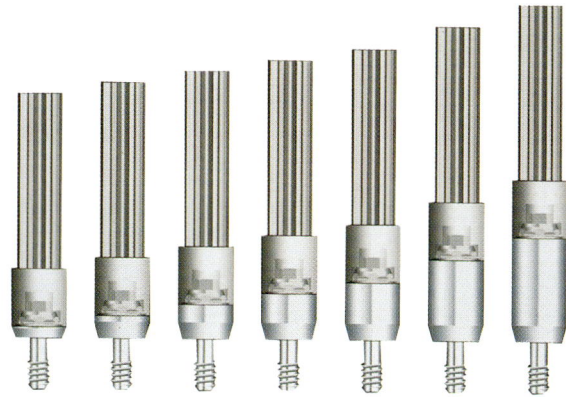

Fig 9-14 The Multi-Unit abutment is available in seven lengths (heights) for each platform.

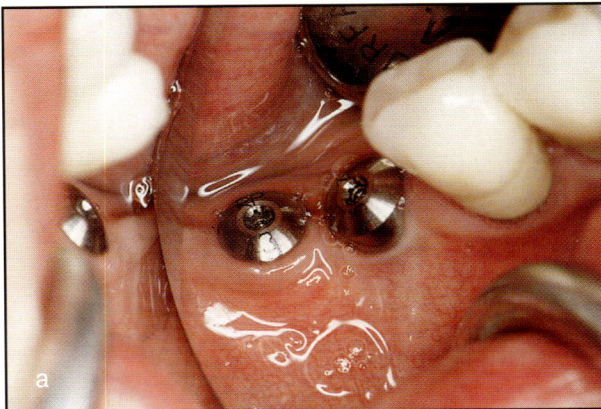

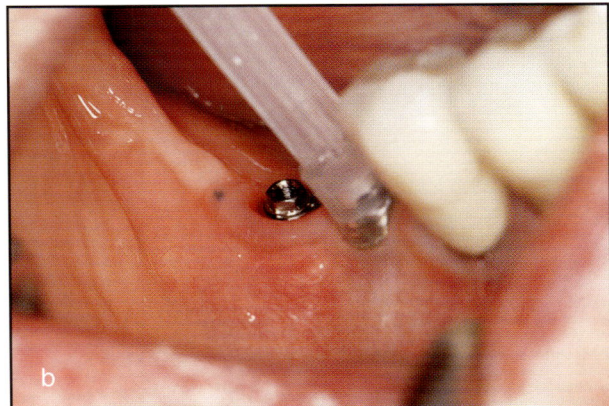

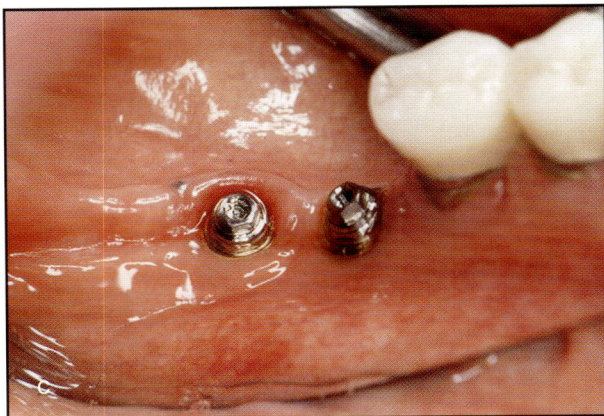

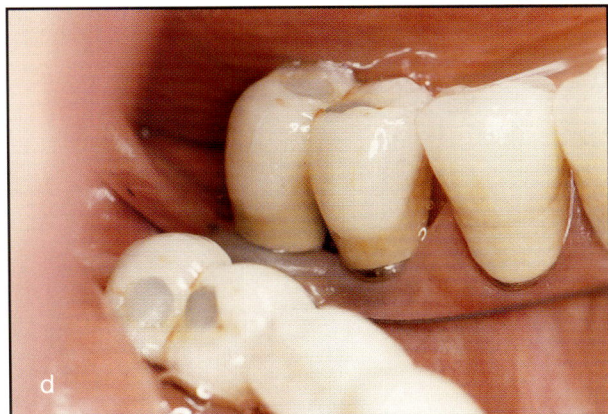

Fig 9-15 *(a)* Healing abutments in place. *(b)* The Multi-Unit abutments positioned with the premounted holder. *(c)* Two Multi-Unit abutments in position. *(d)* Permanent two-unit fixed partial denture (porcelain-fused-to-gold) in place.

Cement-retained fixed partial dentures

An increased interest in cemented implant-supported restorations has recently been noticed. The use of the CeraOne abutment and cementation of the crown have caused few problems, and the results reported have been good (for example, Andersson et al 1995).

The introduction of preparable titanium abutments (TiAdapt) has made the cementation of implant-supported supraconstructions possible. When the cementing technique is used, the location of the screw-access holes becomes unimportant, and disangulation of the implant can be corrected by preparation of the abutment. Another advantage of this technique is that the cement layer will partly compensate for eventual misfit of the framework. TiAdapt or Procera abutments can be selected for multi-unit restorations with the same protocol used for single crowns.

All-in-One technique

A milling technique to fabricate the titanium framework has recently been developed and marketed. This All-in-One technique has the following significant improvements compared with the traditional casting technique:

1. The framework has better fit.
2. The framework is one solid piece, without any welding joints.
3. The cost of the titanium material is lower than the cost of the gold alloy.
4. Titanium is used in the framework, as well as in the implant pillar (implant + abutment).
5. The framework can be used on all platforms and with all types of abutments. Porcelain or acrylic resin can be added to the framework.
6. The framework can be used at the implant level.

7. The new technique does not require any changes in the clinical sequence.

In addition, the clinical procedures are in line with the standard protocol for the cast framework.

Figure 9-16 illustrates the All-in-One technique. After the try-in of the tooth setup (see Fig 9-16a), a resin framework is fabricated by the technician (see Fig 9-16b). This framework, together with the cast, is sent to the factory, where the cast and framework are scanned using a laser (see Fig 9-16c). The position and angulation of the implants and abutments are scanned into a computer, together with the outer surfaces of the resin framework. These data are processed and transferred to a milling machine that fabricates the framework in one solid piece (see Figs 9-16d to 9-16f). Following try-in of the framework (see Fig 9-16g), porcelain or acrylic resin can be added to the titanium framework. Finally, the supraconstruction is connected to the implants (see Figs 9-16h and 9-16i). Ongoing clinical studies in Sweden using the All-in-One technique have demonstrated successful results.

Conclusions

Many different treatment options with many different components exist in implant prosthodontics today. Choices among them must aim for the rational use of the components for the majority of patients treated, ease in handling, a safe and fast clinical procedure, and an economically favorable outcome for both patient and dentist. The components and techniques used also must not jeopardize the treatment results achieved using the Brånemark system over the years. In a limited number of patients the standard choices are not enough, and a custom-designed approach is useful.

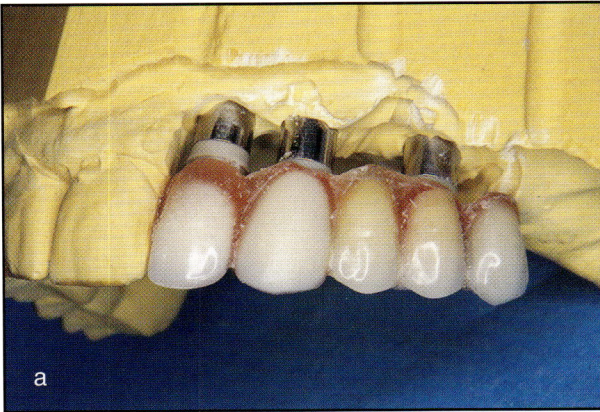

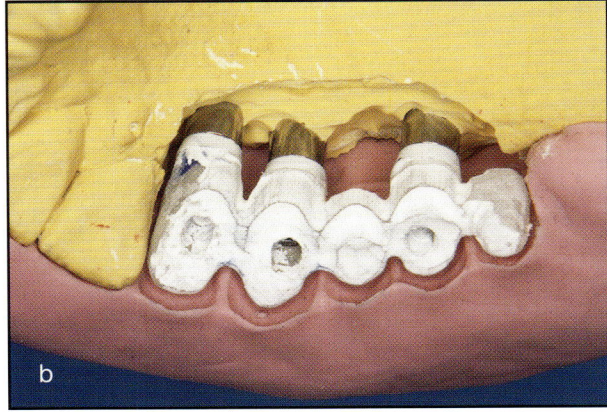

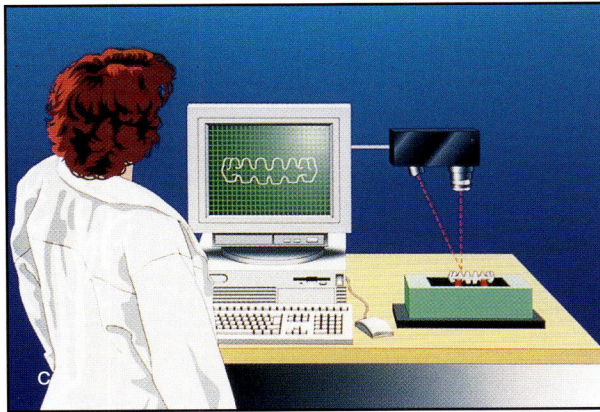

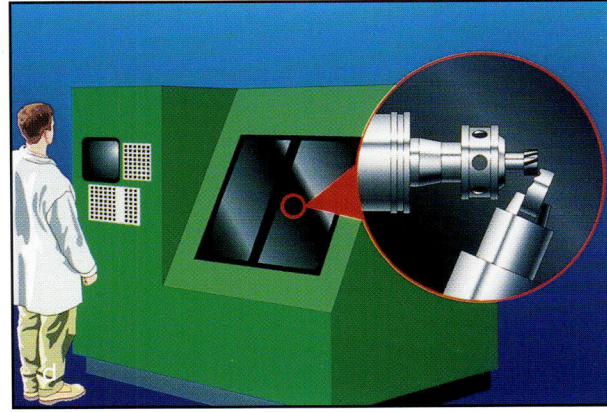

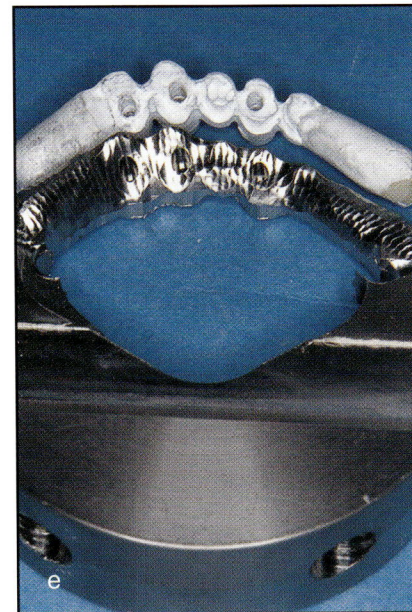

Fig 9-16 *(a)* Try-in of the tooth setup. *(b)* Resin framework fabricated using the tooth setup as a guide. *(c)* Resin framework and model scanned using a laser. *(d)* Machine milling the titanium framework in one solid piece. *(e)* Resin framework, the milled titanium framework, and the original piece of titanium.

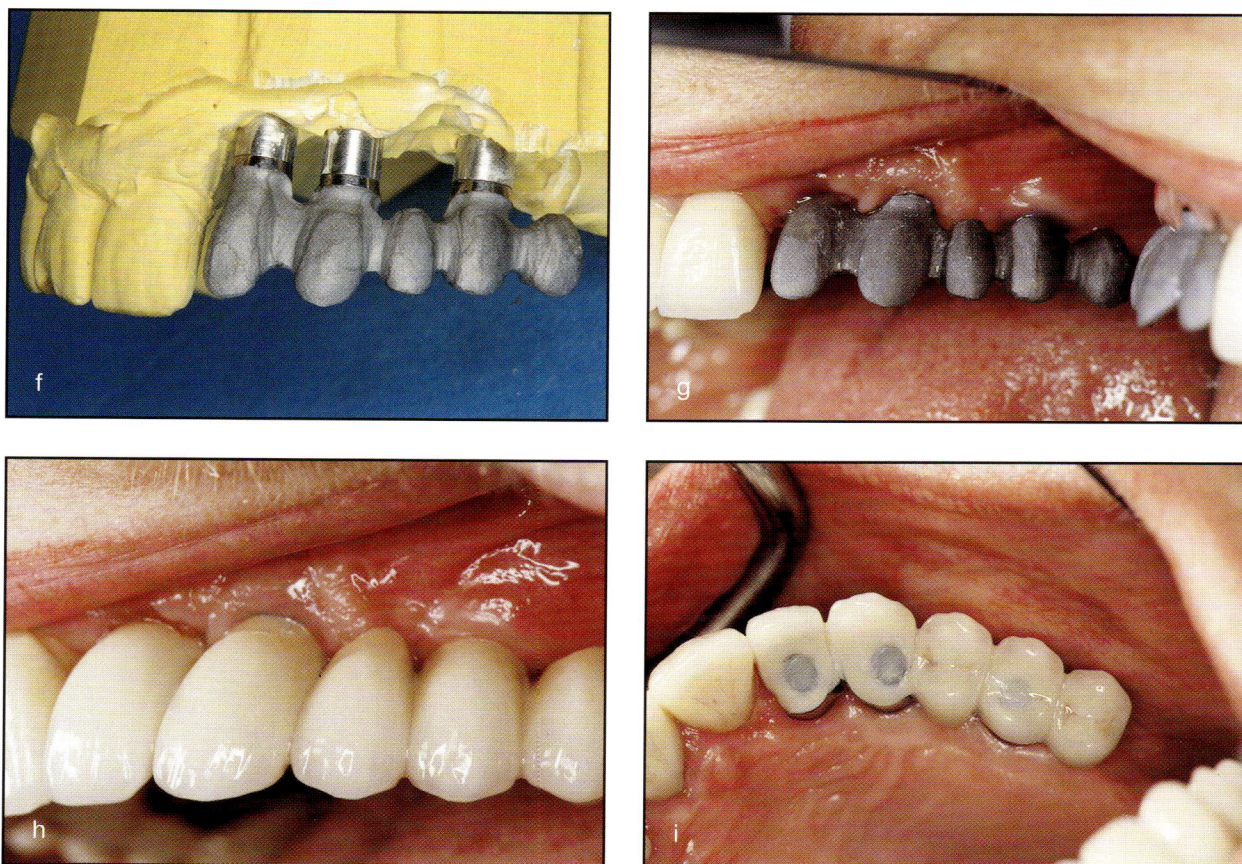

Fig 9-16 *(f)* Try-in of the titanium framework on the working cast. *(g)* Clinical try-in of the titanium framework. *(h)* Clinical buccal aspect of the five-unit All-in-One fixed partial denture with porcelain used as the veneering material. *(i)* Occlusal aspect of the five-unit fixed partial denture.

References

Abrahamsson I, Berglundh T, Glantz PO, Lindhe J. The mucosal attachment at different abutments: An experimental study in dogs. J Clin Periodontol 1998;25:721–727.

Abrahamsson I, Berglundh T, Lindhe J. The mucosal barrier following abutment dis/reconnection. J Clin Periodontol 1997;24:568–572.

Andersson B, Ödman P, Lindvall A-M, Lithner B. Single-tooth restorations on osseointegrated implants: Results and experiences from a prospective study after 2–3 years. Int J Oral Maxillofac Implants 1995;10:702–711.

Henry P, Laney WR, Jemt T, Harris D, Krogh PHJ, Polizzi G, et al. Osseointegrated implants for single-tooth replacement: A prospective 5-year multicenter study. Int J Oral Maxillofac Implants 1996;11:450–455.

Jemt T, Pettersson P. A 2-year follow-up study on single implant treatment. J Prosthet Dent 1993;21:203–208.

Chapter 10

One-stage Surgery and Early Functional Loading

Ingvar Ericsson, LDS, Odont Dr

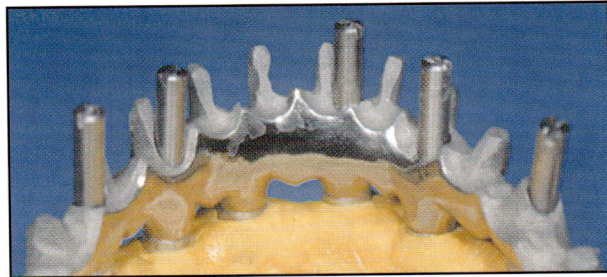

The Brånemark implant system was introduced 30 to 35 years ago (Brånemark et al 1969), and the principle of osseointegration, or "direct anchorage of an implant by the formation of bony tissue around the implant without the growth of fibrous tissue at the bone-implant interface" (Dorland's 1994), was emphasized (Albrektsson et al 1986; Albrektsson 1993). This implant methodology provided not only a scientific foundation for implant stability but also predictable long-term clinical success (see, for example, Adell et al 1981, 1990; Ericsson et al 1986, 1990; Jemt et al 1989; van Steenberghe et al 1990; Jemt and Lekholm 1993, 1995; Lekholm et al 1994).

One-stage Surgery

The Brånemark implant system was originally designed to be a two-stage system and prescribes that the fixtures be submerged during the initial healing phase. The reasons for this approach are *(1)* to minimize the risk of infection, *(2)* to prevent apical migration of mucosal epithelium along the titanium surface, and *(3)* to minimize the risk for undue early loading of the implant (Brånemark et al 1969, 1977).

Published reports, however, have described a successful treatment outcome using a one-stage surgical protocol with the Brånemark system (Ericsson et al 1994; Henry and Rosenberg 1994; Bernard et al 1995; Becker et al 1997; Hermans et al 1997; Collaert and De Bruyn 1998; Friberg et al 1999). These clinical observations are in agreement with some experimental histologic studies (Gotfredsen et al 1991; Ericsson et al 1996; Abrahamsson et al 1996, 1999). Furthermore, Ericsson et al (1997) reported that the marginal bone level at implants placed anteriorly in the edentulous mandible and supporting fixed supraconstructions is stable at 12 to 60 months, irrespective of whether the implants are placed according to a one- or two-stage surgical protocol.

Becker et al (1997) reported on 135 Brånemark implants placed according to the one-stage surgical protocol (that is, 3 to 6 months of healing before loading). The implants were placed in the maxilla as well as the mandible. The implant survival rate during the first year of observation following loading was 95% to 96%. It should be noted that in this group of patients, 32 single-tooth replacements were included (Becker W, Becker BE, Israelson H, Lucchini JP, Handelsman M, Ammons W et al, personal communication, 1997).

Collaert and De Bruyn (1998) treated 85 patients with partially edentulous mandibles (n = 35) or completely edentulous mandibles (n = 50) by means of fixed supraconstructions retained by Brånemark implants. A total of 330 implant pillars were placed. Out of these 330 implants, 211 were placed according to the one-stage protocol (that is, 3 to 4 months of healing before loading) and 119 according to the traditional two-stage protocol. A somewhat higher percentage of failures was reported in the partial than the completely edentulous situation irrespective of whether the implants were placed using a one- or two-stage surgical approach. The overall implant survival rate, during the observation period of up to 2 years, was reported to be approximately 95%. The authors concluded that "a 1-stage surgical approach with normally submerged-type Brånemark implants can be as predictable as the common 2-stage procedure in the completely and partially edentulous mandible."

Hermans and coworkers (1997) treated 13 patients for edentulism in the mandible by means of implants placed in a one-stage surgical procedure. The follow-up period was 3 years, and "the cumulative failure rate reached for the single step operative technique was 1.9%." In other words, a similar treatment outcome was obtained for the one-stage technique and the traditional, submerged technique. Bernard et al (1995) placed 10 implants according to a one-stage surgical technique in five edentulous mandibles. After the initial 3-month healing period, the implants served as retainers for overdentures. No implant failures or peri-implant soft or hard tissue complications were reported.

In the clinical studies previously cited, the original dentures most often were adjusted and relined by a soft tissue conditioner 1 to 2 weeks after implant placement to minimize unfavorable functional loading. However, during the initial healing period, implants placed according to a one-stage surgical procedure will be directly and unpredictably loaded to some extent during function via the adjusted and relined denture. Furthermore, such loading might be unfavorable for the implants, as the deformation pattern of complete denture base material during functional conditions has been found to be complex and unpredictable (Glantz and Stafford 1983).

Despite this fact, Brånemark implants placed according to a one-stage surgical procedure demonstrated the same success rate as implants placed according to the original two-stage procedure (Ericsson et al 1994, 1997; Bernard et al 1995; Becker et al 1997; Hermans et al 1997; Collaert and De Bruyn 1998). In other words, "an initial and direct loading of implants piercing the mucosa via the adjusted and relined denture obviously does not jeopardize a proper osseointegration of the fixtures" (Ericsson et al 1997). Such a statement is in agreement with clinical data reported by Henry and Rosenberg (1994), who concluded that "controlled immediate loading of adequately installed, nonsubmerged implants, by reinsertion of a modified denture, does not appear to jeopardize the process of osseointegration in the anterior mandible." Favorable loading conditions are achieved through a rigid fixed supraconstruction (Glantz, Strandman, Svensson et al 1984;

Glantz, Strandman, and Randow 1984). It is therefore reasonable to believe that a successful treatment outcome could also be achieved when rigid appliances are connected to the implants soon after their placement (early functional loading).

Early Functional Loading

Based on the information in the previous discussion, Randow et al (1999) were interested in comparing the outcome of oral rehabilitation of edentulous mandibles by fixed supraconstructions connected to implants placed according to either (1) a one-stage surgical procedure and immediate loading or (2) the original two-stage concept, with the working hypothesis that there are no differences in treatment outcome between the two methods. A total of 88 implants were placed in 16 patients according to the one-stage protocol and loaded via a fixed appliance within 20 days. The implants placed according to the original protocol were loaded approximately 4 months after implant placement. At the time of delivery of the fixed appliances, all patients were radiographically examined, and this examination was repeated at the 18-month follow-up visit. The analysis of the radiographs revealed that during the 18-month observation period, the mean loss of bone support amounted to approximately 0.5 mm around the implants irrespective of whether they were exposed to early loading or not (Figs 10-1a, 10-1b, and 10-2a). All implants were found to be clinically stable at all observation intervals. The authors concluded that it is "possible to successfully load titanium dental implants immediately following installation via a permanent fixed rigid cross-arch supraconstruction. However, such a treatment approach has so far to be strictly limited to the inter-foramina area of the edentulous mandible."

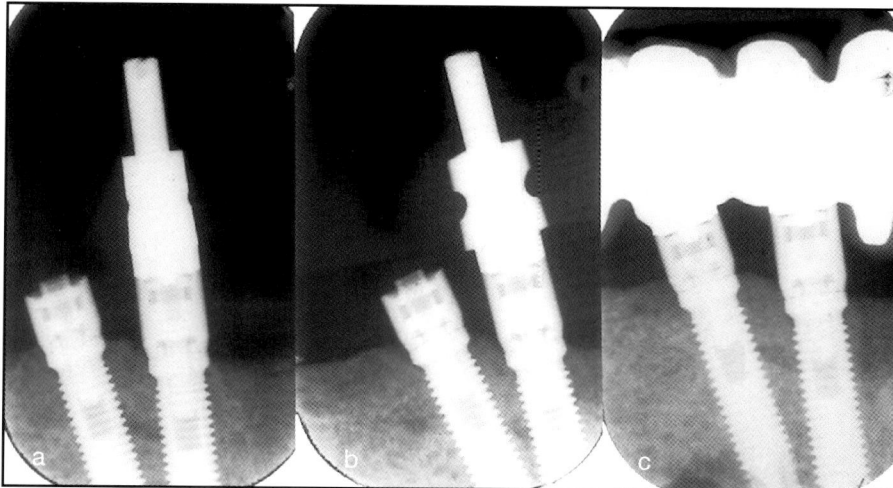

Fig 10-1 Marginal bone level around implants placed according to the one-stage surgical protocol with early loading. (a) Condition at time of placement. (b) Condition at the 18-month follow-up examination. (c) Condition at the 60-month follow-up examination.

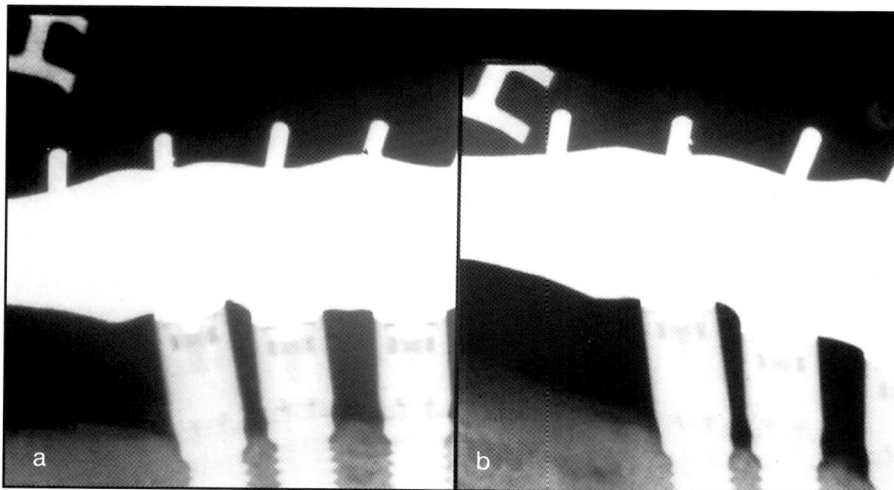

Fig 10-2 Marginal bone level around implants placed and loaded according to the original protocol. (a) Condition at the 18-month follow-up examination. (b) Condition at the 5-year follow-up examination.

Ericsson et al (2000) followed the patients for another 3.5 years (that is, up to 60 months). Analysis of radiographs disclosed that during this 42-month observation period, the average bone change was within the same range (0.2 mm) around implants placed in one surgical session with early loading and around implants placed according to the traditional protocol (Figs 10-1c and 10-2b; see also Figs 10-1b and 10-2a). Furthermore, the authors reported that none of the implants failed during the observation interval, and the stability of the implants increased with time.

In two publications, Schnitman and co-workers (1990, 1997) reported on 63 Bråne-mark system implants placed in 10 patients (Fig 10-3). Of these 63 implants, 28 were placed and "immediately loaded to support an interim fixed bridge." Of these 28 implants, 4 failed. The remaining 35 implants, which were placed according to the original two-stage protocol, osseointegrated properly and were still functioning. In other words, the survival rate for the immediately loaded implants in the two studies mentioned was approximately 85%. However, it must be emphasized

Fig 10-3 Treatment approach by Schnitman and coworkers (1990, 1997). Five to six implants were placed in the anterior mandible between the foramina, and one of these implants close to the midline had abutment connection immediately following placement. The remaining implants were submerged, and abutments were connected 3 to 4 months later. In addition, distal to the exit of and above the nerve-vessel bundle, one short implant was placed bilaterally using a one-stage surgical technique. Thus, three implants were exposed in the oral cavity and immediately connected to an interim fixed partial denture. Three to four months later the permanent fixed partial denture was fabricated and attached to all available implants.

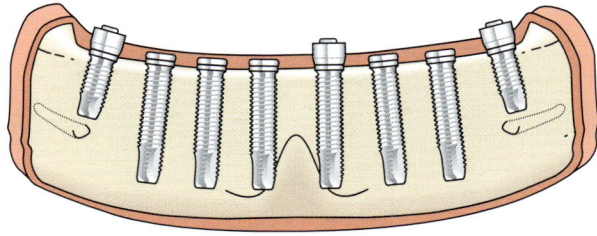

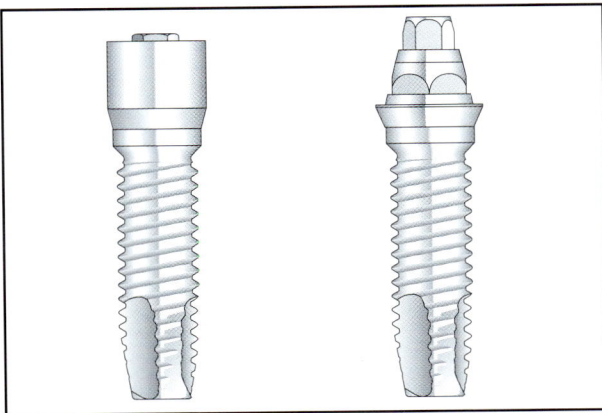

Fig 10-4 Two Brånemark two-piece implant pillars: Implant plus standard abutment *(left)* and implant plus MirusCone abutment *(right)*.

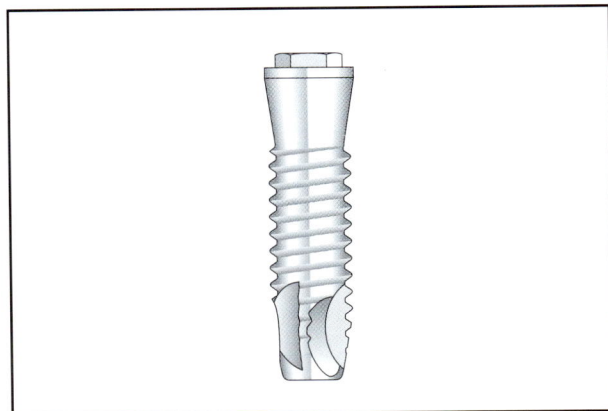

Fig 10-5 Brånemark conical implant, which can be used as a one-piece implant pillar.

that Schnitman et al (1997) reported on a 10-year outcome. The survival rate for the submerged implants was 100% in both studies. Furthermore, Balshi and Wolfinger (1997) applied a treatment approach for the edentulous mandible similar to that of Schnitman et al (1997). They reported that 80% (32 out of 40) of the immediately loaded Brånemark system implants survived over the observation period and concluded that their "preliminary results have been favorable, with all patients functioning with a fixed implant prosthesis from the day of first-stage surgery."

When using the one-stage surgical protocol in combination with early functional loading, it is possible to use either the common implant pillar (a two-piece implant pillar consisting of implant plus standard abutment or implant plus MirusCone abutment) (Fig 10-4) or the conical implant (Fig 10-5). This conical implant is designed with a 3.5-mm conical part coronal to the threads. In other words, the conical part pierces the mucosa when the threads are anchored into the jaw bone and thus serves as a one-piece implant pillar (Fig 10-6). Figure 10-7 illustrates the described

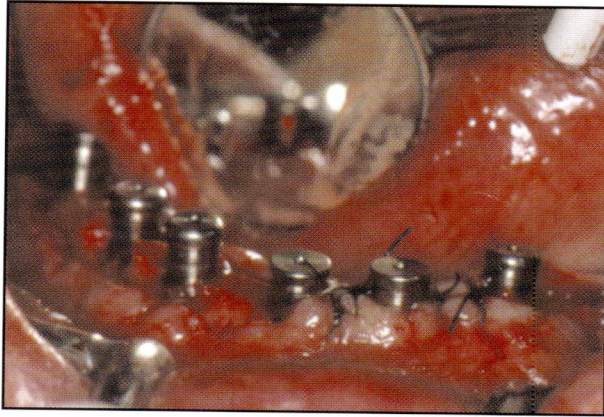

Fig 10-6 Clinical condition immediately following implant placement and during adaptation and suturing of the flaps.

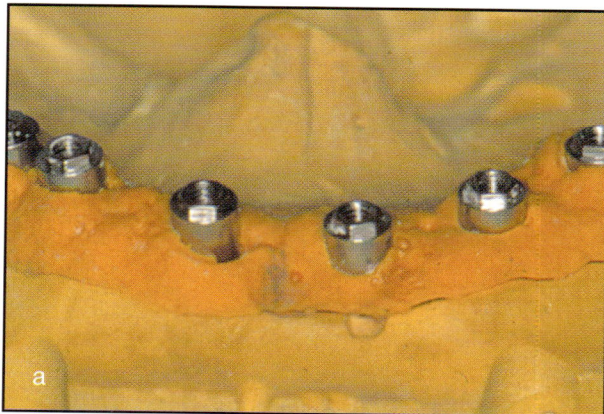

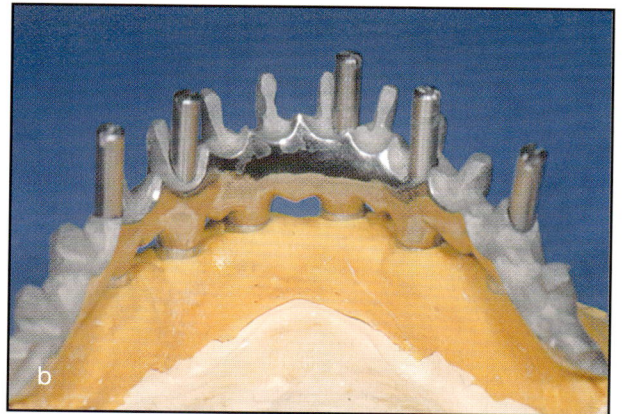

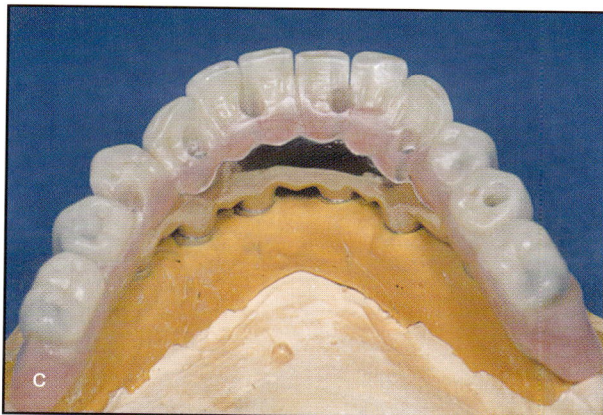

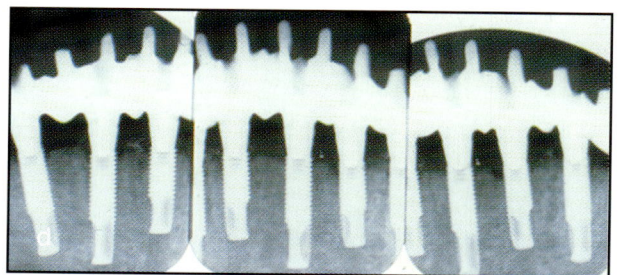

Fig 10-7 (a) Stone cast with implant replicas. (b) Titanium All-in-One framework. (c) Cross-arch prosthetic restoration. (d) Condition immediately following connection of the cross-arch prosthetic restoration.

treatment approach in an edentulous mandible. The total treatment time, from implant placement to delivery of the permanent fixed partial denture, using the Procera All-in-One framework, is 5 to 7 days.

To further challenge the original protocol for Brånemark system implant placement, a study was designed to evaluate the treatment outcome using the one-stage protocol and immediate loading for single-crown restorations (Ericsson et al 1999). The study was designed as a pilot study and performed at the Dental Faculties at Malmö and Umeå University in Sweden. Fourteen patients were treated according to the following protocol. After placement of the implant, an impression was immediately taken. A provisional crown in light central occlusion and with no lateral load contacts was fabricated and connected within 24 hours. Three to six months later, the provisional crown was replaced by a permanent one. During the same period, eight patients with single-tooth losses were treated according to the standard protocol. These patients served as controls. Radiographs were taken at the 6- and 18-month follow-up examinations. Two of the immediately loaded implants were lost during the observation period (3 and 5 months following placement, respectively; survival rate of approximately 85%). A similar mean loss of supporting bone (about 0.1 mm) was observed in this group of patients compared with a control group treated according to the traditional protocol. Thus, the marginal bone level changes observed in the Malmö and Umeå University study agree with figures reported by Randow et al (1999) and Ericsson et al (2000), which lends further support to the feasibility of applying such a treatment approach in single-tooth restorations.

Further Evolution

Brånemark Novum concept

Recently, Brånemark et al (1999) reported on a new method for implant treatment of the edentulous mandible: "The new protocol involves prefabricated components and surgical guides, elimination of the prosthetic impression procedure and attachment of the permanent bridge on the day of implant placement." Fifty patients were followed for 6 months to 3 years after completion of rehabilitation. Three implants failed to integrate and three implants were lost during the observation period, resulting in an overall survival rate of 98% and a prosthetic survival rate of 98%. The average bone loss matches figures reported for the original protocol and "did not exceed 0.2 mm per year when calculated from the 3-month examination." The data reported by Brånemark et al (1999) are in line with those reported above.

Future advances

Nobel Biocare has introduced new drilling and torque equipment (OsseoCare) that, through its graphic display, facilitates the clinical evaluation of bone quality. Furthermore, resonance frequency assessment (Meredith 1997) performed immediately after implant placement helps the clinician decide whether or not to use the early functional loading concept. Such a decision, based on both bone quality and implant stability, is thus individualized for each implant—the "individual functional loading" concept.

Conclusions

Well-controlled experimental studies (Ericsson et al 1996) and clinical studies (for example, Ericsson et al 1994, 1997; Henry and Rosenberg 1994; Bernard et al 1995; Becker et al 1997; Hermans et al 1997; Collaert and De Bruyn 1998) have clearly demonstrated that the one-stage surgical procedure is applicable to the originally designed two-stage Brånemark system. In addition, Schnitman et al (1997), Balshi and Wo finger (1997), and Randow et al (1999) have suggested that it is justifiable not only to adopt the one-stage surgical procedure for Brånemark system implant placement but also to expose such implants to immediate or early functional loading when they are placed in the edentulous mandible. In addition, Ericsson et al (2000) concluded on the basis of a 5-year follow-up study that "the marginal bone level change is within the same range around implants installed according to the 1-stage surgical procedure and early loaded as around implants installed and loaded according to the original 2-stage protocol. Furthermore, this concept with its overall favorable results could initiate a paradigm shift regarding the treatment approach for the edentulous mandible." Such a treatment concept can perhaps also be valid for single-tooth replacements when a full-arch occlusal support is available (Ericsson et al 1999). However, an ultimate prerequisite for applying such a treatment protocol seems to be good initial implant stability.

References

Abrahamsson I, Berglundh T, Moon I-S, Lindhe J. Peri-implant tissues at submerged and non-submerged titanium implants. J Clin Periodontol 1999;26: 600–607.

Abrahamsson I, Berglundh T, Wennström J, Lindhe J. The peri-implant hard and soft tissues at different implant systems: A comparative study in the dog. Clin Oral Implants Res 1996;7:212–219.

Adell R, Eriksson B, Lekholm U, Brånemark P-I, Jemt T. A long-term follow-up study of osseointegrated implants in the treatment of totally edentulous jaws. Int J Oral Maxillofac Implants 1990;5:347–359.

Adell R, Lekholm U, Rockler B, Brånemark P-I. A 15-year study of osseointegrated implants in the treatment of the edentulous jaw. Int J Oral Surg 1981;6:387–416.

Albrektsson T. On long-term maintenance of the osseointegrated response. Aust Prosthodont J 1993;7(suppl):15–24.

Albrektsson T, Zarb G, Worthington P, Eriksson RA. The long-term efficacy of currently used dental implants: A review and proposed criteria of success. Int J Oral Maxillofac Implants 1986;1:11–25.

Balshi TJ, Wolfinger GJ. Immediate loading of Brånemark implants in edentulous mandibles: A preliminary report. Implant Dent 1997;6:83–88.

Becker W, Becker BE, Israelson H, Lucchini JP, Handelsman M, Ammons W, et al. One-step surgical placement of Brånemark implants: A prospective clinical multicenter study. Int J Oral Maxillofac Implants 1997;12:454–462.

Bernard J-P, Belser UC, Martinet J-P, Borgis SA. Osseointegration of Brånemark fixtures using a single-step operating technique: A preliminary prospective one-year study in the edentulous mandible. Clin Oral Implants Res 1995;6:122–129.

Brånemark P-I, Breine U, Adell R, Hansson B-O, Ohlsson Å. Intra-osseous anchorage of dental prostheses, I. Experimental studies. Scand J Plast Reconstr Surg 1969;3:81–100.

Brånemark P-I, Engstrand P, Öhrnell L-O, Gröndahl K, Nilsson P, Hagberg K, et al. Brånemark Novum: A new treatment concept for rehabilitation of the edentulous mandible: Preliminary results from a prospective clinical follow-up study. Clin Implants Dent Rel Res 1999;1:2–16.

Brånemark P-I, Hansson BO, Adell R, Breine U, Lindström J, Hallén O, et al. Osseointegrated implants in the treatment of the edentulous jaw: Experience from a 10-year period. Scand J Plast Reconstr Surg 1977;16(suppl):1–132.

Collaert B, De Bruyn H. Comparison of Brånemark fixture integration and short-term survival using one-stage or two-stage surgery in completely and partially edentulous mandibles. Clin Oral Implants Res 1998;9:131–135.

Dorland's Illustrated Medical Dictionary, ed 28. Philadelphia: Saunders, 1994:1198.

Ericsson I, Glantz P-O, Brånemark P-I. Tissue integrated implants ad modum Brånemark in the rehabilitation of partially edentulous jaws. In: Laney WR, Tolman DE (eds). Tissue Integration in Oral, Orthopedic and Maxillofacial Reconstruction. Chicago: Quintessence, 1990:174–187.

Ericsson I, Lekholm U, Brånemark P-I, Lindhe J, Glantz P-O, Nyman S. A clinical evaluation of fixed-bridge restorations supported by the combination of teeth and osseointegrated titanium implants. J Clin Periodontol 1986;13:307–312.

Ericsson I, Nilner K, Klinge B, Glantz P-O. Radiographical and histological characteristics of submerged and nonsubmerged titanium implants: An experimental study in the Labrador dog. Clin Oral Implants Res 1996;6:20–26.

Ericsson I, Nilson H, Lindh T, Nilner K, Randow K. Immediate functional loading of Brånemark single tooth implants: An 18 month clinical pilot study. Clin Oral Implants Res 1999;11:26–33.

Ericsson I, Randow K, Glantz P-O, Lindhe J, Nilner K. Some clinical and radiographical features of submerged and non-submerged titanium implants. Clin Oral Implants Res 1994;5:185–189.

Ericsson I, Randow K, Nilner K, Petersson A. Some clinical and radiographical features of submerged and non-submerged titanium implants: A 5-year follow-up study. Clin Oral Implants Res 1997;8:422–426.

Ericsson I, Randow K, Nilner K, Petersson A. Early functional loading of Brånemark dental implants: A 5-year follow-up study. Clin Implants Dent Rel Res 2000;2:70–77.

Friberg B, Sennerby L, Lindén B, Gröndahl K, Lekholm U. Stability measurements of one-stage Brånemark implants during healing in mandibles: A clinical resonance frequency analysis study. Int J Oral Maxillofac Surg 1999;28:266–272.

Glantz P-O, Stafford GD. Clinical deformation of maxillary complete dentures. J Dent 1983;11:224–230.

Glantz P-O, Strandman E, Randow K. On functional strain in fixed mandibular reconstructions, II. An in vivo study. Acta Odontol Scand 1984;42:269–276.

Glantz P-O, Strandman E, Svensson SA, Randow K. On functional strain in fixed mandibular reconstructions, I. An in vitro study. Acta Odontol Scand 1984;42:241–249.

Gotfredsen K, Rostrup E, Hjörting-Hansen E, Stoltze K, Budtz-Jörgensen E. Histological and histomorphometrical evaluation of tissue reactions adjacent to endosteal implants in monkeys. Clin Oral Implants Res 1991;2:30–37.

Henry P, Rosenberg I. Single-stage surgery for rehabilitation of the edentulous mandible: Preliminary results. Pract Periodontics Aesthet Dent 1994;6:15–22.

Hermans M, Durdu F, Herrmann I, Malevez C. A single-step operative technique using the Brånemark system: A prospective study in the edentulous mandible [abstract]. Clin Oral Implants Res 1997;8:437.

Jemt T, Lekholm U. Implant treatment in edentulous maxillae: A 5-year follow-up report on patients with different degrees of jaw resorption. Int J Oral Maxillofac Implants 1995;10:303–311.

Jemt T, Lekholm U. Oral implant treatment in posterior partially edentulous jaws: A 5-year follow-up report. Int J Oral Maxillofac Implants 1993;8:635–640.

Jemt T, Lekholm U, Adell R. Osseointegrated implants in the treatment of partially edentulous patients: A preliminary study on 876 consecutively placed fixtures. Int J Oral Maxillofac Implants 1989;4:211–217.

Lekholm U, van Steenberghe D, Herrmann I, Bolender C, Folmer T, Gunne J, et al. Osseointegrated implants in the treatment of partially edentulous jaws: A prospective 5-year multicenter study. Int J Oral Maxillofac Implants 1994;9:627–635.

Meredith N. On the clinical measurement of implant stability and osseointegration [thesis]. Göteborg: Univ of Göteborg, Sweden, 1997.

Randow K, Ericsson I, Nilner K, Petersson A. Immediate functional loading of Brånemark implants: An 18-month clinical follow-up study. Clin Oral Implants Res 1999;11:8–15.

Schnitman PA, Wöhrle PS, Rubenstein JE. Immediate fixed interim prostheses supported by two-stage threaded implants: Methodology and results. J Oral Implantol 1990;16:96–105.

Schnitman PA, Wöhrle PS, Rubenstein JE, Silva JD, Wang N-H. Ten year results for Brånemark implants immediately loaded with fixed prostheses at implant placement. Int J Oral Maxillofac Implants 1997;12:495–503.

van Steenberghe D, Lekholm U, Bolender C, Folmer T, Henry P, Herrmann I, et al. The applicability of osseointegrated oral implants in the rehabilitation of partial edentulism: A prospective multicenter study on 558 fixtures. Int J Oral Maxillofac Implants 1990;5:272–281.